SPINAL CORD INJURY DESK REFERENCE

Guidelines
for
Life Care Planning and Case Management

Terry L. Blackwell, Ed.D.
James S. Krause, Ph.D.
Terry Winkler, M.D.
Steven A. Stiens, M.D.

Demos Medical Publishing, Inc., 386 Park Avenue South, New York, New York 10016

Library of Congress Cataloging-in-Publication Data

Spinal cord injury desk reference : guidelines for life care
planning and case management/Terry L. Blackwell ... [et al.].
    p. ; cm.
   Includes bibliographical references and index.
   ISBN 1-888799-49-8 (pbk. : alk. paper)
   1. Spinal cord–Wounds and injuries. 2. Spinal cord–Wounds
and injuries–Patients–Rehabilitation. 3. Long-term care of the sick.
4. Quality of life.
   [DNLM: 1. Spinal Cord Injuries–rehabilitation. 2. Long-Term Care.
3. Patient Care Planning. 4. Quality of Life. WL 400 S75773 2001]
I. Blackwell, Terry L.
  RD594.3 .S66533 2001
  617.4′82044–dc21   00-065790

CONTENTS

Preface

Injuries to the spinal cord can produce myriad disabilities. For many people, spinal cord injury (SCI) is catastrophic and has personal consequences that are much more complex than the potential loss of feeling and movement. In addition to the physical impact of injury, individuals must make social, vocational, economic, and emotional adjustments following SCI. SCI often requires significant use of assistive personnel beyond the family structure, community resources, applied technology assistance, and psychosocial supports; this requires a program of highly coordinated and integrated lifetime follow-up and care management services.

This need for a continuum of care presents great challenges to health care professionals as well as to individuals with SCI and their families. Life care planning, which entered into the rehabilitation scene in the late 1970s and early 1980s, has proved to be one way of meeting this challenge by providing an organized framework of services, recommendations, and requirements for long-term care management. By using a consistent methodology to assess the individual needs of the person with SCI, the life care plan (LCP) helps health care professionals as well as the person with SCI acquire a comprehensive understanding of the immediate and long-term care requirements necessary to maximize productivity and independence.

Spinal Cord Injury Desk Reference answers the need to have a single reference that both contains information about and serves as a reminder of areas central to the life care planning process for persons with SCI. It offers practitioners a single, easy-to-use resource that summarizes — in a clear, understandable way with easily accessible references — a body of studies and research on SCI that have important implications for life care planning and case management.

This text is an introduction to the basic aspects of SCI, including epidemiology, functional classification, and complications related to aging with a disability. In addition, it covers functional outcomes, potential associated costs, long-term management and care considerations, model LCP guidelines, and legislative, organizational, and agency resources.

Although the text was written primarily for life care planning and case management practitioners, it can also be useful to other professionals who may be involved with the long-term care and management needs of people with SCI. Included in this group are primary and speciality care physicians, nurses, rehabilitation counselors, therapists, insurers/HMOs, attorneys, governmental agencies, disability organizations, and educators, as well as those with SCI and their families.

In using this text, it is important to keep in mind that as research in the area of SCI grows, so will the available resources and information. We have tried to make this text broad in scope and current; however, new information and resources constanty become available. Readers must realize that, when discussing SCI, a subject that involves continually evolving research related to the continuum of care, it is necessary to keep abreast of new developments to remain current and competent in their role as life care planners or case managers for SCI. Our primary goal is to provide information and recommendations that both practitioners and individuals with SCI may use to become informed in addressing the long-term care and management needs.

In summary, *Spinal Cord Injury Desk Reference* provides a quick, easy-to-understand, comprehensive, evidence-based reference for health care practitioners who formulate life care plans for persons with SCI. We have incorporated several features to facilitate use by practitioners; including a variety of reference materials containing information that should prove useful for SCI life care planning and case management. As a final note, the information provided in this text is general in nature and, as such, direct application to a specific individual should not be assumed. Instead, life care planning and case management practitioners would best be served by utilizing this text a as guide from which to incorporate their professional knowledge, judgment, and ethical responsibilities to meet the challenge of addressing the unique long-term care needs of individuals with SCI. It is our hope this text will provide readers with tools and insights for competently addressing the long-term consequences of SCI.

Terry L. Blackwell
James S. Krause
Terry Winkler
Steven A. Stiens

Acknowledgments

The writing of this book was made possible by the help of many individuals. We are especially indebted to Lisa Busby, Susan Charlifue, Jennifer Coker, Paul Deutsch, Tyron Elliott, Logan Foley, Doris Guglielmo, Katherine Hoover, Angeliki Kampitsis, Julie Kitchen, Laura Cheney Krause, Melanie Lattin, Henry McCarthy, Meagan Minvielle, Irmo Marini, Tanya Rutherford, Diana Schneider, Kathryn Shannon, David Slovak, Randall Thomas, and Roger Weed whose helpful input improved this publication.

A special appreciation is extended to the following publishers, organizations, and agencies for their generosity in allowing us to use their ideas and materials for incorporation in this book: American Spinal Injury Association, Arkansas Spinal Cord Commission, Aspen Publishers, Demos Medical Publishing, Department of Veterans Affairs, Elliott and Fitzpatrick, National Spinal Cord Injury Association, National Spinal Cord Injury Statistical Center, Paralyzed Veterans of America, Research and Training Center on Independent Living, University of Kansas, Uniform Data System for Medical Rehabilitation, and the University of Alabama at Birmingham.

Terry L. Blackwell
James S. Krause
Terry Winkler
Steven A. Stiens

Authors

Terry L. Blackwell, Ed.D., Associate Professor of Rehabilitation Counseling, Department of Rehabilitation Counseling, Louisiana State University Health Sciences Center, New Orleans, Louisiana. Prior to his appointment as an associate professor at Louisiana State University Health Sciences Center, Dr. Blackwell was in private practice in Montana and worked throughout the United States specializing in catastrophic rehabilitation and life care planning, consultation, and training. Dr. Blackwell sits on the editorial boards of several rehabilitation journals and has authored or co-authored a number of general books and articles in the areas of job analysis, forensic rehabilitation, ethics, and life care planning.

James S. Krause, Ph.D., Behavioral Scientist, Shepherd Center, Atlanta, Georgia. Dr. Krause has been involved in research in long-term outcomes after spinal cord injury (SCI) for more than a decade. He has published multiple articles on aging, employment, quality of life, secondary conditions, and mortality after SCI. Prior to committing all his time to research, Dr. Krause spent four years working as a staff psychologist in a large SCI rehabilitation hospital. His clinical focus included adjustment counseling, alcohol and drug treatment, and prevention of secondary conditions. Dr. Krause uses his research and clinical background to assist in the development of life care plans and to provide expert testimony in SCI cases by predicting long-term complications, prospects for return to gainful employment, and life expectancy.

Terry Winkler, M.D., Board Certified Physical Medicine and Rehabilitation and Spinal Cord Injury Medicine Physician, private practice, Springfield, Missouri. In his practice, Dr. Winkler specializes in traumatic and acquired brain injury, spinal cord injury, amputations, and life care planning. He holds academic appointments as Clinical Associate Professor at the University of Florida, Gainesville, and Clinical Professor at Louisiana State University Health Sciences Center, New Orleans, Louisiana. In addition, Dr. Winkler serves on committees that review grants on spinal cord injury research for the Paralyzed Veterans of America and the National Institute on Disability and Rehabilitation Research. He has several publications in the area of life care planning.

Steven A. Stiens, M.D., Associate Professor of Rehabilitation Medicine, University of Washington, Seattle, Washington, and Attending Spinal Cord Medicine Physician at VA Puget Sound Health Care System, Harborview Medical Center and University Hospital. Dr. Stiens provides person-centered SCI rehabilitation and primary care as well as training and education for medical students, residents, and SCI fellows. He has published numerous scientific articles and chapters on a wide range of SCI-related topics including neurogenic bowel, psychosocial adaptation, cardiovascular disease, gastrointestinal dysfunction, and mechanisms of neurologic recovery. In addition, Dr. Stiens has developed a variety of training films and educational materials on SCI.

Life Care Planning and Spinal Cord Injury

Few events are as challenging and life-altering as traumatic spinal cord injury (SCI). Any damage to the spinal cord can result in a large variety of functional problems. SCI affects virtually every body system, presenting the injured individual with the prospect of long-term major disability and major disruption of activities and participation in relationships that have defined him or her as an individual. After injury and acute rehabilitation, persons with SCI must direct their ongoing health maintenance and personal care needs. This requires significant support of assistive personnel beyond the family structure, use of community resources, applied technology assistance, and psychosocial supports that work within an interdisciplinary matrix of preventive and rehabilitative services (Blackwell, Weed, & Powers, 1994; Whiteneck et al., 1993; Whiteneck, Tate, & Charlifue, 1999). In addressing the comprehensive needs dictated by onset of disability, it is important that individuals with SCI also develop the autonomy and self-determination necessary to be able to manage their health and direct themselves toward attaining life goals.

Traditionally, the identification and integration of long-term health and personal care needs and programs were not addressed in the SCI rehabilitation process outside of the Model SCI Care Systems programs and Department of Veterans Affairs (VA) Regional SCI Centers. As a consequence, when life care planning entered the rehabilitation scene in the late 1970s and early 1980s it brought with it a consistent methodology for analyzing the extent of disability and the resulting long-term needs of individuals who had sustained a severe injury such as a SCI (Deutsch & Raffa, 1981). A life care plan (LCP) provides consistency of assessment techniques, organization of cost and resource information, and an analysis of supportive research and literature to identify services, treatment, and equipment that will enhance long-term quality of life and allow a person with SCI to maximize both functional potential and self-dependence (Deutsch & Sawyer, 1999). The LCP is the first step in determining the need for resources; case management then works to assist the individual with SCI to manage these resources.

In general, individuals with SCI and their families are not prepared to deal with the long-term physical, emotional, and economic consequences of the injury. Further, with the issue of resource allocation being an ongoing concern, there is a need to coordinate the variety of services necessary to support the lifestyle requirements of persons with SCI throughout their life. The LCP, therefore, provides a summary of the step-by-step process for addressing areas such as equipment needs, supplies, pharmaceuticals, therapeutic modalities, education, attendant care services, and medical follow-up for persons with SCI. The LCP highlights critical stages of development wherein particular services or programs may need to be implemented. It provides an organized framework of supportive services, recommendations, and requirements for long-term, self-directed disability management and care (Deutsch, 1990). By identifying the continuum of care necessary for the successful life adjustment of a person with SCI, the LCP sets out criteria to optimize an individual's physical functioning, facilitate social independence, minimize

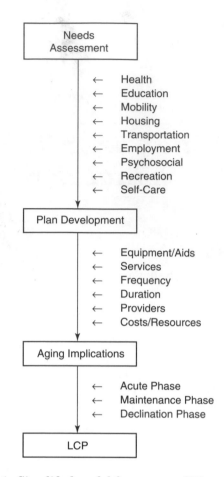

Figure 1-1. Simplified model for process of life care planning.

medical complications, enhance emotional adaptation, and promote reintegration into the community.

Figure 1-1 summarizes specific areas that are typically addressed in developing a comprehensive LCP for an individual with SCI. The following chapters and appendices provide more detail on specific strategies for assessing, planning, and addressing an individual's long-term care and management needs.

Although life care planners come from a range of disciplinary backgrounds, some shared basic areas of knowledge are necessary as a prerequisite to life care planning. These include practical knowledge and understanding of: (Blackwell et al., 1994; Deutsch, 1990; Weed, 1999)

- Literature and research related to SCI
- Medical and psychological aspects and sequelae of SCI and co-morbid conditions
- Typical goods and services needed by individuals with SCI
- Impact of disability on family members and/or significant others
- Medical, psychological, and rehabilitation terminology as it relates to the life care planning process
- Differences between pediatric disability needs and adult disability needs
- Ongoing implications of SCI throughout the individual's lifespan and within various environments
- Various resources to address the long-term needs of persons with SCI
- How to research and develop the information and resources necessary for an individualized, geographically appropriate LCP that fosters self-directed management and care

NATURE OF SPINAL CORD INJURY

Damage to the spinal cord can result in a loss of function, such as mobility or sensation. Frequent causes of damage are trauma (motor vehicle accidents, falls, acts of violence, recreational sporting events, etc.) or disease (cancer, spinal cord vascular disease, and other nontraumatic spinal cord diseases) (Thurman, Sniezek, Johnson, Greenspan, & Smith, 1995). The spinal cord does not have to be severed for a loss of function to occur. In fact, the spinal cord is intact in most people with traumatic SCI, but the damage to it results in loss of function (National Spinal Cord Injury Association [NSCIA], 1996).

The *spinal cord* is the major bundle of nerves that carries impulses to and from the brain to the rest of the body. The brain and the spinal cord make up the *central nervous system (CNS)*, while motor and sensory nerves outside the CNS make up the *peripheral nervous system (PNS)*. Surrounding the spinal cord is a ring of bones called *vertebrae*. The spinal cord lies within the spinal canal formed by the vertebrae of the spinal column (back bones). Thirty pairs of sensory and motor nerves originate in the spinal cord — 8 cervical (neck), 12 thoracic (chest), 5 lumbar (lower back), and 5 sacral (tailbone) — and exit between adjacent openings in the vertebrae (DeLisa & Stolov, 1981). Each spinal nerve is numbered to correspond to the number of the vertebrae near which it exits from the spinal canal, except for the cervical segments where there are eight nerves and only seven vertebrae (see Figure 1-2).

SCI can result in varying degrees of neurologic impairment (e.g., motor and/or sensory loss) depending on where and to what extent the spinal cord is injured (Stover & Fine, 1986). In general, the higher in the spinal column the injury occurs, the more dysfunction a person experiences. Cervical SCIs usually result in loss of function in the arms and legs; injuries in the thoracic region usually affect the chest and the legs; and injuries to the lumbar and sacral vertebrae generally result in some loss of function in the hips and legs (DeLisa & Stolov, 1981; Hu & Cressy, 1992).

In addition to a loss of sensation or motor function, individuals with SCI may also experience other changes. For example, they may experience dysfunction of the bowel and bladder (Glickman & Kamm, 1996; Stiens, Bierner-Bergman & Formal, 1997; Stone, Nino-Murica, Wolfe, & Perkash, 1990). Sexual functioning is frequently impacted (Stiens, Westheimer, & Young, 1997). While men with SCI may have fertility problems, women's fertility is generally not affected (Baker & Cardenas, 1996; Sipski & Alexander, 1992). High level injuries (C1–C4) can result in a loss of many involuntary functions including the ability to breathe, necessitating breathing aids such as mechanical ventilators or diaphragmatic pacemakers (McKinley, Jackson, Cardenas, & DeVivo, 1999). There are many other effects of SCI, some of which may include low blood pressure, inability to regulate blood pressure effectively, reduced control of body temperature, inability to sweat below the level of injury, and chronic pain (Loubser & Donovan, 1996; NSCIA, 1996; Ragnarsson, Hall, Wilmot & Carter, 1995).

NEUROLOGIC CLASSIFICATION OF SPINAL CORD INJURY

Persons with SCI are classified according to the neurologic level of injury by determining the preservation or absence of sensory and motor function. A broad distinction is often made between lesions above and below the first thoracic segments of the spinal cord (Stover et al., 1986). *Tetraplegia* refers to impairment or loss of motor and/or sensory function in the cervical segments of the spinal cord because of damage of neural elements within the spinal canal. Tetraplegia results in

Vertebrae   Spinal Nerves

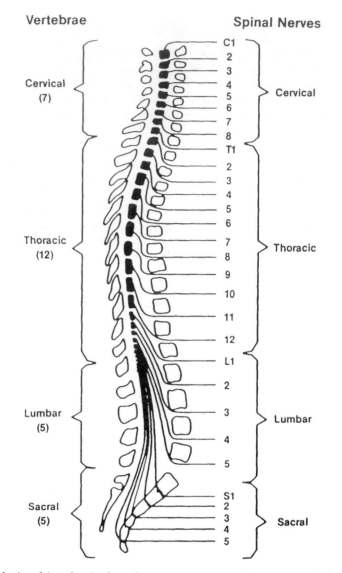

Figure 1-2. Relationship of spinal cord, spinal nerves, and vertebrae. (From *Spinal Cord Injury: The Facts and Figures* by Stover & Fine, p. 26. Birmingham: University of Alabama at Birmingham, 1986. Reprinted with permission.)

impairment of function in the arms as well as in the trunk, legs, and pelvic organs. *Paraplegia* refers to impairment or loss of motor and/or sensory function in the thoracic, lumbar, or sacral (but not cervical) segments of the spinal cord, secondary to damage of neural elements within the spinal canal. With paraplegia, arm function is spared but, depending on the level of injury, the trunk, legs, and pelvic organs may be involved (American Spinal Injury Association [ASIA], 1996).

Another factor affecting the degree of neurologic impairment is the neurologic *extent* of injury. The injury is classified as *complete* if there is no functional motor and sensory preservation in the lowest sacral segments (S4–S5). An *incomplete* injury implies that there is partial preservation of sensory and/or motor functions below the neurologic level, including the lowest sacral segments (ASIA, 1996; Waters, Adkins, & Yakura, 1991).

This information is valuable in predicting the recovery of functional ability, determining the need and effectiveness of various treatment interventions, and developing a comprehensive rehabilitation plan of services (Consortium for Spinal Cord Medicine, 1999a; Ditunno, Stover, Murray, & Ahn, 1992; Waters, Adkins, Yakura, & Sie, 1993).

Neurologic Examination

The neurologic examination allows a physician to classify SCI into broad categories and types. The neurologic level of SCI is determined by the motor and sensory examination that identifies the most caudal (lowest) segment of the spinal cord with normal sensory and/or motor function on both sides of the body. The recommended neurologic assessment follows the classifications published in the *International Standards for Neurological and Functional Classification of Spinal Cord Injury, Revised 1996* (ASIA, 1996), endorsed by the American Spinal Injury Association (ASIA) and the International Medical Society of Paraplegia (IMSOP).

Neurologic examination of sensation includes the 28 *dermatomes* (nerve roots that receive sensory information from the skin areas) for sensitivity to pin prick and light touch. In addition, the motor levels are tested in the 10 paired *myotomes* (groups of muscles) with the motor level defined by the lowest key muscle that has a grade of at least 3, providing the key muscles represented by segments above that level are normal (grade 4 or 5) (ASIA, 1996). The sensory and motor level are evaluated for both right and left sides and recorded on the summary chart (Figure 1-3) with a level of injury assigned and classified as complete or incomplete. With a complete injury there is neither sensation nor motor function in the lowest sacral segment. An incomplete injury has partial preservation of sensation and/or motor function below the neurologic level of injury and includes the lowest sacral segment. Sacral sensation includes sensation at the anal mucocutaneous junction as well as deep anal sensation. Motor function is considered incomplete if there is voluntary contraction of the external anal sphincter upon digital examination.

The greatest proportion of motor and sensory recovery tends to occur within the first six months of injury and typically plateaus at the end of one year (Ditunno et al., 1992; Waters, Yakura, Adkins, & Sie, 1992; Waters et al., 1993; Waters, Adkins, Yakura, & Sie, 1994a; Waters, Adkins, Yakura, & Sie, 1994b). Consequently, it is feasible to begin to base initial rehabilitation and life care planning efforts on the individual's predicted one-year recovery status for purposes of identifying self-care and equipment needs. In many cases, depending on completeness of the injury, this information can be extrapolated with a high degree of accuracy by a physician specializing in physical medicine and rehabilitation or spinal cord injury medicine.

Neurologic Extent of Injury

The ASIA Impairment Scale (adapted from the classification scheme introduced by Frankel et al., 1969) uses the findings from the neurologic examination to describe the neurologic extent of injury. Although the ASIA Impairment Scale is the current scheme for defining the neurologic extent of injury, many individuals with SCI remain classified with the earlier Frankel terminology. Table 1-1 outlines the functional categories of the ASIA Impairment Scale and the corresponding Frankel Grading System categories.

Clinical Syndromes

Also included in the neurologic assessment of individuals with incomplete injuries is the classification of clinical syndromes. Injuries to the spinal cord may result in commonly recognized syndromes if the damage is confined to limited areas of the cord. Incomplete SCIs that occur with some degree of frequency have been defined according to the following neurologic presentations.

Anterior cord syndrome is caused by damage primarily in the anterior two-thirds of the spinal cord and is related to vascular insult. The lesion produces variable loss of motor function and of sensitivity to pain and temperature, while preserving proprioception (position sense). Anterior cord syndrome has the least favorable prognosis of all the partial cord injury syndromes in terms of functional recovery.

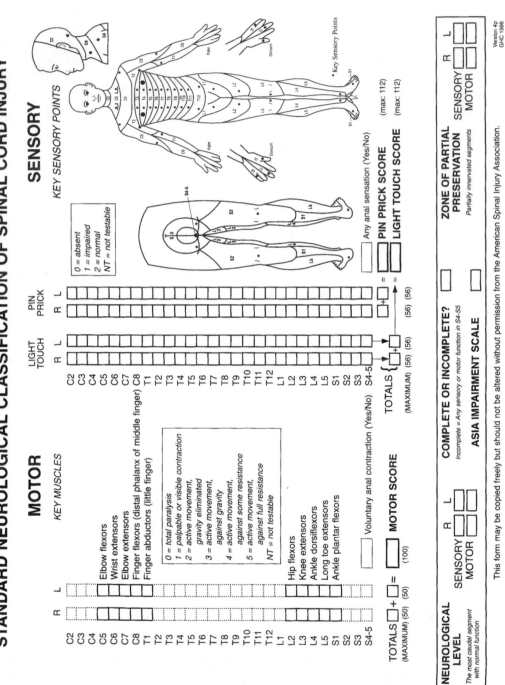

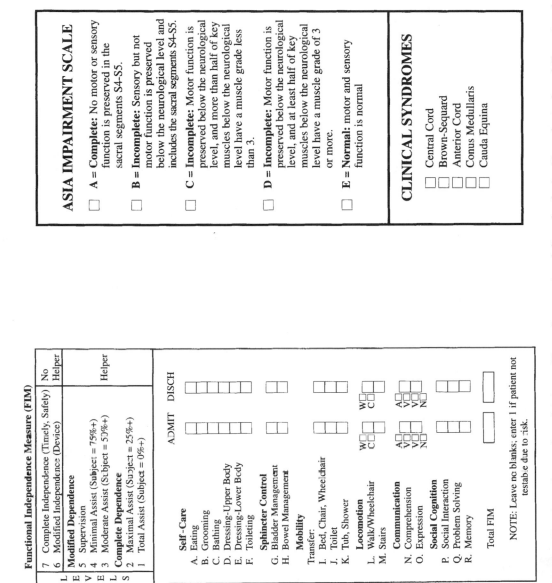

ASIA IMPAIRMENT SCALE

☐ **A = Complete:** No motor or sensory function is preserved in the sacral segments S4-S5.

☐ **B = Incomplete:** Sensory but not motor function is preserved below the neurological level and includes the sacral segments S4-S5.

☐ **C = Incomplete:** Motor function is preserved below the neurological level, and more than half of key muscles below the neurological level have a muscle grade less than 3.

☐ **D = Incomplete:** Motor function is preserved below the neurological level, and at least half of key muscles below the neurological level have a muscle grade of 3 or more.

☐ **E = Normal:** motor and sensory function is normal

CLINICAL SYNDROMES

☐ Central Cord
☐ Brown-Sequard
☐ Anterior Cord
☐ Conus Medullaris
☐ Cauda Equina

Functional Independence Measure (FIM)

L — 7 Complete Independence (Timely, Safely) — No Helper
E — 6 Modified Independence (Device)

V — **Modified Dependence** — Helper
E — 5 Supervision
L — 4 Minimal Assist (Subject = 75%+)
— 3 Moderate Assist (Subject = 50%+)

S — **Complete Dependence**
— 2 Maximal Assist (Subject = 25%+)
— 1 Total Assist (Subject = 0%+)

ADMIT   DISCH

Self-Care
A. Eating
B. Grooming
C. Bathing
D. Dressing-Upper Body
E. Dressing-Lower Body
F. Toileting

Sphincter Control
G. Bladder Management
H. Bowel Management

Mobility
Transfer:
I. Bed, Chair, Wheelchair
J. Toilet
K. Tub, Shower

Locomotion
L. Walk/Wheelchair
M. Stairs

Communication
N. Comprehension
O. Expression

Social Cognition
P. Social Interaction
Q. Problem Solving
R. Memory

Total FIM

NOTE: Leave no blanks; enter 1 if patient not testable due to risk.

Figure 1-3. Standard neurologic classification of spinal cord injury. (From *International Standards for Neurological and Functional Classification of Spinal Cord Injury, Revised 1996.* American Spinal Injury Association (ASIA), 1996. Reprinted with permission.)

Table 1-1. ASIA Impairment Scale/Frankel Grading System

Grade	ASIA	Frankel
A	Complete: No motor or sensory function is preserved in the sacral segments S4–S5.	Complete: No sensory or motor function is preserved below the level of lesion.
B	Incomplete: Sensory but not motor function is preserved below the neurologic level and includes the sacral segments S4–S5.	Incomplete: Preserved sensation only. Preservation of any demonstrable sensation, excluding phantom sensations. Voluntary motor function is absent.
C	Incomplete: Motor function is preserved below the neurologic level, and more than half of key muscles below the neurologic level have a muscle grade less than 3.	Incomplete: Preserved motor (nonfunctional). Preservation of voluntary motor function which performs no useful purpose except psychologically. Sensory function may or may not be preserved.
D	Incomplete: Motor function is preserved below the neurologic level, and at least half of key muscles below the neurologic level have a muscle grade of 3 or more.	Incomplete: Preserved motor (functional). Preservation of voluntary motor function which is useful functionally.
E	Normal: Motor and sensory function is normal.	Complete Recovery: Complete return of all motor and sensory function, but still may have abnormal reflexes.

Brown-Sequard syndrome results from hemitransection or injury to the spinal cord with resultant loss of motor function on the same side as the lesion and contralateral loss of pain and temperature sensation. Brown-Sequard syndrome is often caused by penetrating trauma or unilateral facet fracture or dislocation. Recovery from this syndrome is generally associated with fairly normal bowel and bladder function. Many people with Brown-Sequard syndrome regain some strength in the lower extremities and may be able to walk, although some functional bracing or ambulatory device may be necessary, such as a cane or crutch.

Cauda equina syndrome results from nerve compression involving one or more of the nerve roots of the lumbar or sacral spine. This syndrome is often associated with unilateral or bilateral leg pain, numbness or paresthesis in the lower extremities, and bowel or bladder incontinence. Cauda equina syndrome is frequently caused by a central lumbar disc herniation. Lesions that produce the syndrome can also be caused by tumors, arteriovenous malformations, and hematomas. The prognosis for cauda equina syndrome is best if a definitive cause is identified and prompt appropriate surgical management occurs.

Central cord syndrome typically results from a cervical cord contusion that causes damage to the grey matter in the interior cord. This injury results in proportionally greater loss of motor function to upper extremities than lower extremities, with variable sensory sparing. Central cord syndrome may result from trauma (especially in older individuals or individuals who have cervical arthritis), spondylitic myelopathy, syringomyelia, or neoplasm. Individuals with this syndrome may achieve functional walking with return of motor and sensory power to the lower extremities and trunk, although the gait may be spastic. However, they tend to have poor recovery of hand function because of the irreversible nature of central grey matter destruction. Individuals with central cord syndrome are usually able to regain bowel and bladder function. Unfortunately, their overall function is limited by upper extremity assistive capacity for gait and activities of daily living (ADLs).

Conus medullaris syndrome results from damage to the grey matter in the spinal cord where the sacral roots emerge, with or without involvement of the lumbar nerve roots. This syndrome is characterized by an areflexic bladder, bowel and, to a lesser degree, lower extremities. Motor and sensory loss in the lower extremities is variable. Conus medullaris syndrome is relatively uncommon compared to other clinical syndromes.

REHABILITATION AND FUNCTIONAL OUTCOMES FOR SPINAL CORD INJURY

Rehabilitation has been defined as the development of a person to his or her fullest physical, psychosocial, vocational/avocational, and educational potential after SCI (DeLisa, Martin, & Currie, 1993; Stiens, Haselkorn, Peters, & Goldstein, 1996). The goals of rehabilitation are to minimize the person's impairments, limitations in performance of activities, and restrictions for participation in various life areas (World Health Organization [WHO], 1999). This process involves a team of professionals with complementary expertise who function together through interdisciplinary interaction to improve the individual's life effectiveness following SCI. The team typically consists of a rehabilitation physician, nurse, physical therapist, psychologist, social worker, occupational therapist, recreation therapist, dietitian, rehabilitation counselor, and other health care professionals as indicated (Stiens & Berkin, 1997).

Once the individual is medically stabilized and able to participate the process of rehabilitation can begin. SCI rehabilitation attempts to use a person-centered approach to review individual's needs and treatment goals (Stewart et al., 1995; Quill & Brody, 1996). Each rehabilitation team member establishes relationships in order to know the individual and formulate person-centered goals. As the individual is evaluated, an initial rehabilitation problem list is developed. This list is a summary of the primary areas of patient limitation that will require focused intervention. The problem list is organized to include the primary diagnosis, which may include the person's injury level and completeness of injury. Next, spine stability is addressed with a problem that documents the placement of internal fixation and the levels it traverses. Further down the list all pertinent diagnoses are noted, especially if the person is currently under treatment. Below diagnoses, impairments are listed, such as neurogenic bowel and bladder. Below that are problems that deal with overcoming various disabilities such as mobility deficits and activities of daily living. Finally, issues that contribute to handicaps are listed as problems. These may range from issues such as adaptation to SCI to social role function, community reintegration, and architectural accessibility. Table 1-2 outlines the essential components of a typical problem list for a person with SCI.

After initial development, the rehabilitation problem list is reviewed and modified by the interdisciplinary rehabilitation team. The results of their individual evaluations of the person with SCI and the goals they derived with the individual to guide rehabilitation are then discussed in interdisciplinary rounds or goal setting

Table 1-2. Rehabilitation Problem List for Individuals with Spinal Cord Injury

- SCI level, ASIA level
- Spine stability
- Other associated diagnoses (e.g., traumatic brain injury, hypertension, etc.)
- Neurogenic skin
- Neurogenic bowel
- Neurogenic sexual dysfunction
- Mobility
- Activities of Daily Living
- Psychosocial function/adaptation
- Financial needs/resources
- Community reintegration
- Educational/Vocational
- Architectural accessibility
- Discharge planning

meetings. These goals drive the process of rehabilitation toward discharge and beyond (Stiens et al., 1996).

The desired global outcome for persons after SCI is the achievement of their fullest potential by identifying and accomplishing goals in their individual lives. Each person-centered outcome is unique and is accomplished by providing a continuum of evaluation and problem-directed services that minimize illness, impairments, disabilities, and handicaps. Outcomes are initially achieved through a process of acute interdisciplinary rehabilitation. Thereafter, continual reevaluation of the person's medical condition and reappraisal of person-centered goals are needed to maximize outcome as the individual continues his or her development and fully participates in relationships and community activities.

Conceptually, rehabilitation of persons with SCI needs to view the experiences of the individual as integrated into a hierarchy of dynamically related natural systems (see Table 1-3). Each level represents an organized dynamic unit that interacts as part of a larger system and subsumes the smaller system (Engel, 1982). The *biopsychosocial model* presented in Table 1-3 conceptualizes a hierarchy of systems that require interventions and the various rehabilitation team members who may be involved in addressing issues at the respective system levels during the process of SCI rehabilitation and subsequent long-term planning efforts (Stiens et al., 1996).

The desired global outcome for persons after SCI is the achievement of their fullest potential by identifying and accomplishing goals in their individual lives. Each person-centered outcome is unique and is accomplished by providing a continuum of evaluation and problem-directed services that minimize illness, impairments, disabilities, and handicaps. Outcomes are initially achieved through a process of acute interdisciplinary rehabilitation. Thereafter, continual re-evaluation of the person's medical condition and reappraisal of person-centered goals are needed to maximize outcome as the individual continues his or her development and fully participates in relationships and community activities.

A primary goal in long-term care planning is to minimize the impact of disability and to limit the occurrence of secondary conditions so that an optimal level of functional independence and quality of life can be maintained throughout the person's lifespan. As the person ages, the likelihood of complications in body systems typically impaired by SCI will increase (Charlifue, Weitzenkamp, & Whiteneck, 1999; McKinley, Jackson, Cardenas, & DeVivo, 1999). Complications of the skin, nervous,

Table 1-3. Biopsychosocial Model of Rehabilitation Interventions

Hierarchy of Systems	Interdisciplinary Rehabilitation	Focus for Interventions; Problem List; LCP
Society	Disability Rights Legislation	Promote Opportunity
Culture	Publication, Education	Promote Acceptance
Subculture	Clergy	Resume Spiritual Roles
Community	Recreation Therapist	Community Reintegration
School	Special Education	Achievement
Employment	Rehabilitation Counselor	Resumption of Vocation
Family	Social Worker	Social Reintegration
Two-Person	Social Worker/Psychologist	Adaptation in Relationships
Person-Experience and Behavior	Psychologist	Adjustment to SCI
Nervous System	Occupational Therapist	Task Reacquisition
Organ/Organ Systems	Physical Therapist	Mobility/Motor Adaptation
Tissue	Rehabilitation Nurse	Illness/Self Management
Cells	Rehabilitation Physician	Diagnosis and Treatment
Organelle	Dietician	Nutrition, Weight, Endurance
Molecular	Pharmacist	Pharmacologic Therapy

Source: From *A Clinical Rehabilitation Course for College Undergraduates Provides An Introduction to Biopsychosocial Interventions that Minimize Disablement* by S.A. Stiens and D. Berkin, p. 463. Copyright © 1997 by American Journal of Physical Medicine and Rehabilitation. Reprinted with permission.

respiratory, musculoskeletal, cardiovascular, gastrointestinal, and genitourinary systems will likely necessitate a change in the previously performed routines for management and care. These new routines, in turn, may create a need for new skill development, equipment, and/or assistance from others. Further, these changes in functional abilities may also impact the individual's lifestyle, family, social, and vocational/avocational roles (Maynard, 1993). Therefore, these aging-related issues must be factored into the long-term care planning strategies for individuals with SCI.

Function, as it relates to SCI, is defined within two contexts. First, it applies to the medical context that defines the impairment of neurologic function (ASIA, 1996). *Impairments* are deficits in organ function or the presence of an organ. Impairment of neurologic function is one of the most objective measures of SCI.

In addition to neurologic measures, function also applies to the rehabilitation context as it relates to altered activities of daily living such as self-care and mobility and to changes in social role functions such as vocational, marital status, and avocational interests (Ditunno, Cohen, Formal, & Whiteneck, 1995). Deficits in task performance at the level of the person are *disabilities*. Because individuals with SCI vary widely in their capabilities, their overall rehabilitative functional outcome depends both on level of injury and residual muscle function along with an interplay of numerous psychological and physical factors (Yarkony, 1994). With rehabilitation, new techniques can be taught and adaptive equipment can be used to enable the person to perform many life activities despite impairments.

Management and Care of Spinal Cord Injury

After injury and acute rehabilitation, persons with SCI must have the knowledge and capability to direct their ongoing health and personal care needs (DeJong, Brannon, & Batavia, 1993). This requires an integration of both preventive and rehabilitative services over the person's lifetime. In addressing these needs, the life care planner must work closely with the individual with SCI, family, physicians, other health care professionals, and consulting specialists. The LCP must emphasize health maintenance, community integration, avocational and vocational development, and social adjustment.

Typically, an annual evaluation is performed to detect deterioration of systems, new diagnoses, and changes in function or equipment needs. This should be completed by an interdisciplinary team of health care professionals knowledgeable in SCI. Special attention must be given to the presentation of new symptoms, a review of medications, laboratory tests, and other evaluations necessary for the aggressive prevention and treatment of secondary complications and the preservation of function. In addition, an evaluation of equipment, particularly wheelchair(s), adaptive equipment, and pressure relief devices is needed along with periodic assessment of psychosocial problems and avocational/vocational goals to determine whether changes caused by age, living conditions, or family relationships will require further adaptation or assistance (Blackwell et al., 1994; Consortium for Spinal Cord Medicine, 1999a; Stover, Hall, DeLisa, & Donovan, 1995; Thomas, 1995).

Common Needs of People with Spinal Cord Injury

Although the spectrum of needs varies from individual to individual, a number of shared characteristics must be considered in developing a LCP for individuals with SCI. DeJong et al.(1993) describe these as follows:

- Persons with SCI are highly vulnerable to a variety of acute conditions such as pressure sores, urinary tract infections, and respiratory tract infections. If left unattended for even short periods of time, these conditions can quickly escalate and become life-threatening emergencies. However, many of these conditions are largely preventable with appropriate medical follow-up and care.

- Once a person with SCI develops an acute condition, the period for recovery and recuperation is frequently longer than for persons in the general population. Further, given the mobility limitations of persons with SCI, participation in selected therapeutic regimes may also be more limited.
- People with SCI are also at a greater risk for developing many chronic health conditions that accompany the aging process. Further, the onset of a new chronic health condition can have a substantial functional consequence. For example, the onset of exertional angina or respiratory insufficiency may require upgrading from a manual wheelchair to a power wheelchair and from a conventional automobile to an adapted van.
- To preserve function, individuals with SCI will need intermittent rehabilitative services and assistive technologies. For example, after years of using a manual wheelchair, the onset of arthritis and upper extremity pain may require the use of a power wheelchair. The need for new equipment may require a rehabilitation evaluation in an inpatient, outpatient, or home setting.
- In contrast to the general population, approximately half of all persons with SCI need some type of assistance with their daily care. This assistance is essential because it allows individuals to lead active and productive lives and to maintain a level of health that may prevent future complications.
- People with SCI who require mechanical ventilation will also require careful monitoring by qualified health care personnel and/or family members. Another necessity is an ongoing assessment by a variety of health care professionals such as respiratory therapists, nurses, and physicians.

Complications Secondary to Spinal Cord Injury

Those with SCI are more vulnerable to certain medical and psychosocial complications during their post-injury lifetimes (Stiens, Bierner-Bergman, & Formal, 1997). Cole (1994) concluded that, once an injury has occurred, the focus is on simultaneous treatment of the injury and prevention of secondary disabilities. Some of the medical complications that increase with age and duration of SCI are bladder infections, gastrointestinal tract problems, pressure sores, respiratory problems, fatigue, and bowel management problems (Anson & Shepherd, 1996; Gerhart, Bergstrom, Charlifue, Menter, & Whiteneck, 1993; Gerhart, Charlifue, Menter, Weitzenkamp, & Whiteneck, 1995; Pentland & Rosenthal, 1995; Stiens, Bierner-Bergman, & Goetz, 1997). These complications can further limit an individual's functional capacity, which in turn leads to an increase in the level of disability (Ravesloot, Seekins, & Walsh, 1997).

Many individuals with SCI will experience pressure sores at some time (Fuhrer, Garber, Rintala, Clearman, & Hart, 1993; Garber, Rintala, Rossi, Hart, & Fuhrer, 1996; Stover & Fine, 1986). Clinical depression is up to five times more prevalent than in the general population and may be a particular problem among racial and ethnic minorities (Kemp, Krause, & Adkins, 1999; Stiens et al., 1997). Urinary tract infections are almost inevitable. Fertility problems affect most men with SCI (Linsenmeyer, 1997; Martinez-Arizala & Brackett, 1994; Sipski, 1997; Szasz, 1992). Pain, contractures, and spasticity are also common occurrences (Centers for Disease Control [CDC], 1990). Treatment for these complications is often costly, as a result of unplanned hospitalizations. Findings from the National Spinal Cord Injury Statistical Center (NSCISC) indicate that after attendant care and household assistance, the costs of hospitalization because of complications of SCI rank second for people with tetraplegia and first among those with paraplegia (Ivie & DeVivo, 1994).

Aside from the direct economic impact, complications secondary to SCI may also exact a high personal toll in terms of disrupting the individual's ability to live independently and productively. In addition to resulting absences from school, work, and family life, complications and resultant hospitalizations can compromise many of the functional gains made during rehabilitation (American Congress of Rehabilitation Medicine, 1993). Because many of the conditions that necessitate hospitalization and loss of productivity may be preventable, particularly those related to pressure sores, urinary tract infections, and psychosocial problems, it is critical that the LCP focus on strategies to prevent complications, to whatever extent is possible.

CONCLUSION

A comprehensive LCP, by providing for effective and efficient medical and health-related professional support systems, as well as attendant or nursing services, should positively influence the issue of complications by reducing their frequency, severity, and cost (Deutsch, 1992). Consequently, a schedule of periodic follow-up assessment is essential to monitor, maintain, and improve the health of persons with SCI and to maximize their opportunities for community integration, avocational and vocational achievement, and psychosocial adjustment.

Systematic assessment by an interdisciplinary team of health care professionals knowledgeable and experienced in SCI treatment and care is essential to the long-term management and care of people with SCI (Whiteneck & Menter, 1993). Routine follow-up must include comprehensive medical, equipment, psychosocial, and avocational and vocational assessments from the patient's perspective and be able to anticipate gender differences and needs as a consequence of SCI.

Although there is presently no research to demonstrate the most appropriate frequencies for follow-up assessments, accumulated research and clinical experience have resulted in a number of evidence-based, general practice guidelines (Whiteneck & Menter, 1993; Consortium for Spinal Cord Medicine, 1997a, 1997b, 1998a , 1998b, 1999a, 1999b; U.S. Preventive Health Services Task Force, 1989; Department of Veterans Affairs [VA], 1994, 1998), available to life care planners and health care professionals (see Appendix O). However, the life care planner and case manager must keep in mind that these guidelines are not fixed protocols that must be followed, but are intended for health care professionals and providers to consider in working with individuals with SCI.

In summary, if the long-term care of SCI is to be effectively managed, strategies to prevent or delay more costly secondary impairments, disabilities, and handicaps, as well as effective methods to intervene and treat these conditions, must be identified and implemented into the LCP (Whiteneck & Menter, 1993). This type of long-range assessment often requires the life care planner or case manager to carefully prepare questions that prompt physicians, health care professionals, and providers into exploring those areas that address long-term issues for the individual with SCI (Blackwell et al., 1994). Some examples of discipline-specific questions that may need to be addressed in this planning phase process are included in Chapter 5.

2

Model for Life Care Planning with Spinal Cord Injury

By providing a comprehensive, interdisciplinary approach that systematically documents the needs of an individual with SCI over his or her life span, the LCP sets out criteria to maximize the individual's function, facilitate social independence, minimize the impact of secondary complications, enhance emotional adaptation, and promote reintegration into the community. The first step in the life care planning process begins with a thorough review of the medical records and a meeting with the individual and family. This is followed by consultation with various health care professionals and treatment team members, as needed, along with subsequent meetings with the individual and family, who are encouraged to take an active role in the needs assessment and plan development process. Once the initial plan is developed and agreed upon, then the life care planner must begin investigating resources, costs, and availability of services for subsequent plan finalization and implementation (Blackwell, Weed, & Powers, 1994).

Although the structure of the finalized plan may vary, several basic features must be included. The LCP must be comprehensive, objective, instructional, and provide information and recommendations that are informative, direct, and clearly understood by all who are involved with subsequent implementation of the plan. In addition, the LCP must be consistent with the individual's clinical needs and should reflect risk factors that have the potential to affect available resources (McCollom, 1999). Knowledge about the person whom the plan will serve is essential to the LCP process. As with acute rehabilitation, the LCP process must be individualized and goal-driven to ensure successful, ongoing adaptation to SCI.

The following sections provide an overview of the primary areas that are typically addressed in developing a comprehensive LCP for an individual with SCI. Each area further identifies general goals and objectives of the LCP, based on contemporary research and perspectives related to best-practice services (Blackwell et al., 1994; Reynolds, 1993). These factors include health, education, mobility, housing, transportation, employment, psychosocial adjustment, recreation, and self care.

Because the LCP is a dynamic document that can be updated and revised as a person moves through the age-related phases and continually adapts to SCI, the following sections are meant as general guidelines to assist the life care planner in anticipating the range of needs that may be present over a person's lifetime as a consequence of SCI. An example of a subsequent LCP for an individual with SCI is presented in Chapter 4.

HEALTH

A person who has sustained a SCI has a number of unique health care issues that require ongoing care and management. A careful program of preventive care will be of significant benefit to the person's general health, physical function, and social

15

and vocational effectiveness. Health promotion for these individuals is the result of interaction between disability management strategies, general health maintenance, and lifestyle practices. As a result, the life care planner must view disability-related health management and general health promotion strategies as equally important components of care when addressing long-term health needs in the LCP (Lanig, Chase, Butt, Hulse, & Johnson, 1996). This focus, in turn, requires an integration of preventive and rehabilitative services and includes care of both acute and chronic complications.

Periodic evaluations are necessary to systematically monitor health status and vulnerability to certain SCI-related complications. These evaluations must focus on function and well-being, equipment needs and assistance, medications and supplies, psychosocial and vocational status, and appropriate diagnostic tests for the body systems at particular risk (Department of Veterans Affairs [VA], 1998; Whiteneck & Menter, 1993). The Department of Veterans Affairs (VA), in published clinical practice guidelines (see Appendix O), recommends routine annual examinations that focus on health maintenance and the detection and prevention of SCI-related complications. The VA emphasizes that a primary function of long-term care for individuals with SCI is the prevention of complication due to disability.

In addressing long-term health care needs, the life care planner must also look at lifestyle alternatives that may be required as a result of age-related changes in impairment and/or functional abilities caused by increasing pain, weakness, and fatigue beyond what is expected for a person's chronologic age. Studies on aging and SCI suggest that health status declines correlate positively to years post-injury, particularly in persons more than 20 years post-SCI, than to chronological age (Krause & Crewe, 1991; Maynard, 1993; Whiteneck, 1993a). In addition, there must be a surveillance strategy to assess the individual's compliance with prescribed treatment, because for many people with SCI, compliance is often problematic for a number of reasons.

Table 2.1. Health Care Needs Assessment

Life Care Plan Goal	Life Care Plan Objectives
The goal of the LCP in addressing a person's long-term health-related needs is to develop a program of health promotion strategies based on research and clinical assessment that incorporates prevention and rehabilitation, positive consumer outcomes, and cost effective, consistent follow-up care and treatment and facilitates opportunities for optimal quality of life within the continuum of health care.	• To incorporate an ongoing systemic evaluation process that prompts consistency in assessment, planning, and treatment. The evaluation process must be based upon a comprehensive, individualized assessment by an interdisciplinary team of health care professionals experienced in the long-term care and treatment of SCI. • To identify and anticipate the need for equipment and resources that will facilitate individual adaptation and achievement of life goals. • To identify time frames, costs, frequency, duration of goods and services, and vendors/service providers for each of the recommendations identified. • To anticipate health care-need changes as a result of aging or duration with SCI. • To assess the appropriateness of the health recommendations with the individual's function, preferences, and lifestyle needs and the relationship of these items to other areas of the LCP, such as education, mobility, housing, transportation, employment, recreation, and self care.

Many age-related medical complications of the skin, respiratory, gastrointestinal, genitourinary, and musculoskeletal systems will necessitate a change in previously performed routines for managing these systems. These changes often create a need for new skill development, new equipment, and/or additional assistance from others (Maynard, 1993). In addition to addressing appropriate age-related alternatives to the individual's psychosocial, environmental, equipment, and attendant care needs, the life care planner must also incorporate respective specialist evaluations and treatment strategies and interventions necessary for providing efficient care.

Essential to the recognition and management of the individual's long-term health care needs is an ongoing systemic evaluation, follow-up, and intervention process by an interdisciplinary team of health care professionals experienced in the area of SCI and a program of education leading to alternative strategies. Although there is currently no research to demonstrate the most appropriate frequency for evaluation strategies, accumulated clinical experience from the Model Systems and VA data suggests that, in general, a person with SCI should be seen for comprehensive medical, equipment, psychological, and social assessments every one to three years (Whiteneck & Menter, 1993; VA, 1998). Obviously, these follow-up assessments may be more frequent as problems are encountered, generalized decline becomes more apparent, or as individuals become unable to monitor themselves effectively.

EDUCATION

The educational level of individuals with SCI becomes a significant factor for future employment. People who improve their educational level post-injury also increase the likelihood of their being employed, with the best outcomes obtained by persons with 16 years of education or more (Dijkers, Abela, Gans, & Gordon, 1995; Krause, 1992b; Krause, 1996; Krause, Sternberg, Maides, & Lottes, 1998). The assumption is that individuals with higher levels of education are more likely to make career adjustments and to find gainful employment in fields where the physical consequence of SCI is not a deterrent to employment success (Berkowitz, Harvey, Greene, & Wilson, 1992).

In addition to increasing the likelihood of obtaining competitive employment, post-injury education and training provide individuals with meaningful and constructive activity, increase the probability of social interaction, and contribute to feelings of self-worth (Walker & Holstein, 1994). Consequently, education is a critical component, whenever feasible, of any long-term planning efforts directed at enhancing post injury avocational or vocational productivity. However, when incorporating educational recommendations into the LCP, the life care planner must also consider the person's age, physical and mental status, level of functional independence, and adjustment to disability, as well as aptitudes, interests, and learning abilities (Donovan, 1981).

In addressing a person's educational needs, the life care planner must also be aware of the pertinent special education and civil rights legislation that relates to both children and adults with SCI. This information should be incorporated into the LCP as appropriate. At present, two primary federal laws form the basis for identifying school district and educational institution obligations and a disabled student's rights to education: the *Individuals with Disabilities Education Act (IDEA)* and Section 504 of the *Rehabilitation Act of 1973*.

IDEA is an educational law that supports special education and related services programming for children with disabilities and guarantees access to public education. Some of the services identified under IDEA that may apply to students with SCI include transportation, physical therapy, occupational therapy, adaptive physical education, psychological and social work services, and rehabilitation counseling. Students with SCI are typically qualified for services under the categories of "orthopedic impairment" or "other health impairment."

Table 2.2. Educational Assessment

Life Care Plan Goal	Life Care Plan Objectives
The goal of the LCP in addressing an individual's educational needs is to optimize the person's vocational and avocation potential and outcomes.	• To assess the individual's past and present functional abilities, aptitudes, educational values, interests, and expectations as these relate to educational goals. • To assess strength, stamina, bowel/bladder management, interpersonal support, adaptive equipment/assistance, transportation, accessibility, and mobility needs as these relate to the ability to successfully participate and complete an educational/training program. • To identify time frames, costs, frequency, duration of services and vendors, programs, and special support services, as appropriate for each of the recommendations identified. • To assess the appropriateness of the recommendations with the individual's function, preferences, and lifestyle needs, and the relationship of these recommendations to other areas of the LCP, such as health, mobility, transportation, psychosocial, employment, and self care.

Section 504 is a civil rights law that guarantees that people with disabilities are not to be discriminated against in any program, including schools, which receives federal funds. As a result, individuals with disabilities who qualify for admission into post-secondary education programs must be provided with services (e.g., modifications, accommodations, or auxiliary aids) that enable them to participate in and benefit from all educational programs and activities (Blackwell et al., 1994). Further information on the two laws is found in Chapter 3.

MOBILITY

Mobility has a profound effect on who a person is and who the person becomes. Basic mobility is central to the independence of people with SCI and key to their participation in family, community, and vocational roles (Triolo et al., 1996; Stiens, 1998c). Consequently, reestablishing and maintaining mobility is critical to the success the individual with SCI achieves in many life goals. Mobility refers to two basic capabilities: travel through the environment and manipulation of the environment. Consideration of the environment is essential for assessment of current and projections of future mobility capabilities. Assessment begins with consideration of the interaction between the person and the environment he/she is currently in (e.g., hospital, transitional living, etc.) and then extrapolating to the environments the individual expects to eventually occupy. Initial assessment by the interdisciplinary rehabilitation team and later by the life care planner should include an analysis of the series of sectors of the environment that surround the individual with SCI (see Figure 2-1).

The environment can be viewed from the perspective of the person with SCI then divided into sectors that surround the individual like shells or spheres (Stiens, 1998c). The *immediate* environment consists of the space that is in direct contact with the person and moves with the individual (e.g., clothes, adaptive equipment). The *intermediate* environment includes the living spaces that have been or could be adapted specifically for the individual with SCI. Typically, this will be the home

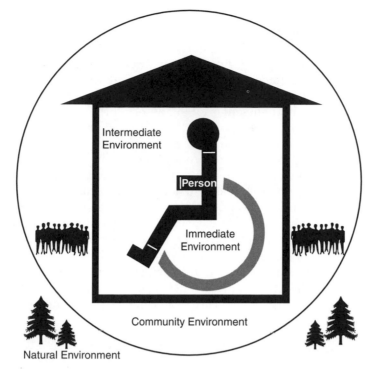

Natural Environment

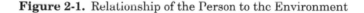

Source: From Personhood, Disablement, and Mobility Technology by S.A. Stiens in *Designing and Using Assistive Technology: The Human Perspective* by D.B. Gray, L.A. Quatrano, and M.L. Lieberman (Eds.), p. 43. Copyright © 1998 by Paul H. Brookes Publishing Co. Reprinted with permission.

Figure 2-1. Relationship of the Person to the Environment

or work space. Next is the *community* environment which is the space modified for public use. The community environment includes sidewalks, streets, public buildings, and adapted parks. Ideally, these areas would be universally accessible allowing all persons to use these spaces. Finally, there is the *natural* environment which is the space that has been minimally changed or left unaltered by man (e.g., lakes, waterways, forests, fields, and mountains that preserve animal habitats) that may or may not be accessible by wheelchair.

Long-term planning begins with the consideration of the individual's mobility in all four sectors of the environment by exploring his or her past utilization of mobility prior to injury. A careful review of the activities the person has done and potentially could do with proper equipment must be carried out as part of the life care planning process. The assessment next needs to consider the environment the person is in or is moving toward. Simple interventions in the immediate environment (i.e., surrounds the person and moves with them) may include items such as clothing that fits well and allows full movement and provides adequate protection from extremes of temperature and sunlight. Other interventions in the immediate environment may involve adaptive devices that are carried, bracing, and a fitted wheelchair. In the intermediate environment (personal home or office) the individual with SCI may be enabled with items such as environmental controls, adaptive furniture, or special appliances. Adaption in the community environment requires education regarding accessibility law and experience utilizing methods for overcoming architectural barriers, such as steps and curbs. This process often requires coordination with other health care professionals and searches for devices that could increase or maintain the individual's independence.

Many people with SCI need adaptive equipment and/or assistance with activities involving mobility, especially bed, wheelchair, toilet, and tub/shower transfers. Wheelchairs are the primary means of mobility for home, school, work, and recreation for most people with SCI. A person's level of functional independence is related directly to his or her ability to complete a variety of wheelchair mobility skills and transfers, with or without the use of special options or adaptions (American Spinal Injury Association [ASIA], 1993; Yasukawa, Stevens, & Ueberfluss, 1994). The selection and prescription of the wheelchair must be based on individual choice and lifestyle needs along with a team process evaluation involving a physiatrist/physician, occupational therapist, and physical therapist to determine which positioning/mobility system best optimizes the person's function.

Cooper, Boninger, and Rentschler (1999) asserted that clinical considerations in determining wheelchair choice must include fit, ease of propulsion, ease of transfers, ability to load in a motor vehicle, maneuverability, and aesthetics. Evidenced-based practice suggest it is extremely important to obtain the best chair possible for an individual with SCI and have it set up properly based on individual needs and lifestyle requirements (Cooper, 1998). Cost should not be the determining factor in evaluating a person's wheelchair needs, because the initial purchase price can be misleading. In a cost analysis study of manual wheelchairs, Cooper et al. (1996) demonstrated that although ultralight wheelchairs may cost approximately four times that of depot or standard wheelchairs, on average the ultralight may last more than ten times as long as the less expensive chair. From these studies the authors concluded that, overall, ultralight wheelchairs are more durable and cost effective than depot wheelchairs for people with SCI who are moderately active. In addition, Cooper et al.

Table 2.3. Mobility Assessment

Life Care Plan Goal	Life Care Plan Objectives
The goal of the LCP in addressing an individual's long-term mobility-related needs is to maximize and maintain independence, safety, and health, in the home and community setting through the use of appropriate adaptive equipment and devices.	• To incorporate an ongoing, interdisciplinary (e.g., physical therapist/occupational therapist, psychiatrist/physician, and rehabilitation equipment specialist) team evaluation process that encourages consistency in assessing the individual's functional status and subsequent prescription for mobility equipment needs. • To identify the environmental factors (home, mode of transportation, terrain, and lifestyle), activities (driving, shopping, food preparation, personal hygiene, child care, airline travel and recreation), and individual factors (socioeconomic status, religious preference, and profession) that influence the selection of appropriate equipment. • To identify the type, model, and accessories for mobility-related equipment, for both primary and backup items, including costs, local vendors, and maintenance/replacement schedules for each items recommended. • To anticipate equipment need changes as a result of aging or duration with SCI, including age-initiated and age-suspended changes. • To assess the appropriateness of the mobility recommendation to the individual's function, preferences, and lifestyle needs, and the relationship of these items to other areas of the LCP, such as health, education, housing, transportation, employment, recreation, and self care.

(1999) noted that neither lightweight nor depot wheelchairs incorporate the adjustability included in the design of ultralight wheelchairs. Wheelchair adjustability for long-term users can increase user mobility and possibly reduce the risk of secondary conditions such as shoulder pain, postural deformities, and repetitive strain injuries (Cooper, 1998; Cooper et al., 1996, 1999).

Many people with paraplegia can transfer independently and use a manual wheelchair. However, some individuals with paraplegia may require a power wheelchair because of activities involving increased energy and time expenditure. Although it is not unusual for some people with lower-level tetraplegia (C6 or below) to be able to use a manual wheelchair, many may choose to use a power wheelchair to save energy and to reach a maximum level of function (Blackwell et al., 1994).

The goal in identifying a person's mobility system, seating, support, and transfer needs in the life care planning process is to achieve as much independence as possible with the least amount of equipment. To maximize functional independence, the equipment should interface with both the user and the environment. Fit and function are critical elements in the selection of appropriate equipment (Galvin & Scherer, 1996; Stiens, 1998c).

The life care planner must keep in mind that, because of pathophysiologic changes associated with aging and SCI, equipment needs change during a lifetime. In general, those functional abilities that required the greatest personal and/or therapeutic effort to achieve in the acute phase of injury are those most likely to be lost as a result of age-related declines in physical capacity. These abilities include mobility and transfer-related activities (Maynard, 1993). As a result, people with incomplete or low-level SCI who may have been accustomed to independent walking with braces or crutches in the years immediately following injury may require a wheelchair after only five or ten years. In addition, individuals who used a manual wheelchair for mobility and were once able to transfer independently may later require a power wheelchair and have additional needs for pressure relief, posture, and seating along with an increased need for assistance with transfers or the use of mechanical or powered lifts and other adaptive equipment (Gerhart, Bergstrom, Charlifue, Menter, & Whiteneck, 1993; Johnson & Whiteneck, 1992; Maynard, 1993; Waters, Sie, & Adkins, 1993).

In anticipating a person's long-term mobility needs the life care planner must also consider issues related to lifestyle and environment (e.g., home, work, school), accessibility, transportability, the individual's ability to perform independent pressure reliefs (persons who lack the motor function to perform push-ups or lean for pressure relief should have a power recline system), and the availability of support systems that can provide the care required to keep a wheelchair functioning safely and appropriately (ASIA, 1993; Burns & Betz, 1999; Cooper, 1998; Formal, Cawley, & Stiens, 1997; Gerhart, 1993; Gerhart, Johnson, & Whiteneck, 1992).

HOUSING

Because the home environment is the base of operations for daily living and vocational pursuits, the importance of access becomes an essential quality of life issue (Jackson, 1994). With more than 90 percent of people with SCI being discharged to private residences following initial rehabilitation, it is imperative that the LCP include the range of modifications, renovations, and adaptive equipment needed to provide the individual with adequately accessible housing (Blackwell et al., 1994; Dijkers et al., 1995). The life care planner must keep in mind that housing needs are different for each individual and cannot be generalized to the disability. Planning must integrate both practical and functional considerations with more subjective qualities such as privacy and visual aesthetics in meeting the individual's needs (Davies & Beasley, 1999). Areas to be considered when assessing an individual's housing needs include general access, circulation/mobility, entry areas, sleeping, bathing/toileting, recreation, and transportation (Jackson, 1994).

In general, three possibilities are available for attaining an accessible home: 1) modifying an existing home; 2) relocating to an existing unit (house, apartment, or mobile home) that meets the individual's needs or that is easily modified; or 3) designing and building a new home to meet the person's needs. In terms of priorities, consideration should initially be given to modifying an existing home if already owned.

Modifications that are typically considered to provide an accessible home environment may include:

- Installation of ramps (with two exits recommended for safety)
- Widening of doorways and halls
- Removal of thresholds between rooms
- Installation of lift/elevator for getting from one level of the home to the other
- Renovating the kitchen with accessible appliances, shelves, and working spaces
- Modifying the bathroom to accommodate a wheelchair and related needs
- Replacing floor coverings
- Lowering light switches
- Renovating plumbing
- Modifying walks and driveways
- Modifying heating and air conditioning
- Incorporating an environmental control unit (ECU) or other adaptive equipment to maximize independence and safety

In addition to obtaining associated costs, the person's age, level of injury, living situation, and prioritization of time and energy for home management activities and unmet training needs are all issues the life care planner must consider when identifying home modifications with the individual and family. Consideration also must be given to providing for an initial and periodic reassessment of the person's living environment to ensure that changing needs are met throughout the aging process.

In terms of independence in home management tasks, individuals with injuries at C8 or lower are typically the best candidates for home modifications. The occupational therapist will often be a resource for help and advice in providing

Table 2.4. Housing Assessment

Life Care Plan Goal	Life Care Plan Objectives
The goal of the LCP in addressing a person's housing needs is to develop a plan that provides a safe, accessible, functional, and convenient environment that enhances the individual's lifestyle.	• To conduct a home evaluation to assess how the individual's lifestyle, function, activities of daily living, support system, equipment/assistance, and safety requirements relate to accessible housing needs. • To identify initial and recurring costs of modifications and equipment, frequency, maintenance and replacement schedules, vendors, service, support, and training needs relevant to use of equipment. • To anticipate changing needs as a result of aging and duration with SCI. • To assess the appropriateness of the housing recommendations with the individual's function, preferences, and lifestyle needs, and the relationship of these recommendations to other areas of the LCP, such as mobility, transportation, and self care.

the initial home evaluation and recommendations for modifications and needed accessories.

Additional assistance and information about community housing and programs may also be available from advisory groups on disability issues, rehabilitation facilities, independent living programs, and respective state protection and advocacy offices that help to maintain the rights of individuals with disabilities. The Rehabilitation Engineering Research Center for Accessible Housing (see Chapter 3) is another useful resource for providing technical assistance, training, and published information on topics for improving the useability, availability, and affordability of housing for people with disabilities. Local contractors can be contacted to obtain cost estimates for necessary modifications once needs have been determined through the initial evaluation (Blackwell et al., 1994).

TRANSPORTATION

Access to and full participation in the community is as important for persons with SCI as is accessibility in the home environment. Transportation is basic to working or going to school and accessing health care services. It is also a necessity in maintaining contact with the community. Transportation services are an unmet need for many individuals with SCI (McAweeney, Forchheimer, & Tate, 1996; Means & Bolton, 1994). Depending on the level of injury, muscle function, and endurance, most people with SCI can drive their own vehicles. For many, the best means of local transportation is by automobile or van (Blackwell et al., 1994).

Although specific transportation needs must be assessed on an individual basis, as a general guideline a person with high-level tetraplegia (above C5) will probably not be considered a driving candidate. Instead, the life care planner should focus on affordable special mass transit or private transportation services. The individual with a C6 level injury may be able to drive a van from a power wheelchair with "sensitive" steering and assistive or standard hand controls. A person with a C7 level injury may be able to drive a car equipped with an automatic wheelchair lift or to drive a van with an adjustable captain's chair, depending on his or her transfer skills and endurance. People with C8 or below injuries typically should be able to

Table 2.5. Transportation Assessment

Life Care Plan Goal	Life Care Plan Objectives
The goal of the LCP in addressing a person's long-term transportation-related needs is to identify geographic-specific transportation services that will maximize independence within the community.	• To incorporate routine SCI team assessments that monitor functional and mobility status as it relates to long-term safety issues, equipment needs, training, licensure, and transportation/vehicle recommendations. • To identify equipment/vehicle needs, accessories, and modifications, costs, maintenance/replacement schedules, and vendors/service providers for each of the recommendations identified. • To anticipate equipment, assistance, and service need changes as a result of aging and duration with SCI. • To assess the appropriateness of the recommendations with the individual's function, preferences, and lifestyle needs and the relationship of these items to other areas of the LCP, such as health, mobility, employment, recreation, and self care.

drive a car with power steering and standard hand controls (Kessler Institute for Rehabilitation, 1996). In the case of young children, the initial transportation needs may be limited to special safety car seats but later may progress to the family's need for a modified van with lift and wheelchair tie downs, as the child grows older and transfer becomes more of an issue (Deutsch & Sawyer, 1993).

As in the identification of other adaptive equipment needs, in addressing an individual's transportation needs the life care planner must consider accessories and modifications (e.g., lifts, door openers, swivel seats, tie downs, raised ceilings, lowered floors, hand controls, etc.), durability, availability, maintenance, and replacement schedules, as well as costs. A driver's evaluation and training, as appropriate, also typically must be incorporated in the LCP for those who will be driving. Specific information about evaluation requirements and training programs can be obtained from each State Department of Motor Vehicles, as well as from various local rehabilitation facilities (Blackwell et al., 1994). Finally, the life care planner must keep in mind that, for long-term planning purposes, the individual's equipment and transportation needs will change, often necessitating a switch to power wheelchairs, modified vans, and lifts due to aging-related issues and disability.

EMPLOYMENT

For many individuals with SCI, employment is more important than it is for the general population because of the psychological and financial adjustments that must be made (Blackwell et al., 1994). Returning to gainful employment has always been a highly valued rehabilitation goal and was once considered synonymous with rehabilitation success (Neff, 1971). An individual with SCI derives significant benefits from being employed, many of which are economic (Blackwell, Millington, & Guglielmo, 1999). For this reason (and others) it is important for the life care planner to assess the likelihood of an individual's return to gainful employment. This includes identifying resources needed to return to work (including funds for further education, transportation, equipment, and assistance, if appropriate), and ensuring that the influence of being or not being employed is assimilated into the life care plan. If compensative employment is not deemed a viable option, it is incumbent on the life care planner to account for the individual's needs to pursue productive avocational activities and to define any associated SCI-specific goods and services related to these needs. Issues of return to employment and earnings capacity will also impact instances where the LCP is a part of litigation.

Life care planners must assess for the probability of return to gainful employment in each LCP. Wherever possible the LCP should incorporate resources necessary to increase the likelihood of employment. This includes assessing whether the individual has a chance of returning to the pre-injury job. If this is not an option, it will be necessary to further assess previous employment and educational history, his or her overall capability for work, the potential for reeducation, and the desire to return to work, to determine whether return to work is a viable option. Obtaining a vocational evaluation may be helpful in this process (Habeck & Lynch, 1997). Because increasing educational level is the single most important factor in returning to employment after SCI, this should also be evaluated in any LCP. Education is costly, but effective. The maximum likelihood of returning to work is positively related to obtaining at least a college degree.

There are many circumstances under which an individual may not be a good candidate for gainful employment. Gainful employment may not be the best alternative if a person's educational level is too low or if he or she lacks the intellectual aptitude to obtain the degree of education needed. Similarly, employment may not be the best option for individuals who are injured late in life. If employment is not deemed a viable option, other types of productive avocational activities should be explored. For example, transportation resources should be identified to perform

Table 2.6. Employment Assessment

Life Care Plan Goal	Life Care Plan Objectives
The goal of the LCP in addressing an individual's employment needs is to maximize the person's return-to-work potential.	• To incorporate an ongoing vocational assessment process throughout the person's work life to ensure appropriate placement and support in a capacity consistent with the individual's changing functions, needs, and goals. • To determine a developmental sequence of services (e.g., vocational evaluation, career counseling and guidance, training/education, work hardening, accessibility, adaptive equipment/assistance, post-placement follow-up/evaluations, etc.) as necessary for employment and support. • To identify time frames, costs, frequency and duration of services, vendors, and providers for each of the employment-related service recommendations. • To evaluate the impact of age, education, severity of injury, race/ethnic, gender, and aging/duration with disability on work life recommendations and needs. • To assess the appropriateness of employment recommendations with the individual's function, preferences, and lifestyle needs and the relationship of these items to other areas of the LCP, such as health, education, mobility, transportation, psychosocial function, and self care.

volunteer work or other recreational activities. For a homemaker, resources should be allocated for appropriate home modification to allow the individual to carry out this role.

It is also necessary to consider that some individuals who return to work may have specials needs because of their SCI. For example, in addition to environmental accommodations, some individuals may need to work shortened work weeks, have flexible hours, or other accommodations related to their health needs.

Assessing the possibility of return to employment is not identical to determining loss of earnings potential, although the two may be related. Even when individuals return to work, they may lose income because they must work fewer hours or must work at jobs that carry fewer economic benefits. Furthermore, because the primary considerations are not necessarily economic in nature, the actual pay derived from a job may be balanced by the cost of job-related expenses (e.g., additional attendant care, transportation, etc.).

Consequently, the key to successful long-term vocational planning for persons with SCI is appropriate professional assistance in the areas of vocational adjustment counseling, career guidance and exploration, training and education, and selective placement with periodic follow-up and reevaluations of feasibility (Habeck & Lynch, 1997). The life care planner also must address issues related to financial disincentives, motivation, attendant care, bowel and bladder independence, environmental accessibility (including public transportation), decreasing strength and stamina, and increasing incidence of medical complications as a consequence of aging with SCI (Blackwell et al., 1994, 1999; Krause, 1992b; Stiens, 1998c; Stiens, Bierner-Bergman, & Goetz, 1997; Trieschmann, 1988).

PSYCHOSOCIAL FUNCTIONING

SCI necessitates major physical and psychosocial adaptations. Some factors that may impact an individual's psychosocial adaptation include changes in roles and responsibilities to perform household and child care tasks; increased need for quality attendant care; reduced mobility resulting in reduction of outings and social contacts; loss of social supports; financial pressures and a lowered standard of living; changes in sexual function; job loss and the resulting loss of social status; increased need for appropriate health care services, accessible and affordable transportation, and housing; and assumption of a stigmatized disabled status (Centers for Disease Control [CDC], 1990; Dijkers et al., 1995; Macleod, 1988). These factors in turn can have a significant impact on the emotional, psychological, and social well-being of the person with injury, and extend to family and friends as they attempt to cope with the lifestyle changes necessitated by SCI (Berkowitz et al., 1992). Further, many of these factors can interact and become both a secondary complication (e.g., suicide, self-neglect, depression, drug and alcohol abuse, impaired productivity) and a mediating factor for health outcomes and quality of life (CDC, 1990).

Several psychological factors must be considered after SCI. First, there are two primary components to an individual's subjective well-being. The first relates to nonclinical outcomes, such as life adjustment and life satisfaction. Multiple components may be measured, each of which relates to a particular area of life (Dijkers, 1997, 1999; Tate, Riley, Perna, & Roller, 1997). For example, Krause (1998) used factor analysis to identify the underlying dimensions of self-reported responses to 20 life satisfaction and 30 problem items, finding seven dimensions: 1) engagement in life, 2) negative affect, 3) health problems, 4) finances, 5) career opportunities — including both vocational and educational, 6) home and family life, and 7) interpersonal/sexual relationships. The primary importance of nonclinical aspects of subjective well-being to life care planning is that counseling may be needed to address particular areas, such as career or vocational, family, or interpersonal counseling. Counseling for these issues must be time-limited and focused, rather than ongoing for years or decades post-SCI.

It is important to recognize that, while there are substantial individual differences in personality among individuals with SCI, some characteristics are more prominent than they are in the general population. For example, Rohe and colleagues (Rohe & Athelstan, 1982, 1985; Rohe & Krause, 1998) identified personality traits that are highly prevalent after SCI. They found that the vocational interests and personality types most common among their study participants were reflective of a rugged outdoors orientation, with a preference for working manually with concrete tasks (Holland's Realistic theme). Individuals with this pattern of interests are not generally outgoing and prefer structure to the abstract. These individuals would generally rather work with things (tools) rather than people. Even though this pattern of interests is often incongruent with the limitation imposed by injury (e.g., a person with high level tetraplegia who is interested in working with his hands), Rohe and Krause (1998) found that these interests were not as likely to change over an 11-year period as that of the general population. It is not surprising to find such common personality traits given the selective nature of SCI itself. SCI is most likely to occur in young males engaging in high-risk behaviors (Taylor, 1967), and alcohol intoxication is often a factor in injury onset (Heinemann et al., 1988, 1991). There is also a great deal of stability in behavior pre- and post-injury (Fordyce, 1964).

It is important to consider personality because it impacts the effectiveness of strategies to elicit information by the life care planner. It is noteworthy that the interests patterns of counselors, life care planners, and case managers is often opposite to that of the client profile just described (based on Holland's typology). Therefore, life care planners working with individuals with SCI must assess the personality of the individual they are working with to develop the most effective LCP.

Proposing ongoing counseling for "adjustment issues" is ineffective with individuals who have the personality type described by Rohe. The LCP will be more effective if interventions or supports are consistent with the individual's personality.

The clinical aspects of subjective well-being may be much more problematic. Clinical depression is the most commonly identified long-term psychosocial consequence of SCI. In a review of research, Elliott and Frank (1996) found the rates of clinical depression much higher among people with SCI.

The emergence of depression, particularly among individuals aging with SCI (Krause, Kemp, & Coker, 1999), must be acknowledged by the life care planner. The onset of depression post-injury is obviously most predictable by a history of depression pre-injury. However, education is also a highly significant predictor of depression, with particularly high levels noted among individuals with less than 12 years of education. If clinical depression appears likely, the LCP should include allocation of resources for at least one episode of clinical depression during the post-injury period. Although treatment of depression is expensive, sometimes requiring six months of treatment and therapy, it is a cost effective means of limiting social isolation and declining health. Fortunately, pilot research at the Research and Training Center on Aging with Spinal Cord Injury at Rancho Los Amigos has found traditional treatment for depression highly successful among individuals with SCI who are living in the community.

In addressing an individual's psychosocial adjustment needs in the LCP, it is important to determine on both a short- and long-term basis the range of services and support that may be needed to ensure that an adequate adjustment to disability is achieved and that the person can reassume a functional role in the community (Stiens, Bierner-Bergman, & Formal, 1997). In pediatric cases, adaptation to disability may also need to address the parents' adaptation to the child's handicap (Gans, 1993). It is especially important that the needs of the long-term caregiver (parents, spouse, significant other) be addressed in the LCP. Combining the roles of spouse and significant other and caregiver places an enormous strain on a marriage or relationship. Whenever possible, the use of attendant care services should be provided to remove the burden of caregiver from the spouse or significant other because the preservation of marriage and relationships is important to the person's long-term wellness.

Table 2.7. Psychosocial Functioning Assessment

Life Care Plan Goal	Life Care Plan Objectives
The goal of the LCP in addressing a person's long-term psychosocial needs is to develop a program of surveillance and supportive interventions to ensure adequate adaptation and well-being for both the individual with SCI and the family, through age-related transitions.	• To incorporate an ongoing, periodic evaluation process that prompts consistency in psychosocial status assessment and treatment. This process must recognize and be sensitive to gender, racial/ethnic- and disability-related issues of people with SCI. • To identify costs, frequency, duration, and providers/services (e.g., individual/family counseling, sexuality counseling, parent skills training, peer support groups, etc.) as recommended in the LCP. • To anticipate service need changes as a result of aging and duration with SCI. • To assess the appropriateness of the psychosocial recommendations with the individual's personality, preferences, and needs, and the relationship of these services to other areas of the LCP such as health, education, employment, recreation, and self care.

Because SCI affects both the individual and family, family adjustment is another area that is frequently an issue after onset of disability and one that must be addressed in the LCP. All family members, including children, will likely have experienced losses and stressors and should have available to them some level of support and assistance. Further, as part of the life care planning process it is imperative that consideration be given to sexual adjustment (Stiens, Westheimer, & Young, 1997), marital/relationship issues, and age-related transition needs as the individual and family move through the maintenance and declination phases of SCI. Consequently, building supports through family, friends, hobbies, church, peer support, and/or appropriate counseling and interventions must become a central focus of the LCP in terms of preventing more serious problems, which can result in increased long-term costs.

RECREATION

Recreational pursuits are critical to the emotional and physical health and well-being of individuals with SCI (PVA, 1997). Recreational activities are highly beneficial for people with SCI. Physical activity stimulates circulation, helps prevent skin breakdown, increases fluid intake, provides for a sense of self-worth and mental health, improves the immune system and overall health, helps provide increased mobility and independence, and supports the individual's construction of an identity after injury (Blackwell et al., 1994; Cooper, 1998; Dattilo, Caldwell, Lee, & Kleiber, 1998; Foreman, Cull, & Kirkby, 1997; Kessler Institute for Rehabilitation, 1996; Lee, Dattilo, Kleiber, & Caldwell, 1996; McAweeney, Forchheimer, & Tate, 1997; Taylor & McGruder, 1996).

Relatively few studies have examined the role of leisure satisfaction in relation to quality of life or life satisfaction for people with SCI (Manns & Chad, 1999). Much of the research that has examined the contribution of leisure to life satisfaction has been conducted with non-SCI and elderly populations (Kinney & Cole, 1992). Kinney and Cole (1992) conducted interviews of 790 individuals with physical disability (23 percent of the study population had SCI) to determine the contributions leisure satisfaction make to a person's overall life satisfaction. The most significant predictor of life satisfaction was found to be leisure involvement and satisfaction. Kinney and Cole further found that leisure involvement can have a positive impact on an individual's psychological and physical health.

Development of an understanding of the leisure lifestyle a person pursues requires a careful and permissive history that attempts not only to identify the activities the individual enjoys but also to uncover aspects of the person's personality that guides his or her enjoyment. Review of past experiences and skills that have been developed for various activities can provide a foundation for intervention. Determination of each individual's medical restrictions, spine stability, impairments, disabilities, and handicaps prepares the recreation therapist and other interdisciplinary rehabilitation team members information to then offer recommendations regarding adaptive techniques, equipment, and therapeutic experiences for the person with SCI. Actual participation in activities generates options for adapted sports or recreation enjoyed previous to injury and offers options for new activities that may provide enjoyment and satisfaction as well. Knowledge of the individual's family constellation, friends, and others who may share in or support activities is essential. The life care planner needs to review the medical history of the person with SCI to identify the type of recreation therapy evaluations that may have been conducted and recommendations for future follow-up. The recreational goals of the individual need to be addressed in the LCP with funding for equipment as needed for the best leisure outcome following SCI.

Given the variety of options, adaptive equipment, and aids available, people with SCI can participate in a number of recreational activities at whatever level they

Table 2.8. Recreational Assessment

Life Care Plan Goal	Life Care Plan Objectives
The goal of the LCP in addressing an individual's long-term recreation needs is to identify activities that will bring personal fulfillment to the person with SCI and maintain and enhance health and well-being.	• To identify available and accessible recreational activities and pursuits that the individual can enjoy and participate in post-SCI, that are consistent with his or her interests, function, and safety needs. • To incorporate a periodic interdisciplinary (e.g., physiatrist/physician, physical therapist/occupational therapist, recreational therapist, etc.) team evaluation process that will assess the person's functional status and changes in recreational pursuits caused by age, living conditions, support systems, new equipment needs/assistance, etc. • To identify costs, and anticipate replacement/maintenance schedules for equipment/modifications, and vendors/service providers for items recommended. • To anticipate equipment need changes as a result of aging and duration with SCI. • To assess the appropriateness of the recreation recommendations with the individual's function, preferences, and lifestyle needs, and the relationship of these items to other areas of the LCP, such as health, mobility, transportation, psychosocial, and self care.

choose. In many cases they can participate in the same recreational activities they enjoyed prior to injury with the help of adaptive equipment and modifications. More detailed information on adaptive sports and recreational activities can be obtained by contacting the appropriate association or organization listed in Appendix N.

In planning these pursuits, the life care planner must work closely with the individual and family so that they make informed, self-directed choices in identifying activities that will bring fulfillment and pleasure. It is important to consider safety of the environment, the methods used to perform the activity, precautions against special injury (e.g., blisters, abrasions, cuts, pressure sores), and the safety standards and specifications of the equipment used. Personal issues such as bowel and bladder management, medications, sitting tolerance, and transportation also must be considered (Blackwell et al., 1994). It is also important for the LCP to incorporate some type of periodic assessment process (e.g., every one to three years) of the person's leisure time and recreational activities, to determine whether changes caused by age, living conditions, or support systems and family relationships require further equipment adaptation or assistance.

SELF-CARE

Many individuals with SCI have a permanent disability that limits mobility, sensation, and other functional abilities. Despite these limitations, many live independent and productive lives. Improved independence and safety, and improved or maintained health, are realistic outcomes for people with SCI when appropriate adaptive equipment and assistance is available and used. On the other hand, increased dependence, increased medical complications, and long-term care costs are some of the predictable outcomes of inappropriate equipment or inadequate levels of assistance (ASIA, 1993; Nosek, 1993).

Although people with SCI are typically discharged to private residences once the acute restoration phase has been completed (Dijkers, Abela, Gans, & Gordon, 1995; Stover & Fine, 1986), many of these individuals often require some assistance from others in activities of daily living (ADLs). These home- and community-based services are most critical to the independence of people with SCI. According to Harvey, Rothschild, Asmann, and Stripling (1990), about two-thirds of those with SCI receive some assistance in one or more activities, such as personal care, meal preparation, laundry, and other in-home activities. Much of this assistance is provided internally by family members, friends, and others rather than from formal service systems. However, as Nosek (1993) asserts, reliance on family members as the primary provider of personal assistance is often inadequate and leads to many adverse effects related to family and lifestyle role changes and economic strain, particularly if the spouse or partner must quit her or his job to assist the individual with a disability. Burnout, fatigue, exhaustion, stress, loss of intimacy, and social isolation are some of the more common consequences cited in situations where the family is primarily responsible for providing assistance (Maynard, 1993; Nosek, 1993; Trieschmann, 1988; Weitzenkamp, Gerhart, Charlifue, Whiteneck, & Savic, 1997). Although studies (Berkowitz, Harvey, Greene, & Wilson, 1992; Berkowitz, O'Leary, Kruse, & Harvey, 1998; DeVivo, Whiteneck, & Charles, 1995) have consistently demonstrated that attendant care and household assistance services represent a sizable share of annual direct costs (particularly among those with cervical-level injuries) following the first year post-SCI, little is known about the amount of care that would optimally be required based on needs rather than resource availability.

In the earlier PSA-DIS study, Berkowitz et al. (1992) found from a prevalence-based sample of 758 individuals with SCI that 65.7 percent of the study participants received some level of assistance with ADLs. As expected, the amount of assistance received varied by level and severity of injury. Individuals with tetraplegia required almost twice as much personal assistance as those with paraplegia. Women with SCI required somewhat more assistance than men. Overall, 72.6 percent of those who provided assistance to persons with SCI did so on voluntary basis.

In subsequent investigation of 500 people past one year post-SCI by Berkowitz et al. (1998), just over half (56.4 percent) of the total study population reported needing assistance with ADLs. Although this total was slightly less than Berkowitz et al. (1992) previous survey (65.7 percent), overall, the number of hours per week had increased from an average of 39.6 to 51.4 (more than a full-time job). Slightly more than two-thirds (69.9 percent) reported that this assistance was provided by an immediate family member, typically either a spouse (34.8 percent) or parent(s) (24.8 percent).

Because of the cross-sectional character of the Berkowitz et al. (1992, 1998) investigations on the level of utilization of personal assistance services by people with SCI, neither study was able to address the changing needs that may occur from aging with disability. Further, they did not take into consideration how additional medical and environmental variables may affect the number of assistance hours needed.

In a collaborative study between Craig Hospital and two British SCI treatment centers, Gerhart, Charlifue, Menter, and Whiteneck (1993) assessed the impact of aging on functional changes in people with long-term SCI. A total of 279 individuals (20 to 47 years post-SCI) participated in this study. Of the study sample, 65 percent had initially sustained thoracic, lumbar, or sacral level injuries, and 77 percent of these individuals and 80 percent of those with cervical level injuries that injuries which were functionally complete (Frankel A, B, or C). The majority of the study participants had been independent following initial rehabilitation. As these people aged many of them experienced functional declines necessitating changes in equipment and assistance (Gerhart et al., 1993). These functional declines often appeared by the time individuals with tetraplegia were in their late 40s, and the early 50s for those with lower level injuries.

In addressing the individual's long-term care needs, the life care planner must recognize that virtually all adaptive equipment items must be replaced periodically. Many of the larger, more expensive items, such as wheelchairs, orthoses, commode chairs, and vehicle modifications, are by virtue of their heavy usage very prone to wear and tear. The actual life expectancy of a piece of equipment is impacted by many factors, including how the piece of equipment is used (e.g., everyday; for work; for recreation; in what weather, geographic, and climatic conditions), the individual's size, weight, activity level, etc. In addition, it is important to anticipate that the individual's needs may change over time, making a wheelchair, bed, or other device that is appropriate now for independence and self care, useless or inappropriate as age combines with disability to create greater dependency (ASIA, 1993).

Accurate estimation of the amount and level (often determined by state regulatory requirements for agency-provided services) of assistance needed to support a person with SCI is of critical importance to the LCP process. As part of the long-term care plan, adequate and appropriate assistance can reduce or prevent many health complications and help individuals with SCI maintain themselves at greater levels of independence and productivity. In addition to looking at the amount of assistance required, the LCP also must focus on a delivery system (individual provider or agency-based) in which the individual and family have the greatest possible choice and control of who provides assistance. Further, the LCP must anticipate service needs provided in a community setting, backup and emergency services, availability in locations other than the home (e.g., school and work), and flexibility of hours.

The importance of individual needs assessment for assistance cannot be overemphasized. It must be developed on a case-by-case basis that is individualized to the unique circumstances, characteristics, and capabilities of each person (Consortium for Spinal Cord Medicine, 1999a). Any projections must be based on the

Table 2.9. Self-Care Assessment

Life Care Plan Goal	Life Care Plan Objectives
The goal of the LCP in addressing a person's long-term self care needs is to develop a plan to maximize the individual's self dependence through provision of appropriate equipment and levels of assistance.	• To incorporate an ongoing, interdisciplinary SCI team evaluation process that prompts consistency in assessment of the individual's functional status and changing equipment, safety, and assistance care needs (e.g., skilled nursing, personal attendant care, homemaking, etc.). • To identify time frames, costs, goods and services, including frequency, duration, maintenance and replacement schedules as well as vendors and service providers for each item recommended. • To anticipate adaptive equipment/assistance need changes as a result of aging and duration with SCI. • To assess the appropriateness of the self care recommendations with the individual's function, preferences, and lifestyle needs and the relationship of these items to other areas of the LCP, such as health, education, mobility, housing, transportation, employment, psychosocial, and recreation.

individual's functional needs and life demands and not merely on diagnostic status or classification. One way to systematically identify the self-care needs and demands of a person with SCI is to obtain contributing information through completion of the Functional Independence Measurement (FIM)™ instrument with different observers (e.g., individual with SCI, family members, and caregivers). Because each of these reporters may represent a different potential bias, it is critical to incorporate other data as well, including medical information and patient factors, social role participation, quality of life, and environmental factors and supports (Consortium for Spinal Cord Medicine, 1999a).

CONCLUSION

SCI is a lifelong condition requiring continuous management to stabilize, diminish, or prevent impairments; avoid or limit secondary complications; and improve and maintain function, independence, productivity, social role, and quality of life. Therefore, the LCP must focus on preventive health maintenance procedures and services with appropriate equipment and applied technology to promote long-term survival and an independence role for the person with SCI. Best practice for assessment of goods and services is based on individual needs and treatment guidelines, as needed to optimize long-term health care, independence, and quality of life, while minimizing the risk of secondary complications. This assessment must be comprehensive, individualized, and performed by an interdisciplinary team of health care professionals experienced in working with individuals with SCI. No one member of the team has the depth of knowledge or range of skills necessary to independently assess or treat an individual with SCI (Consortium for Spinal Cord Medicine, 1999a).

Treatment guidelines must incorporate systematic evidence-based studies and clinical application of populations that best describe the individual with SCI. Although there is a growing body of high-quality, well-defined research for SCI populations, these data should never be used to project individual needs as dictated by onset of injury. Although supportive research and literature can assist health care providers and individuals with SCI to make informed decisions regarding long-term planning considerations, it is still imperative that the LCP be developed around the unique needs of the individual with SCI.

3

Resources and Legislation Related to Spinal Cord Injury

The primary function of the life care planner is to identify long-term needs that have resulted from the onset of a SCI. As stated throughout the previous chapters, life care planners must be concerned with developing needs-based rather than cost-driven plans. This is central to the life care planning process. However, there may be circumstances where the life care planner is asked to step out of his or her distinct role of needs assessment and into case management. Unlike pure life care planning, this role requires the life care planner to assist in identifying funding and other resources, as well as to develop priorities in the needs assessment based on available resources. Life care planners working on cases in active litigation or other mediation must avoid stepping outside their primary role until after settlement or arbitration has been completed. At that point, the life care planner may assist in resource allocation. This chapter is intended to assist the life care planner with this task.

IDENTIFYING RESOURCES

Over the years, people with SCI have moved from the role of *patient* to the role of *consumer*. As consumers, people with SCI need information and services that will help them to live as independently as possible (McColl & Rosenthal, 1994; Research and Training Center on Independent Living [RTC/IL], 1994). This need has become evident through the advent of a number of consumer-driven research projects such as those funded by the World Institute on Disability, Paralyzed Veterans of America, the American Paralysis Association, and the Spinal Cord Society. The findings from these projects and a culmination of consumer disability group efforts resulted in the passage of the 1990 Americans with Disabilities Act (Corbet, 1995).

The goal of the LCP is to maximize the individual's physical, mental, social, and vocational function within the constraints of disability and environmental barriers. Therefore, the life care planner and case manager must be able to identify and coordinate various service providers, insurance companies, local health care providers, state and federal funding agencies, and various voluntary or non-profit agencies and organizations. Identifying and coordinating these resources with the individual and his or her family is necessary to develop a comprehensive plan that assists in making appropriate choices relevant to the best use of resources over the long-term continuum of care needed to maintain overall quality of life (Sims, Manley, & Richardson, 1993).

Figure 3-1 is a breakdown of the various sources for sponsors of care for individuals with SCI. These data were extrapolated from the National Spinal Cord Injury Statistical Center (NSCISC). The results should be interpreted with caution, because some of the sponsors, such as the Department of Veterans Affairs (VA)

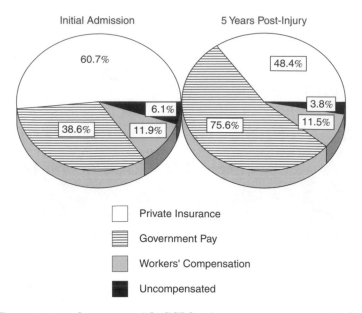

Figure 3-1. Percentages of persons with SCI having common sponsors[a] of care at initial admission and five years post injury[b].
[a]Private Insurance includes Health Maintenance Organizations, CHAMPUS (TRICARE) or other private insurance.
Government Pay includes Medicare, Medicaid, VA, county medical, public health service, vocational rehabilitation, or other government payor.
Uncompensated includes self-pay, indigent, or other private funds.
[b]Percentages do not sum to 100 because many individuals have more than one sponsor.
(From the Economic Impact of Spinal Cord Injury, M.J. DeVivo, G.G. Whiteneck, and E.D. Charles in *Spinal Cord Injury: Clinical Outcomes from the Model Systems*, S.L. Stover, et al., p. 255. Aspen Publishers, Inc., 1995. Reprinted with permission.)

and Health Maintenance Organizations (HMOs), may be underrepresented in the National SCI Database.

Further, in considering the various sponsors of care, the life care planner or case manager must recognize that many private sector health insurance plans, such as indemnity plans and HMOs, are more likely to pay for goods and services during the acute phases of SCI, while a public sector health plan, such as Medicaid, is more likely to pay for goods and services along the continuum of SCI, although at a more restricted level of coverage (DeJong, Brannon, & Batavia, 1993).

In addressing the continuum of comprehensive long-term needs for persons with SCI, the life care planner or case manager must have a practical understanding of how to research and develop the information and resources necessary for an individualized, geographically appropriate LCP that fosters self-directed management and care. At times, this planning process may require developing creative alternatives for funding sources and services to maintain the needs-driven focus that is central to a LCP.

The following sections outline a number of basic resources that may serve as a starting point to assist life care planners and case managers and individuals with SCI to increase their knowledge and understanding of the information and services related to LCP development and implementation.

In addition, this chapter reviews key legislation, public resources, major funding sources, and consumer organizations that may be used in addressing the person's long-term continuum of care needs. It is imperative that life care planners and case managers view these resources as only a starting point for enhancing the knowledge necessary to adequately address the comprehensive long-term planning needs of individuals with SCI.

MODEL SPINAL CORD INJURY PROGRAM

The Model Spinal Cord Injury program is a delivery, demonstration, evaluation, and research program funded and managed by the National Institute on Disability and Rehabilitation Research (NIDRR), Office of Special Education and Rehabilitative Services, U.S. Department of Education. NIDRR evolved from a single research and demonstration project in 1970 into 16 regional Model Systems at the present time. Established to examine costs, treatment, outcomes, complications, and other factors related to SCI, the Model Systems provide a comprehensive, interdisciplinary service delivery system in which medicine, rehabilitation engineering, and the social sciences work with the primary consumer — the person with SCI — to achieve his or her maximum potential through individual empowerment, independence, and community integration. These Model Systems work together to demonstrate improved care, participate in independent and collaborative research, provide continuing education relating to SCI, and maintain a national database. Since 1984, the National Spinal Cord Injury Statistical Center (NSCISC) at the University of Alabama at Birmingham has been responsible for supervising and directing the collection, management, and analysis of the world's largest database on SCI.

To qualify for designation as a Model System and to receive funding from NIDRR, rehabilitation programs must use and evaluate a SCI treatment prototype based on providing continuity of care through the development of four areas within a system (Federal Register, 1999). Model SCI Systems must:

1. Establish a multidisciplinary system of providing rehabilitation services specifically designed to meet the special needs of individuals with SCI, including emergency medical services, acute care, vocational and other rehabilitation services, community and job placement, and long-term community follow-up and health maintenance.
2. Participate in national studies of SCI by contributing to the National SCI Database and by other means.
3. Conduct a significant and substantial research program in SCI that will contribute to the advancement of knowledge in one of the following areas: 1) employment outcomes; 2) maintaining health and function; 3) technology for access and function; or 4) independent living and community integration.
4. Provide for the widespread dissemination of research and demonstration findings to other Model Systems, rehabilitation practitioners, researchers, individuals with SCI and their families, and other public and private organizations involved in SCI care and rehabilitation.

The information collected by the Model Systems is disseminated through presentations for professionals and individuals with SCI and families; newsletters; papers in clinical and research journals; data summaries supplied to government agencies and other interested parties; consumer-based literature; and in a variety of written materials and media. The information generated by the Model Systems can be quite useful in understanding and addressing the long-term needs and implications of individuals with SCI. Additional information is available on the Web at www.ncddr.org/mscis.

The 16 Model SCI Systems that are funded for the 2000–2005 Project Period are:

Model Spinal Cord
  Injury System
University of Alabama
  at Birmingham
Birmingham, AL
Model Spinal Cord
  Injury System
Rancho Los Amigos
  National
  Rehabilitation Center
Downey, CA
Northern California
  Model Spinal Cord
  Injury System
Santa Clara Valley
  Medical Center
San Jose, CA
Rocky Mountain
  Regional Spinal Cord
  Injury System
Craig Hospital
  Englewood, CO
University of Miami
  Model Spinal Cord
  Injury System
University of Miami
Miami, FL
Georgia Regional Model
  Spinal Cord Injury
  Care System
Shepherd Center, Inc.
  Atlanta, GA

Special Projects and
  Demonstrations for
  Spinal Cord Injuries
Boston University
  Medical Center
  Hospital
Boston, MA
University of Michigan
  Model Spinal Cord
  Injury System
University of Michigan
Ann Arbor, MI
Missouri Model Spinal
  Cord Injury System
University of
  Missouri — Columbia
Columbia, MO
Northern New Jersey
  Model Spinal Cord
  Injury System
Kessler Institute for
  Rehabilitation
West Orange, NJ
Mount Sinai Spinal
  Cord Injury Model
  System
Mount Sinai Medical
  Center
New York, NY

Model Spinal Cord Injury
  System
Thomas Jefferson
  University Philadelphia,
  PA
Model Spinal Cord Injury
  System
The Institute for
  Rehabilitation and
  Research
Houston, TX
Missouri Model Spinal Cord
  Injury System
University of
  Missouri — Columbia
Columbia, MO
VCU/MCV Spinal Cord
  Injured Model System
Virginia Commonwealth
  University/Medical
  College of Virginia
Richmond, VA
Northwest Regional Spinal
  Cord Injury System
University of Washington
  School of Medicine
Seattle, WA

REHABILITATION RESEARCH AND TRAINING CENTERS (RRTCS)

In addition to the Model Systems program, the NIDRR also sponsors a number of Rehabilitation Research and Training Centers (RRTCs) that conduct research and training activities aimed at producing new knowledge to improve rehabilitation methodology and service delivery systems for persons with disabilities. Each RRTC provides for dissemination of information and research activities through a variety of formats that may include training and presentations, research-based journal articles, manuals, information packets, videotapes, slide series, and books. The targeted groups for these activities include health care professionals, consumers, third party payors, and community groups. The following RRTCs may assist the life care planner and case manager to identify further research-based, informational resources directed at better understanding and altering the course of disability for persons with SCI.

RRTC on Secondary Conditions of Spinal
  Cord Injury
University of Alabama at Birmingham
Birmingham, AL
RRTC on Aging with Spinal Cord Injury
Los Amigos Research and Education
  Institute, Inc.
Downey, CA

RRTC on Personal Assistance Services
World Institute on Disability
Oakland, CA
RRTC on Rural Rehabilitation
  Services
University of Montana
Missoula, MT

REHABILITATION ENGINEERING RESEARCH CENTERS (RERCS)

The Rehabilitation Engineering Research Centers (RERCs) are supported by the NIDRR to conduct programs of advanced engineering or technical research to develop and test new engineering solutions to problems associated with disability. Each Center is affiliated with a rehabilitation setting that provides an environment for cooperative research and for the development of rehabilitation technologies into rehabilitation practice. The Centers' additional responsibilities include developing systems for the exchange of technical and engineering information and improving the distribution of technological devices and equipment to individuals with disabilities. As with the Model Systems and the RRTCs, the following RERCs can be another valuable resource for the life care planner or case manager when addressing long-term care needs of individuals with SCI.

RERC on Applications of Technology to
  the Rehabilitation of Children with
  Orthopedic Disabilities
Los Amigos Research and Education
  Institute, Inc.
Downey, CA
RERC on Telerehabilitation
Catholic University of America
Washington, DC
RERC in Prosthetics and Orthotics
Northwestern University
Chicago, IL
RERC for Ergonomic Solutions for
  Employment
University of Michigan
Ann Arbor, MI
RERC on Assistive Technology for Older
  Persons with Disabilities
State University of New York (SUNY) at
  Buffalo
Buffalo, NY

RERC on Universal Design and the
  Built Environment at Buffalo
State University of New York
  (SUNY) at Buffalo
Buffalo, NY
RERC on Universal Design and the
  Built Environment
North Carolina State University
  Center for Universal Design
Raleigh, NC
RERC on Wheeled Mobility
University of Pittsburgh
Pittsburgh, PA
RERC on Information Technology
  Access
University of Wisconsin
Madison, WI
RERC on Telecommunication
  Access
University of Wisconsin Trace
  Center
Madison, WI

RURAL HEALTH RESEARCH CENTERS (RHRCS)

The federal Office of Rural Health Policy, of the Health Resources and Services Administration, U.S. Department of Health and Human Services, presently funds five Rural Health Research Centers (RHRCs). These centers can also serve as resources for life care planners and case managers when addressing the health care issues of individuals with SCI who live in rural communities.

Maine Rural Health Research Center
University of Southern Maine
Portland, ME
Project Hope Walsh Center for Rural
    Health Analysis
Bethesda, MD
University of Minnesota Rural Health
    Resource Center
Institute for Health Services Research
Minneapolis, MN

North Carolina Rural Health Research
    Program
Sheps Center for Health Services
    Research
Chapel Hill, NC
WWAMI Rural Health Research
    Center
University of Washington
Seattle, WA

DEPARTMENT OF VETERANS AFFAIRS (VA)

The Department of Veterans Affairs (VA) provides a full range of long-term care and benefit services for veterans with SCI. Through the Regional SCI Centers, the VA provides acute care to approximately 400 newly injured veterans annually and more than 15,000 persons with chronic SCIs. The VA serves approximately 7 percent of the total U.S. SCI population (Department of Veterans Affairs, 1999). Individuals with service-connected disabilities are given priority.

In addition to providing acute and long-term care services, the VA also provides funding to researchers in VA hospitals throughout the country to conduct research on all aspects of SCI, from the development of new assistive devices to improved treatment for SCI-related health problems. The VA research program consists of four distinct research services.

- Medical Research Service supports basic and clinical studies that advance knowledge leading to improvement in the prevention, diagnosis, and treatment of diseases and disabilities.
- Rehabilitation Research and Development focuses on promoting healing and improving quality of life for veterans with disabilities in need of prosthetic devices, sensory aids, and mobility assistance.
- Health Services Research and Development examines the impact of organization, management, and financing of health care services on the delivery, quality, cost, and outcomes of care.
- The Cooperative Studies program conducts multihospital, randomized clinical trials for new medical therapies.

In fiscal year 1998, the VA allocated over $7 million dollars to fund 62 projects dealing specifically with SCI. Non-VA funding to VA investigators for 114 additional projects totaled almost $6 million dollars. An additional 180 projects with no specific funding were directed toward various aspects of SCI.

From a clinical perspective, the VA was the first to provide organized medical management services to individuals with SCI. Because of its responsibility to provide care to veterans, the VA has provided services to the population of persons with SCI who have been living with their disabilities for a large portion of their lives. Given its long history of research and clinical experience with people who have chronic SCI, the VA can be a valuable resource for long-term care needs information. In addition, the VA can offer a continuum of long-term care services to veterans with SCI.

There are currently 23 VA Regional Spinal Cord Injury Centers, located in the following cities:

Long Beach, CA

Palo Alto, CA

San Diego, CA

Miami, FL

Tampa, FL

Augusta, GA

Hines, IL

Roxbury, MA

St. Louis, MO

East Orange, NJ

Albuquerque, NM

Bronx, NY

Castle Point, NY

Cleveland, OH

San Juan, PR

Memphis, TN

Dallas, TX

Houston, TX

San Antonio, TX

Hampton, VT

Richmond, VA

Seattle, WA

Milwaukee, WI

SPINAL CORD INJURY ASSOCIATIONS AND ORGANIZATIONS

The following associations and organizations are involved in a variety of SCI-related topics, including research, treatment, empowerment, and education. In addition, several of these organizations function as a consumer-driven clearinghouse of information on a wide range of topics, including personal care and lifestyles, legislation, self-help devices, equipment, transportation, employment, education, and activities of daily living. They can also serve as a resource in providing referrals to local contacts for self-help and advocacy services.

American Association of Spinal Cord
  Injury Nurses
75-20 Astoria Boulevard
Jackson Heights, NY 11370
(718) 803-3782

American Association of Spinal Cord
  Injury
Psychologists and Social Workers
75-20 Astoria Boulevard
Jackson Heights, NY 11370
(718) 803-3782

American Paralysis Association
500 Morris Avenue
Springfield, NJ 07081
(800) 225-0292

American Paraplegia Society
75-20 Astoria Boulevard
Jackson Heights, NY 11370
(718) 803-3782

American Spinal Injury Association
  (ASIA)
345 East Superior Street, Room 1436
Chicago, IL 60611
(312) 908-1242

National Spinal Cord Injury
  Association
8701 Georgia Avenue, Suite 500
Silver Spring, MD 2091
(800) 962-9629 (helpline)

Paralyzed Veterans of America
PVA Spinal Cord Research Foundation
801 18th Street NW
Washington, DC 20006
(800) 424-8200

Spinal Cord Society
Wendell Road
Fergus Falls, MN 56537
(218) 739-5252

MAJOR FUNDING SOURCES

The long-term costs of SCI can be reduced by providing cost effective services and assistive devices to help persons with SCI increase their capacities to live independently and productively. However, individuals with SCI often lack adequate access to these services and assistive devices because of financial constraints

(Batavia, 1990). As a consequence, the life care planner or case manager must be able to provide guidance on how these long-term needs can be met through the use of a variety of available sources. Some of the major sources of funding assistance for long-term care services of people with SCI are outlined below. Each source has different eligibility criteria and specific rules regarding the types of goods and services that can be covered and purchased. Often more than one source may be required to obtain the services needed. Because state and federal rules and regulations change constantly and can vary from state to state, the life care planner or case manager must confirm the status of the information with respective programs, agencies, or other sources.

Medicare

Legislative / Legal Basis

Title XVIII of the Social Security Act. Medicare has two parts: Mandatory hospital insurance (Part A) and Optional medical insurance (Part B).

Eligibility

Persons who are 65 years of age or older and have paid into the Social Security system for a minimum of 40 quarters or 10 years; or, under 65 years of age but disabled enough to qualify for Social Security Disability Insurance (SSDI) for at least 24 months are eligible for Medicare benefits.

Service Coverage Policies

Part A covers the costs of hospitalization (full cost for days 1 through 60 after deductible is met; full cost for days 61 through 90 after coinsurance is met); skilled nursing care (covers 100 percent of first 20 days of each benefit period, days 21 through 100 are covered once the coinsurance is met); home health care, and hospice care. Part B is an optional program that covers physician and outpatient care, medical supplies, and other medical services. Medicare covers few services at the chronic end of the continuum of health care needs.

Equipment Payment Policies

Durable medical equipment (DME) such as wheelchairs (a copayment of 20 percent is required from the individual). Medicare will not pay for equipment which has the primary purpose of enhancing functional status or fostering independence, any equipment covered by Medicare must be considered "medically necessary."

For More Information

Health Care Financing Administration
6325 Security Boulevard
Baltimore, MD 21207
(410) 786-3000

Medicaid

Legislative / Legal Basis

Title XIX of the Social Security Act.

Eligibility

Categorically needy persons who are eligible for Aid to Families with Dependent Children (AFDC) or Supplemental Security Income (SSI) programs are eligible for Medicaid. Some states cover medically needy individuals whose incomes, after deducting medical expenses, fall below the income threshold.

Service Coverage Policies

Medicaid must cover the following services if they are determined to be medically necessary for all categorically needy persons: inpatient hospital services; outpatient hospital services; lab and x-ray services; services in a skilled nursing facility; early and periodic screening, diagnosis, and treatment; family planning; physician; and home health services. Other services, many of which are of concern to persons with SCI, may be provided at the option of the state.

Equipment Payment Policies

These policies vary from state to state but "medical necessity" is a critical factor for payment. State payment for equipment generally follows Medicare policies. Most states pay for home medical equipment (HME) and many pay for prosthetics and orthotics. A growing number of states are paying for augmentative communication equipment.

For More Information

Contact the local State department of social or human services. Local Medicaid administrators are usually local, regional, or county social services agencies, human resources agencies, health department, or community hospitals.

Federal/State Rehabilitation

Legislative / Legal Basis

Rehabilitation Act of 1973 and Amendments (Title I)
   Title I — Vocational Rehabilitation (VR) Services
   Title VI — Supported Employment
   Title VII — Independent Living

Eligibility

To qualify, an individual must be a working age person who is disabled and has some potential to benefit from the provision of services. The emphasis is on persons with severe disabilities. Other Titles of the Rehabilitation Act stress independent living and supported employment where vocational potential is not the determining factor.

Service Coverage Policies

Title I may offer the following services while the individual participates in rehabilitation: medical, psychological, and vocational evaluations; counseling, guidance, and work-related services; vocational and other training services; physical and mental restoration services; maintenance; occupational licenses, tools, equipment, and initial stocks and supplies; transportation; rehabilitation technology and telecommunication services; transition, on-the-job, and other related personal assistance services. Title VI provides for supported employment services. Title VII provides the following no-cost core services: information on and referral to locally accessible housing, transportation, employment opportunities, individuals available to serve as personal care attendants; independent living skills training; peer counseling; and, both individual and community advocacy to improve opportunities for increased independence.

Equipment Payment Policies

Equipment that is justified as expediting the goal of vocational placement is covered. Usually purchases are reserved for clients who are at least job ready (Title I). In many states rehabilitation agencies retain ownership of the equipment.

For More Information

For additional information on available resources, contact the appropriate state department of rehabilitation services, typically listed as the Department or Office of Rehabilitation Services or the Department of Vocational Rehabilitation Services.

Plan for Achieving Self-Support (PASS)

Legislative / Legal Basis

1980 Amendments to the Social Security Act.

Eligibility

The plan provides an income and/or resource exclusion that allows a person who is blind or disabled and receiving SSI to set aside income and/or resources for a work goal such as education, vocational training, or starting a business.

Service Coverage Policies

A PASS is different for each person and can be used for almost any expense that helps to achieve an individual's vocational goal. Financial assistance is available for up to four years for one PASS. The initial plan can be approved for a period of 18 months, with extensions available for 12 and 18 months, respectively.

Equipment Payment Policies

Individuals can set aside funds to purchase work-related equipment, such as a computer or other assistive devices.

For More Information

To learn more about PASS services, contact a local Social Security representative or consult the Social Security Administration (SSA) booklet entitled the *Red Book on Work Incentives: A Summary Guide to Social Security and Supplemental Security Income Work Incentives for People with Disabilities* (1999).

Special Education

Legislative / Legal Basis

Individuals with Disabilities Education Act (IDEA) (P.L. 101-476), formerly the Education for All Handicapped Persons Act (P.L. 94-142).

Eligibility

Children with disabilities aged birth through 21 are eligible under this Act. Although qualified students are eligible for services through age 21, states are not obligated to provide services beyond age 18, if it is inconsistent with state law, court ruling, or practice.

Service Coverage Policies

IDEA requires that state and local school districts make a free, appropriate public education (FAPE) available to all eligible children with disabilities, in the least restrictive environment. The school must have available and must consider a full range of educational alternatives, related services, and assistive technology.

Some of the services identified under IDEA that could apply to students with SCI may include transportation; physical and occupational therapy; adaptive physical education; counseling services; home trainer services; social work services in school; and rehabilitation counseling. The major instrument used to document that the student qualifying for special educational services receives an appropriate and individualized education is the Individualized Education Plan (IEP). The IEP is developed by a team of professionals, with input from the student's parents. It is reviewed annually and procedures are established to ensure an impartial hearing in the case of a dispute.

Equipment Payment Policies

Equipment that is justified as expediting educational goals of students is covered under the Act. IDEA is also responsible for meeting the family support needs of families with preschool aged children. In many states equipment is owned by and remains at the student's school.

For More Information

For additional information, contact the appropriate State Education Department and the Office of Protection and Advocacy.

Department of Veterans Affairs (VA)

Legislative / Legal Basis

Title 38 of the U.S. Code.

Eligibility

Eligibility for VA services is determined by the veteran's service and financial status. Category A includes service connected veterans or nonservice connected veterans but with income below $15,000 if single or $18,000 with dependent: Category B includes veterans not in Category A but with annual income below $20,000 if single or $25,000 with dependent; Category C is all other veterans.

Service Coverage Policies

VA benefits may be available to individuals who have served in the Armed Forces. Benefits may include nonservice connected disability payments available to wartime veterans who become permanently and totally disabled and qualify for the benefit. The VA may pay an additional amount for use of an attendant in certain cases. Medical assistance in a VA medical facility is open to any veteran who qualifies.

Equipment Payment Policies

Equipment is paid for when deemed part of the overall medical or rehabilitation intervention, which is dependent upon eligibility status. The VA pays for such equipment as sensory aids, prosthetic and orthotics, and mobility and transportation equipment, when deemed necessary.

For More Information

Additional information on all veterans' benefit program is available through the Department of Veterans Affairs at (800) 827-1000.

DISABILITY RIGHTS LEGISLATION

Persons with SCI have rights, guaranteed by law, to education, employment, inclusion, and integration in society. As a consequence, the life care planner or case manager must be familiar with pertinent disability legislation and be able to educate individuals with SCI and their families, so that they are aware of the rights and benefits guaranteed under these laws (Danek et al., 1996).

The following is a brief overview of some of the major federal legislation that ensures equal opportunity for people with disabilities. These laws ensure that the disabled can achieve their full potential as productive, participating members of society. Much of the information in this section was derived from *A Guide to Disability Rights Laws* (1996) published by the U.S. Department of Justice. A more detailed discussion of these laws can be obtained by contacting the respective agencies and organizations listed below.

Americans with Disabilities Act (ADA)

The ADA prohibits discrimination on the basis of disability in employment, state and local government, public accommodations, commercial facilities, transportation, and telecommunications. It also applies to the U.S. Congress.

To be protected by the ADA, a person must have a disability or have a relationship or association with an individual with a disability. An individual with a disability is defined by the ADA as a person who has a physical or mental impairment that substantially limits one or more major life activities, a person who has a history or record of such an impairment, or a person who is perceived by others as having such an impairment. The ADA does not specifically name all impairments that are covered.

ADA Title I: Employment

Title I requires employers with 15 or more employees to provide qualified individuals with disabilities an equal opportunity to benefit from the full range of employment-related opportunities available to others. For example, it prohibits discrimination in recruitment, hiring, promotion, training, pay, social activities, and other privileges of employment. It restricts questions that can be asked about an applicant's disability before a job offer is made and it requires that employers make reasonable accommodation to the known physical or mental limitations of otherwise qualified individuals with disabilities, unless it results in undue hardship. Religious entities with 15 or more employees are covered under Title I.

Title I complaints must be filed with the U.S. Equal Employment Opportunity Commission (EEOC) within 180 days of the date of discrimination, or 300 days if the charge is filed with a designated state or local fair employment practice agency. Individuals may file a lawsuit in federal court only after they receive a "right-to-sue" letter from the EEOC.

Charges of employment discrimination on the basis of disability may be filed at any EEOC field office. Field offices are located in 50 cities throughout the U.S. and are listed in most telephone directories under "U.S. Government." The appropriate EEOC field office in a specific area can be obtained by contacting:

(800) 669-4000 (voice)
(800) 669-6820 (TTY)

Information on EEOC enforced laws can be obtained by calling:

(800) 669-3362 (voice)
(800) 800-3302 (TTY)

Information on how to accommodate a specific individual with a disability can be obtained by contacting:

Job Accommodation Network
918 Chestnut Ridge Road, Suite 1
Morgantown, WV 26506
(800) 526-7234 (voice/TTY)
(800) 232-9675 (voice/TTY)

ADA Title II: State and Local Government Activities

Title II covers all activities of state and local governments regardless of the government entity's size or receipt of federal funding. Title II requires that state and local governments give people with disabilities an equal opportunity to benefit from all of their programs, services, and activities (e.g., public education, employment, transportation, recreation, health care, social services, courts, voting, and town meetings).

State and local governments are required to follow specific architectural standards in the new construction and alteration of their buildings. They also must relocate programs or otherwise provide access in inaccessible older buildings, and communicate effectively with people who have hearing, vision, or speech disabilities. Public entities are not required to take actions that would result in undue financial and administrative burdens. They *are* required to make reasonable modifications to policies, practices, and procedures where necessary to avoid discrimination, unless they can demonstrate that doing so would fundamentally alter the nature of the service, program, or activity being provided.

Complaints of Title II violations may be filed with the Department of Justice within 180 days of the date of discrimination. In certain situations, cases may be referred to a mediation program sponsored by the Department. The Department may bring a lawsuit where it has investigated a matter and has been unable to resolve violations. Further information on filing a complaint can be made by contacting:

Disability Rights Section
Civil Rights Division
U.S. Department of Justice
P.O. Box 66738
Washington, D.C. 20035-6738
(800) 514-0301 (voice)
(800) 514-0383 (TTY)

Title II may also be enforced through private lawsuits in federal court. It is not necessary to file a complaint with the Department of Justice or any other federal agency or to receive a "right-to-sue" letter before going to court.

ADA Title II: Public Transportation

The transportation provisions of Title II cover public transportation services, such as city buses and public rail transit (e.g., subways, commuter rails, Amtrak). Public transportation authorities may not discriminate against people with disabilities in the provision of their services. They must comply with requirements for accessibility in newly purchased vehicles, make good faith efforts to purchase or lease accessible used buses, remanufacture buses in an accessible manner, and, unless it would result in an undue burden, provide paratransit where they operate fixed-route bus or rail systems.

Paratransit is a service where individuals who are unable to use the regular transit system independently (because of a physical or mental impairment) are picked up and dropped off at their destinations. Questions and complaints about public transportation should be directed to:

Federal Transit Administration
U.S. Department of Transportation
400 Seventh Street Southwest
Washington, DC 20590

Documents and Questions	(202) 366-1656 (voice)
	(202) 366-4567 (TTY)
Legal questions	(202) 366-1936 (voice/relay)
	(202) 366-9306 (voice)
	(202) 755-6787 (TTY)
Complaints	(202) 366-2285 (voice)
Enforcement	(202) 366-0153 (TTY)

ADA Title III: Public Accommodations

Title III covers businesses and nonprofit service providers that are public accommodations, privately operated entities offering certain types of courses and examinations, privately offered transportation, and commercial facilities. Public accommodations are private entities who own, lease, lease to, or operate facilities such as restaurants, retail stores, hotels, movie theaters, private schools, convention centers, doctors' offices, homeless shelters, transportation depots, zoos, funeral homes, day care centers, and recreation facilities — including sports stadium and fitness clubs. Transportation services provided by private entities are also covered by Title III.

Public accommodations must comply with basic nondiscrimination requirements that prohibit exclusion, segregation, and unequal treatment. They also must comply with specific requirements related to architectural standards for new and altered buildings; reasonable modifications to policies, practices, and procedures; effective communication with people with hearing, vision, or speech disabilities; and, other access requirements. Additionally, public accommodations must remove barriers in existing buildings where it is easy to do so without much difficulty or expense, given the public accommodation's resource.

Courses and examinations related to professional, educational, or trade-related applications, licensing, certifications, or credentialing must be provided in a place and manner accessible to people with disabilities, or alternative accessible arrangements must be offered.

Commercial facilities, such as factories and warehouses, must comply with the ADA architectural standards for new construction and alteration.

Complaints of Title III violations may be filed with the Department of Justice. In certain situations, cases may be referred to a mediation program sponsored by the Department. The Department is authorized to bring a lawsuit where there is a pattern or practice of discrimination in violation of Title III or where an act of discrimination raises an issue of general public importance. Title III may also be enforced through private lawsuits. It is not necessary to file a complaint with the Department of Justice (or any other federal agency) or to receive a "right-to-sue" letter before going to court. Additional information on filing a complaint can be made by contacting:

Disability Rights Section
Civil Rights Division
U.S. Department of Justice
P.O. Box 66738

Washington, DC 22035-6738
(800) 514-0301 (voice)
(800) 514-0383 (TTY)

ADA Title IV: Telecommunications

Title IV addresses telephone and television access for people with hearing and speech disabilities. It requires common carriers (telephone companies) to establish and maintain interstate and intrastate telecommunications relay services (TRS) 24 hours a day, seven days a week. TRS enables callers with hearing and speech disabilities who use text telephones (TTYs or TDDs) and callers who use voice telephones to communicate with each other through a third-party communications assistant. The Federal Communications Commissions (FCC) has set minimum standards for TRS services. Title IV also requires closed captioning of federally funded public service announcements. Further information about TRS can be gained by contacting:

Federal Communications Commission
1919 M Street Northwest
Washington, DC 20554

Documents and Questions   (202) 418-0190 (voice)
    (202) 418-2555 (TTY)
Legal questions   (202) 418-2357 (voice)
    (202) 418-0484 (TTY)

Fair Housing Act

The Fair Housing Act, as amended in 1988, prohibits housing discrimination on the basis of race, color, religion, sex, disability, familial status, and national origin. Its coverage includes private housing, housing that receives federal financial assistance, and state and local government housing. It is unlawful to discriminate in any aspect of selling or renting housing or to deny a dwelling to a buyer or renter because of disability of that individual, an individual associated with the buyer or renter, or an individual who intends to live in the residence. Other covered activities include, for example, financing, zoning practices, new construction design, and advertising.

The Fair Housing Act requires owners of housing facilities to make reasonable exceptions in their policies and operations to afford people with disabilities equal housing opportunities. For example, a landlord with a "no pets" policy may be required to grant an exception to this rule and allow an individual who is blind to keep a guide dog in the residence.

The Fair Housing Act also requires landlords to allow tenants with disabilities to make reasonable access-related modifications to their private living space, as well as to common use spaces. (The landlord is not required to pay for the changes.) The Act further requires that new multifamily housing with four or more units be designed and built to allow access for persons with disabilities. This includes accessible common-use areas, doors that are wide enough for wheelchairs, kitchens and bathrooms that allow a person using a wheelchair to maneuver, and other adaptable features within the units.

Complaints of Fair Housing Act violations may be filed with the U.S. Department of Housing and Urban Development. Additional information, including how to file a complaint, can be obtained by contacting:

Office of Program Compliance and Disability Rights
Office of Fair Housing and Equal Opportunity
U.S. Department of Housing and Urban Development
451 Seventh Street Southwest, Room 5242
Washington, DC 20140

Further information can also be obtained by calling the Fair Housing Information Clearinghouse at:

(800) 343-3442 (voice)
(800) 483-2209 (TTY)

Air Carrier Access Act

The Air Carrier Access Act prohibits discrimination by air carriers against qualified individuals with physical or mental impairments. It applies only to air carriers that provide regularly scheduled services for hire to the public. Requirements address a wide range of issues including boarding assistance and certain accessibility features in newly built aircraft and new or altered airport facilities. People may enforce rights under the Air Carrier Access Act by filing a complaint with the U.S. Department of Transportation or by bringing a lawsuit in federal court. Further information, including how to file a complaint, can be obtained by contacting:

Department Office of Civil Rights
Office of the Secretary
U.S. Department of Transportation
400 Seventh Street S.W.
Washington, DC 20590
(202) 366-4648 (voice)
(202) 366-8538 (TTY)

or

Aviation Consumer Protection Division, C-75
U.S. Department of Transportation
400 Seventh Street S.W.
Washington, DC 20590
(202) 366-2220 (voice)
(202) 755-6787 (TTY)

Rehabilitation Act of 1973

The Rehabilitation Act of 1973 prohibits discrimination on the basis of disability in programs conducted by federal agencies, programs receiving federal financial assistance, federal employment, and in the employment practices of federal contractors. The standards for determining employment discrimination under the Rehabilitation Act are the same as those used in Title I of the Americans with Disabilities Act.

Section 501

Section 501 requires affirmative action and nondiscrimination in employment by federal agencies of the executive branch. To obtain more information or to file a complaint, employees should contact their agency's Equal Employment Opportunity Office.

Section 503

Section 503 requires affirmative action and prohibits employment discrimination by federal government contractors and subcontractors with contracts of more than $10,000. Additional information on Section 503 can be obtained by contacting:

Office of Federal Contact Compliance Programs
U.S. Department of Labor
200 Constitution Avenue N.W.
Washington, DC 20210
(202) 219-9423 (voice/relay)

Section 504

Section 504 states that "no qualified individual with a disability in the United States shall be excluded from, denied the benefits of, or subjected to discrimination under" any program or activity that either receives federal financial assistance or is conducted by any executive agency or the U.S. Postal Service.

Each federal agency has its own set of Section 504 regulations that apply to its own programs. Agencies that provide federal financial assistance also have Section 504 regulations covering entities that receive federal aid. Requirements common to these regulations include reasonable accommodation for employees with disabilities; program accessibility; effective communication with people who have hearing or vision disabilities; and accessible new construction and alterations. Each agency is responsible for enforcing its own regulations. Section 504 may also be enforced through private lawsuits. It is not necessary to file a complaint with a federal agency or to receive a "right-to-sue" letter before going to court.

Further information on how to file Section 504 complaints with the appropriate agency can be obtained by contacting:

Disability Rights Section
Civil Rights Division
U.S. Department of Justice
P.O. Box 66738
Washington, D.C. 20035-6738
(800) 514-0301 (voice)
(800) 514-0383 (TTY)

Individuals with Disabilities Education Act (IDEA)

The Individuals with Disabilities Education Act (IDEA) (formerly called P.L. 94-142 or the Education for All Handicapped Children Act of 1975) requires public schools to make available to all eligible children with disabilities a free, appropriate public education in the least restrictive environment appropriate to their individual needs. IDEA requires public school systems to develop appropriate Individualized Education Programs (IEPs) for each child. The specific special education and related services outlined in each IEP reflect the individualized needs of each student.

IDEA also mandates that particular procedures be followed in the development of the IEP. Each student's IEP must be developed by a team of knowledgeable persons and must be reviewed at least annually. The team includes the child's teacher; the parents, subject to certain limited exceptions; the child, if determined appropriate; an agency representative who is qualified to provide or supervise the provision of special education; and other individuals at the parents' or agency's discretion.

If parents disagree with the proposed IEP, they can request a due process hearing and a review from the state educational agency, if applicable in that state. They also can appeal the state agency's decision to state or federal court. Additional information can be obtained by contacting:

Office of Special Education Programs
U.S. Department of Education
330 C Street S.W., Room 3086
Washington, DC 20202
(202) 205-5507 (voice)
(202) 205-9754 (TTY)

Architectural Barriers Act

The Architectural Barriers Act (ABA) requires that buildings and facilities that are designed, constructed, or altered with federal funds, or leased by a federal agency, must comply with federal standards for physical accessibility. ABA requirements are limited to architectural standards in new and altered buildings and in newly leased facilities. They do not address the activities conducted in those buildings and facilities. Facilities of the U.S. Postal Service are covered by the ABA. Additional information or filing a complaint can be made by contacting:

The U.S. Architectural and Transportation Barriers Compliance Board
1331 F Street N.W., Suite 1000
Washington, DC 20004-1111
(800) 872-2253 (voice)
(800) 993-2822 (TTY)

Ticket to Work and Work Incentives Improvement Act of 1999

The Ticket to Work and Work Incentives Improvement Act of 1999 is the most recent law affecting Social Security programs. This law amends the Social Security Act to expand the availability of health care coverage for working individuals with disabilities. It establishes a Ticket to Work and Self-Sufficiency Program in the Social Security Administration to provide SSDI and SSI disability beneficiaries with a choice of providers for vocational rehabilitation and employment-related services. This program will use a voucher system (i.e., "ticket"), which allows beneficiaries to obtain services through Employment Networks that will be established through the U.S. The Employment Networks will be both private organizations and public agencies that have agreed to work with Social Security to provide vocational rehabilitation and employment-related services under this program.

The Ticket to Work and Work Incentives Improvement Act was signed into law December 1999 and will be phased in nationally over a three-year period beginning January 1, 2000, with the first "tickets" issued early in 2001. The law also includes several enhancements to Medicaid and Medicare that are effective October 1, 2000. Under this Act, states will have the option to provide more Medicaid coverage for workers with disabilities. The law also provides for continuation of Medicare coverage for working individuals with disabilities. It lengthens from 4 years to 8 1/2 years the period for which SSDI beneficiaries who return to work can continue to receive reduced-cost Medicare coverage. In addition, the Act enables individuals with disabilities to reestablish eligibility for Social Security disability benefits on an expedited basis if their attempts to return to work prove unsuccessful.

Additional information can be obtained by contacting a local Social Security office or the Social Security Administration, Office of Disability at (410) 965-8046 (voice)/(410) 966-6210 (TTY).

Other Sources of Disability Rights Information

Regional Disability and Business Technical Assistance Centers
2323 South Shepherd, Suite 1000
Houston, TX 77019
(800) 949-4232 (voice/TTY)
(713) 520-5785

U.S. Department of Justice
Office of Assistant Attorney General
Civil Rights Division
P.O. Box 65808
Washington, DC 20035-5808
(202) 514-2151
(202) 514-0293

IMPLICATIONS FOR LIFE CARE PLANNING AND CASE MANAGEMENT

At times, the life care planning process may require the development of creative alternatives to typical funding sources and services to meet a long-term continuum

Table 3-1. Potential Resources and Service Providers

Potential Resources	Health	Education/ Employment	Mobility	Housing	Transportation	Psychosocial Support	Recreation	Self-Care
Private Health Insurance	X		X			X		X
Medicare	X		X			X		
Medicaid	X		X		X	X		X
State Vocational Rehabilitation Agencies		X	X		X	X		
Workers' Compensation	X	X	X	X	X	X		X
Public Health Departments	X							
Public Hospitals/Clinics	X					X		
Private Hospitals	X					X		
Mental Health Centers						X		
Nonprofit Agencies	X							
SSDI Work Incentives		X						
SSI Work Incentives		X	X		X			X
Special Education Programs		X						
State Employment Agencies		X						
Private Employment Agencies		X						
Scholarships/Student Loans		X						
Financing		X						
Personal/Employer Tax Incentives		X						
U.S. Department of Housing and Urban Development				X				
Local Housing Authorities				X				
Local Public Transit Authority					X			
Department of Veterans Affairs	X	X	X	X	X	X	X	X
Independent Living Centers				X	X	X		X
Low Cost Mortgage Programs				X				
Churches, Charities, Service Organizations					X	X	X	
Chamber of Commerce							X	
Wheelchair Sports Organizations							X	
State Sport Associations							X	
Paralyzed Veterans of America	X		X	X	X	X	X	X

of needs. The first step in the allocation of resources for people with SCI is to determine for which funding sources and services an individual may be eligible. There are a number of federal, state, and local programs available to assist persons with disability.

For example, Social Security Disability Insurance (SSDI) and Supplemental Security Income (SSI) are programs for which an individual may qualify to receive financial assistance for general living expenses and health care services. If the person is a veteran, he or she may be eligible for financial and support services through the Department of Veterans Affairs (VA). County or state departments of social services may provide public assistance and support services to people with disabilities and their families. State departments of vocational rehabilitation may assist persons with the purchase of equipment, counseling, training and education, transportation, job placement, and other forms of assistance intended for vocational rehabilitation. Voluntary and charitable organizations at the national, state, and local levels (Catholic Charities, Lutheran Social Services, Jewish organizations, United Way, Easter Seals, etc.) can provide information and services as well. In addition, there are a number of groups or organizations, such as the Paralyzed Veterans of America, various disability advocacy groups, and others that work to ensure that eligible individuals receive the benefits to which they are entitled.

The process of identifying and accessing resources is often a long and arduous task, involving a number of contacts and follow-up inquiries at the national, state, and community levels (Blackwell et al., 1994). Table 3-1 is a summary of potential resources and service providers that the life care planner or case manager may consider in this process (Consortium for Spinal Cord Medicine, 1999c; Rintala, 1997). This is not an exhaustive list, but rather a starting point from which life care planners and case managers can expand their base of information and resources for addressing an individual's long-term needs.

CONCLUSION

To adequately address the comprehensive long-term needs of individuals with SCI, it may be necessary to draw upon a variety of funding and service resources. Assisting with resource allocation for the individual with SCI shifts the focus of the life care planner's role from one of needs identification to a case management role of bringing the individual together with appropriate resources. To fill these roles requires basic information and an expansive sense of service delivery. In the process of assisting the person with SCI to access resources, it is more important for the life care planner or case manager to have a few reliable means of entering systems that provide information, expertise, and assistance than it is to try to be knowledgeable about the single best source for all possible situations. SCI treatment centers; government programs and agencies; private, state, and national SCI and IL organizations; and advocacy and referral services are good starting points. However, it is reasonable to expect to make a number of contacts and inquiries in subsequent searches for information and assistance. A good deal of patience, courtesy, and persistence is required for this time-consuming task of resource identification and access.

4

Sample Life Care Plan for Spinal Cord Injury

LIFE CARE PLAN REPORT

Re:	Brett E. Smith
Date of Birth:	5/3/56
Date of Injury:	7/3/97
Dates of Client Interviews/Evaluation:	5/14/98–8/27/99
Date of Report:	9/1/99

REFERRAL AND BACKGROUND INFORMATION

Brett E. Smith, a 43-year-old former sawmill worker was referred to Louisiana State University Health Sciences Center, Vocational Assessment and Counseling Clinic, by Mr. John Stevens of Lee, Howard & Stevens of Great Falls, Montana. The purpose of this referral is to develop a Life Care Plan to assess the extent to which Mr. Smith has incurred disabling conditions secondary to a work-related accident on 7/3/97, in which he sustained multiple fractures and lacerations, with a subsequent diagnosis of complete C6 tetraplegia (ASIA A).

The Life Care Plan is a comprehensive, multidisciplinary approach which systematically addresses the medical and nonmedical needs of a person with a catastrophic injury and projects the costs of needed goods and services over the person's estimated lifespan. Along with the costs associated with the disabling condition, replacement schedule and frequency of treatment are outlined. The Life Care Plan is specific to the person and is not generalized to a type of injury or disability. It is a dynamic approach in that, as the individual's circumstances change as part of the aging process with disability, the plan can be updated to reflect the current situation. Vocational implications and job alternatives available post-accident are also identified.

At the time of the accident Mr. Smith was 41 years old, working as a lay-up line operator for Rocky Mountain Manufacturing (Northern Division), and living with his wife and their daughter in a house he owned in Whitefish, Montana. At this time Mr. Smith continues to live with his wife and daughter in Whitefish. Mr. Smith has not worked since the time of the injury.

The client was born in Rapid City, South Dakota, and lived there until moving to Whitefish with his family when he was approximately a junior in high school. His parents are retired and continue to live in Whitefish. Mr. Smith's mother is age 71. His father, age 74, held various jobs during his work life. The client's parents' most recent work prior to retirement was owning and operating a restaurant in Whitefish.

Mr. Smith has two older brothers and one older sister. His oldest brother, age 50, is married and lives in Sioux Falls, South Dakota, where he is an instructor at the University of South Dakota. His other brother, age 49, is married, lives in Whitefish, and recently retired. He worked at Blackfeet Industries as a vocational evaluator prior to retirement. Mr. Smith's sister is age 45, married, and lives in Kalispell, Montana. At this time she is working part-time (one to two days a week) for a chiropractor but in the fall may possibly return to her previous work as a receptionist at a law firm.

Mr. Smith is married to his first wife of 17 years, Sandy, age 39, and this is the first marriage for both. At the time of her husband's injury Ms. Smith was working full-time as a receptionist at a title company in Whitefish and earned $7 an hour. She has not been employed since 7/3/97. The couple have one daughter, age 14.

The client denies any history of arrests or convictions. He also denies any history of learning, behavior, or attention disorders in his family.

EDUCATION AND TRAINING

Mr. Smith reports he attended primary, secondary, and high school through his junior year in Rapid City. He graduated from Glacier High School in Whitefish in 1974 and describes his grades as having been "pretty much average, Bs and Cs." He relates he did best in math and did not particularly dislike any subjects other than possibly government.

A review of academic records reflects from grades nine through 12 his grades were typically in the B to C range.

The client has not participated in any other formal academic training to date. He did not hold in the past nor does he now hold any professional/vocational licenses, certifications, or registrations.

MILITARY SERVICE

Following high school Mr. Smith was in the U.S. Navy from 1975 to 1979 and received an honorable discharge with the rank of E-5. He worked as a machinist mate, primarily on submarines, repairing mechanical equipment such as hydraulic systems and air conditioning systems. He was stationed in Hawaii and had one overseas tour of duty to Japan, Okinawa, the Phillipines, and Hong Kong. He did not incur any service connected disabilities.

VOCATIONAL HISTORY

Mr. Smith's work experience has essentially been limited to that of sawmill worker. From 1979 to the time of injury (7/3/97) he worked for Rocky Mountain Manufacturing in Whitefish. His job title was lay-up line operator; however, he was also trained to be an alternate quality control inspector and stock rustler. He was working as a stock rustler the day of the accident. Mr. Smith was paid a base rate of $12.50 an hour plus bonuses; however, he reports his typical wages averaged $21.50 an hour. He relates he worked full-time with occasional overtime and usually worked the day shift.

The only other employment Mr. Smith reports is prior to the entering the military he helped in the restaurant his parents owned in Whitefish.

PRE-INJURY MEDICAL HISTORY

Other than an appendectomy in 1981 and a subdural hematoma in 1994, Mr. Smith denies any history of significant illnesses, injuries, hospitalizations, or surgeries prior to the 7/3/97 injury. The client relates he had no residual problems following treatment for the subdural hematoma. He has no known allergies.

Mr. Smith reports the only time he smoked cigarettes was for a couple years when he was in the service. He notes he very rarely drinks alcohol and he denies any history of treatment for chemical/substance abuse.

Medical records reflect a history of spontaneous, nontraumatic subdural hematoma over the right hemisphere, which presented with headache on awakening on 2/1/94. He had no history of head trauma, bleeding history, or familial history, but had a cold a week prior to admission. The hematoma was treated with right frontal and parietal burr holes by Jerry Mann, M.D., on 2/4/94. Mr. Smith missed six weeks of work following the procedure. Records reflect he never developed neurological findings and was in good health and taking no regular medication at the time of injury in 7/97.

POST-INJURY MEDICAL HISTORY SUMMARY

On 7/3/97 Mr. Smith slipped and fell into a pit while working for Rocky Mountain Manufacturing in Whitefish. He was immediately taken by ambulance to the Emergency Room at the Kalispell Regional Hospital in Kalispell where he was admitted and the following surgical procedures were performed: a carpectomy C6, disk excision C5-6 and C6-7; interbody fusion/arthrodesis C5-7 with a long iliac crest bone graft replacing the lost discs in the destroyed vertebral body; Synthes plating C5-graft-7; repair of large right stellate parietal scalp laceration; and repair of right knee laceration. He also underwent reduction for a posterior right hip comminuted acetabular fracture with subsequent dislocation. Also noted was a nondisplaced right elbow fracture.

Once he was stabilized medically, Mr. Smith was discharged from the Kalispell Regional Hospital on 7/10/97 and transferred to St. Jude's Institute of Rehabilitation in Spokane, Washington. While at St. Jude's his right hip repeatedly subluxed and a routine cervical film several days after admission showed some slippage of the bone plug and backing out of one of the cervical screws. Therefore, he was discharged from St. Jude's on 7/25/97 and admitted to the Columbus Medical Center in Spokane for surgery. On 7/31/97 he underwent a recontouring and repositioning of the bone strut with C5-7, using an Orion anterior cervical plating and on 8/3/97 he underwent an open reduction, internal fixation of the right pelvis.

Mr. Smith was discharged from the Columbus Medical Center on 8/16/97 and readmitted to St. Jude's that same day. While hospitalized at St. Jude's he received intense rehabilitation services, including a neuropsychological evaluation which showed no evidence of significant problems with attention, concentration, information processing, or memory. He was discharged from St. Jude's to his home in Whitefish on 10/19/97. Discharge therapies included physical therapy and occupational therapy three times a week and nursing care to help with catherizations.

Once he returned home Mr. Smith was followed by James B. Stone, M.D., and Mary K. Jones, M.D. He participated in a full outpatient program including physical therapy three times a week and occupational therapy three times a week. He received skilled nursing care twice daily and personal care attendant services daily. Mr. Smith also received speech therapy for approximately one month for problems related with voice dysfunction and swallowing problems. Case management services were also provided. Housing problems were present because of accessibility issues and he and his family moved to a temporary residence in Whitefish. Because it was determined that it would cost more to renovate his home to make it accessible than it would to construct a new accessible house, a new home was built on one acre of land on the outskirts of Whitefish and the family moved into it in 12/98.

In 1/99 Mr. Smith was admitted to the Craig Hospital in Englewood, Colorado, for a 10-day inpatient spinal cord injury evaluation. He underwent physical therapy, occupational therapy, driving evaluations, and vocational rehabilitation consult while at Craig Hospital. Patient education and instruction was provided and equipment needs were specified. Mr. Smith was evaluated for his right hip dislocation and it was recommended that he does not need to undergo any surgical intervention for his hip dislocation. The possibility of tendon transfer procedures was indicated; he was referred for further follow-up once he returned home regarding casting and hand therapy to work on an extension program for better range of motion of the IP joint to improve coordination and tenodesis. Mr. Smith was seen by family services and recreational therapy. A medication change was also recommended, because his white blood count was depressed secondary to medication he had been taking for chronic suppression of urinary tract infection.

POST-INJURY COMPLICATIONS

Mr. Smith's rehabilitation was initially delayed because of the need for additional surgeries and the need for hip precautions related to the hip dislocation and fracture. He saw an orthopedic surgeon in 12/97 regarding his right hip and at that time the doctor also noted an anterior cruciate deficient right knee. The doctor recommended continuation of physical therapy. Some question of hip instability continued, especially regarding transfers and assisted standing, however, evaluation at Craig Hospital determined no surgical procedures were indicated. Mr. Smith reports he was told at Craig Hospital that his hip cannot be repaired but "all the damage has been done" and they do not think he can hurt it any further. The client notes he has to buy a larger size of pants to get them pulled up past his hip and he adds that although he does not feel pain in his hip he does hear a popping sound. Mr. Smith reports his right knee is not a particular problem now, although he adds his "whole right leg is screwed up."

Initial rehabilitation was also delayed because of a right radial fracture resulting in precautions and inability to work on bed mobility and transfers. Mr. Smith reports no specific problems with his right forearm/elbow at this time.

Initially, cervical spine stability was also questionable and Mr. Smith was evaluated several times by a neurosurgeon regarding this. In 1/98 the doctor noted Mr. Smith was doing quite well and there was no sign of neurologic deterioration. Because the fusion was seen to be stable, there was no indication for further surgery.

Following surgery in 7/97 Mr. Smith developed a very weak, breathy quality to his voice and was found to have right vocal cord paralysis related to a recurrent laryngeal nerve injury. He received speech therapy for voice dysfunction and problems swallowing and in 2/98 it was noted the quality of his voice was improving but he continued to have problems swallowing. In 3/7/98 a video esophogram was found to be virtually normal. After approximately one month, speech therapy was discontinued and he was not seen as being in danger of significant aspiration. He states his swallowing "has gotten pretty good" and he does not see this as a significant problem. He notes he no longer receives speech therapy services.

Mr. Smith's voice has somewhat of a breathy, soft quality but he is understandable at all times. Mr. Smith states his doctor has told him he "will never get my God-given voice back" but there would be an improvement. On 2/4/99 the doctor noted he has mild return to function of his right vocal cord but it has not completely compensated. The doctor reports a surgical procedure (medialization laryngoplasty) would provide improved functioning of the vocal cord and allow better vocalization with more strength and clarity; however, the doctor is leaving it up to Mr. Smith regarding whether he will undergo such a surgery.

Mr. Smith had urinary tract infections in 10/97 and 11/97, which were apparently related to a lack of adequate fluid intake. These infections cleared with medication. Another urinary tract infection occurred in 3/98, which was treated with medication and cleared by 4/98. In 11/98 Mr. Smith was taken to the Kalispell Hospital Regional Emergency Room because he was having shortness of breath, weakness, fever, and blood in his urine after having his Foley catheter replaced that morning. His breathing returned to normal and he was treated with medication, discharged, and followed for treatment of a urinary tract infection (antibiotics for 10 days). Mr. Smith reports he had a fifth urinary tract infection in 5/99, which cleared after approximately 10 days of taking antibiotics.

Spasticity, particularly in his legs, and which interferes with sleep at night, has remained an ongoing problem. Mr. Smith reports he continues to experience spasticity in his legs and generating to his abdomen at this time, primarily while lying down in the evenings. He also experiences some spasticity in his hands during the day time.

While hospitalized at St. Jude's Mr. Smith developed a deep vein thrombosis bilaterally, which was treated with Coumadin. Problems with swollen feet and occasional dizziness have been ongoing. In 10/98 Mr. Smith was hospitalized because of right leg swelling and erythema, which occurred after an extended car ride (five hours). He was found to have an extensive deep vein thrombosis in his right leg; it was treated with medication and he was discharged three days later on Coumadin with restrictions of no lower body exercises in therapies.

At this time Mr. Smith continues to wear Ted hose at all times. He also wears an abdominal binder when he is wearing sweatpants. He relates he does not need to wear the binder if he is wearing jeans. Mr. Smith reports at this time that problems with shortness of breath and dizziness have gotten much better because his blood pressure is now more stabilized. He notes he experiences episodes of shortness of breath and/or dizziness primarily only when he is doing substantial physical activity or it is hot. Mr. Smith does note that while he was in Colorado in 8/99 prior to surgery he "passed out" for several minutes.

Mr. Smith developed a decubiti on his right heel in 11/97, which cleared by 2/98. In 3/98 he was noted to have a Grade 2 decubiti on his right ischium, which required an increase in skilled nursing visits and bed rest for approximately four months. Out-patient therapies were essentially stopped as a consequence of being homebound. In 5/98 the ischial decubiti was noted to be healed; however, he had developed a Grade 2 decubiti on his coccyx, the result of a transfer to a commode chair, which required approximately three months to heal. In 9/98 he had some skin irritation in his coccyx area over the previous decubiti; this closed by 11/98. Mr. Smith reports he has had no other incidences of decubiti and relates that using an air bed and a lift has helped greatly with problems in this area. The client also notes he has some problems with ingrown toenails but this situation is monitored by nursing care and treated as needed with Betadyne and has not resulted in any further complications.

Mr. Smith reports he experiences substantial stiffness in his back on a constant basis and he states "it feels like my upper body is one big block." He notes that at the time he was discharged from St. Jude's his upper body felt much better than it does at this time. The client reports he experiences pain or discomfort whenever he is up in his wheelchair and the only relief he finds is when he is lying flat on his back. He expresses that this pain is difficult to describe but states it feels "like a pinched nerve or something" or a burning sensation. He reports experiencing a burning sensation in his lower back, buttocks, and into his thighs. Mr. Smith relates he has not received any instruction in pain management techniques or relaxation techniques, such as biofeedback, and he would be interested in doing so. However, Mr. Smith adds that he has not yet discussed the above-described pain symptoms with his physician. Mr. Smith also notes his neck aches occasionally, especially if he is looking downward. He is doing exercises at home for neck pain at this time.

Mr. Smith saw Erwin C. Thomas, Ph.D., psychologist, in 11/97 and another time in the early part of 1998. In 2/98 records reflect concerns over the Smiths' adaptation to injury remained. Mr. Smith began seeing Tony L. Cook, Ph.D., psychologist, in 2/99 and continues to see him at this time. The client reports he has not received any further psychological services other than those he received while hospitalized on various occasions. Mr. Smith was involved with a local spinal cord injury support group in the past but this group has since become inactive. Ms. Smith received individual counseling from Linda Logan, MA, LPC, on a weekly basis from 11/98 to 5/99.

RECORDS REVIEWED

Joan D. Abbott, Adjuster, Ponder & Associates, Inc.; correspondence; 7/26/98

Raymond T. Bennett, DDS; examination report; 8/29/97

Central Imaging (Robert J. Falk, M.D., William E. Summers, M.D., Don A. Cummins, M.D., William D. Kane, M.D., Richard A. Berg, M.D., Robert B. Hardy, M.D., Peter J. Bowls, M.D., Jacob W. Morgan, M.D.); peripheral venous examination whole body bone scan venous study, x-rays, CT; 7/11/97–10/2/97

Peter C. Colin, DDS; examination/progress notes; 7/24/97–9/13/97

Tony L. Cook, Ph.D.; counseling notes; 2/11/99–4/30/99

Columbus Medical Center, Spokane, Washington; consultation reports, progress notes, diagnostic studies (including x-rays, pathology, laboratory, rhythm strips, etc.), operative reports, radiation therapy treatment summary, physician consultation, physician's orders, admission forms, consent forms, advance directives, pre-op information & care, pre-operative checklist, pre-op teaching, patient/family education documentation record, standards of care plans, anesthetic record, anesthesia pre- and post-op standing orders, PCA order form, anesthesia progress notes, post-op cervical disc, doctor's orders, pain management flow sheet, surgical services intra-op record, pulmonary diagnostics, post-op assessment, interdisciplinary therapy evaluation, nursing discharge summary, multidisciplinary care conference, neurologic observation record, patient progress record, pressure/vascular ulcer evaluation/treatment flow sheet, laminectomy check, post-procedure and laminectomy check, Braden scale for predicting pressure sore risk, neuro-science center assessment flowsheet, clinical records, parenteral nutrition orders, parenteral fluids, parenteral nutrition charting sheets, diabetes record, Heparin sliding scale, anticoagulants, I.V. access flow sheet, medication records, therapy progress notes, therapy treatments, physical therapy treatments, weekly summary physical therapy, occupational therapy progress notes, respiratory therapy, blood transfusion record; 7/25/97–8/16/97

Country Pharmacy; record of prescriptions; 11/14/97–5/21/98

Craig Hospital, Denver, Colorado; admission records, consent form, inpatient history summary, history and physical, hand clinic note, laboratory reports, radiology reports, physicians' orders & progress notes, trending form, medication administration records, nursing admission assessment, patient/family conference nursing summary, nursing care flow sheets, patient functional assessment, patient care plan, patient education flow sheets, assignment of insurance benefits, physical therapy progress notes, physical therapy initial/conference/discharge re-eval note, physical therapy functional checkout, goniometry testing, upper extremity evaluation, muscle evaluation, OT/PT sensory test, family service note, psychological service progress notes, therapeutic recreation progress note/conference note, patient education tests, radiology reports, physical therapy initial/conference/discharge/re-eval note, family service note, independent driver van recommendations, occupational therapy progress notes, occupational therapy initial/conference/discharge/re-eval note, occupational therapy functional independence measure, team conference, rehabilitation engineering note, patient equipment prescriptions, prescription/purchase order authorizations, SCI discharge instructions, discharge summary, responses to life care planning needs questions; 1/13/99–4/8/99

Jonathan L. Demmons, M.D.; office report 9/12/97–10/5/97

Andrew Engstrom, M.D., Kalispell Regional Hospital; MRI, video esophagram; 2/19/98–2/29/98

Michael B. Fox, Kalispell Regional Hospital; radiology reports; 1/2/98

Glacier County Home Health Agency; verbal orders/progress reports, summary of RN's regimen, treatment plan, case conference recertification forms, home health certification and plan of care, addendum, wound assessment with plan of care, nursing care plans, occupational therapy initial evaluation, speech therapy evaluation, physical therapy initial evaluation, team conference forms, therapy notes, medication sheets, verbal order/progress notes, home health visit slip/physical therapy note, physical therapy initial evaluation, discharge summary; 10/30/97–6/29/99

Glacier Public Schools; transcripts; 1971–1974

Melinda Green, RN, Home Health Service; status reports, contact report; 6/30/97–2/20/98

John Hillyard, M.D.; examination/progress notes; 12/5/97

Carrie Howard, RN, Home Health Service/Community Wellness; correspondence, team meeting minutes, case manager progress reports, medical status reports, cost analysis; 5/20/98–5/5/99

Perry C. Howard, M.D.; correspondence, authorization request; 11/11/97–2/21/98

IRS; W-2 forms; 1990–1997

Bert F. James, M.D.; correspondence; 3/26/99

Mary K. Jones, M.D.; progress notes, addendum to plan of treatment, home health certification and plan of care, verbal orders, prescription, correspondence; 7/15/97–4/29/99

Kalispell Regional Hospital; emergency room report, pre-hospital patient form, procedure report, history and physical, operative report, x-ray reports, laboratory reports, physician's progress records, medication administration records, IV flow sheets, graphic, admission history discharge planning, nursing physical assessment, nursing documentation records, patient care plans, respiratory therapy notes, physician's orders, admission and discharge forms, discharge summary, consultation report, transfer summary, discharge orders, discharge summary instructions, home ergonomic evaluation, 7/3/97–5/22/99

Kalispell Regional Hospital Outpatient Occupational Therapy, Troy Terrell, OTR, John Marra, OTR, Kathy Wright, OTR; progress and treatment notes; 7/18/98–4/30/99

Kalispell Regional Hospital Outpatient Physical Therapy, Kent Smyth, P.T.; initial evaluation, progress notes, status report, progress and treatment notes, correspondence; 10/10/97–4/30/99

Linda Logan, MA, LPC; counseling notes, authorization for release of information; 11/18/98–6/11/99

Medi-Day; functional activities charts [not dated]

Montana State Ambulance Trip Report, 7/3/97

NorthMont; in-home services program, service delivery records, personal care services plan/physician approval, personal care services plan/physician order, progress notes; 10/22/97–7/14/99

Northwestern Care, Inc; progress notes, prescription, billing worksheet; 7/3/97–9/17/98

Cory H. Olson, M.D.; examination notes 11/14/97–2/4/99

Outpatient Rehab, Summit Health & Fitness, Mary Lewis, MS, CCC-SP, Troy Terrell, OTR; short term admission/assessment & progress record, physician orders/plan of treatment, voice re-evaluation, initial evaluation, daily treatment test results, therapy summary, speech pathology report; 11/4/97–2/4/99

Robin B. Quinnell, RN, CCM, Community Wellness/The Summit; correspondence, case management progress report, team meeting minutes; 5/20/99–7/3/99

Ronald E. Roberts, M.D.; radiology report; 10/5/97

St. Jude's Rehabilitation Institute, Spokane, Washington; admission form, nursing care, physicians' orders, history and physical, discharge summary, discharge summary addendum, physicians' profile current medication, laboratory reports, daily treatment record physical therapy, daily treatment record occupational therapy, conference meeting minutes, correspondence, prescriptions, equipment list, consultation reports, radiology reports, reports of compatibility testing, neuropsychological evaluation, physician progress notes, patient progress records; 7/10/97–10/6/97

Tom B. Sawyer, Law Offices of Wren, Conners, Kelly & Black; correspondence; 10/8/98

Michael L. Simms, MS, CRC, Vocational Rehabilitation Counseling; correspondence, case status reports, on-site job analysis, vocational rehabilitation retraining plan; 8/1/98–7/18/99

James B. Stone, M.D.; interval histories, correspondence, response to LCP questions, team meeting minutes, prescriptions; 10/9/975/19/99

Western Montana Medical Services; correspondence; 7/8/99

FUNCTIONAL ABILITIES

Information regarding Mr. Smith's present condition was obtained through interviews with Mr. Smith and his wife, and questionnaires and contacts with physicians and other health care personnel who have treated or evaluated Mr. Smith since his injury.

Physical

Mr. Smith has significant limitations/restrictions for activities involving sitting, standing, walking, lifting, carrying, pushing, pulling, climbing, stooping, balancing, kneeling, crouching, crawling, reaching, handling, fingering, feeling, and stamina/endurance. He is also limited in talking because of decreased volume at distances. No limitations are indicated for seeing, hearing, tasting, and smelling.

Cognitive/Behavioral

Although Mr. Smith apparently experienced a brief episode of loss of consciousness following injury there is no indication of residuals from a brain injury. Neuropsychological testing performed in 9/97 indicates intellectual functioning in the average range with abilities in attention, concentration, memory, information processing, and problem solving falling within the normal range. Mr. Smith is seen as having complete functional independence in both expressive and comprehensive communication, social interaction, problem solving, and memory.

There is a consistent indication of difficulties with depression and psychosocial adjustment. Mr. Smith has tended to isolate himself and be socially withdrawn since the time of his injury. He reports he avoids leaving home for fear of getting into difficult situations and he dislikes being in any type of crowds. The client's marital and family life have changed substantially, as has his ability to participate in the vocational and recreational activities he pursued prior to injury.

Mr. Smith belongs to the Faith Lutheran Church and he reports before the injury he went to church on an occasional basis. He relates the last time he went to church was on Christmas Eve in 1997 but "people crowded around" and he became very uncomfortable. He describes this situation as having been overwhelming so he no longer goes out and has a very restricted social life. Mr. Smith notes his wife went to church regularly before his injury but she now goes less frequently. Mr. Smith relates he has gone out to a few movies but went to matinees rather than evening shows because he prefers to avoid crowds.

Environmental

Significant limitations or restrictions are present for the environmental conditions of extreme changes of temperature, inside, outside, heat, cold, and wet/humidity because of problems with overheating and chilling easily and mobility issues. Restrictions are present for exposure to fumes, odors, dusts, mists, gases, and chemicals because Mr. Smith should avoid respiratory irritants. Limitations are also present for activities involving moving mechanical parts, operating automotive equipment, and exposure to unprotected heights, noise, and vibration.

Work

Mr. Smith's ability to work is limited as described by the physical limitations previously outlined in this report.

On 4/8/99 Robert M. Linnell, M.D., of Craig Hospital noted that it is doubtful Mr. Smith could work full-time; however, he noted he may be able to work part-time by beginning four hours at a time and increasing as able. The doctor indicated maximum medical improvement had not yet been reached and projected it will be reached in approximately six months.

ACTIVITIES OF DAILY LIVING

The client reports at this time that he normally arises between 7 A.M. and 8 A.M. and retires between 10 P.M. and 10:30 P.M. Mr. Smith reports that because transfers are difficult, and he now needs to keep his right arm elevated following tendon transfer surgery, he is typically up in his wheelchair all day. He notes he typically naps one or two times during the day, while in the wheelchair, for 15 to 30 minutes at a time. Mr. Smith relates he independently does weight shifts at approximately 30 minute intervals. He states he monitors his own skin condition for as much of his body as he can see and his wife and attendant monitor the rest of his body. He notes he has a hand-held skin inspection mirror but is unable to use it effectively because he cannot flex or turn adequately.

Self-Care

Eating — Mr. Smith is able to eat most foods independently with set-up and adaptive equipment. However, he does need assistance with cutting meat, because he does not have the adaptive equipment to do this himself (Minimal Assist/Modified Independence).

Grooming — He is able to shave some areas of his face independently with set-up and adaptive equipment, however, he is not able to reach all the areas of his face. He is independent in brushing his teeth with set-up and adaptive equipment. His attendant washes and combs his hair. He can comb his hair by having the handle of the comb pushed inside his wheelchair glove (Moderate Assist/Modified Independence).

Bathing — He uses a shower/commode chair and a roll-in shower and needs assistance wheeling in and out of the shower. With the use of adaptive equipment he is independently able to wash his face and chest but requires assistance with bathing the rest of his body (Total Assist/Moderate Assist).

Upper Body Dressing — Mr. Smith requires assistance with pulling his shirt overhead and down in back and he is dependent with fasteners (Moderate Assist/Minimal Assist).

Lower Body Dressing — He needs assistance with putting on and taking off his pants, socks, and shoes. He has no adaptive clothing at this time (Total Assist).

Bladder Management

Current bladder program consists of an indwelling Foley catheter, which is changed one time monthly. This program is subject to change because he may return to an intermittent, external catheter program depending on the outcome of the tendon transfer surgery. Mr. Smith reports his health care providers have advised him they would prefer intermittent catheterization to decrease the chance of urinary tract infections, and he may switch back to this program depending on the hand function he regains following tendon transfer surgery.

Mr. Smith requires assistance to attach the leg bag and tubing. He is able to independently empty the leg bag if he is wearing sweat pants and has a velcro adaptation on the leg bag straps; if he is wearing jeans he requires assistance with this. He notes his wife assists him with his bladder program (Maximal Assist/Moderate Assist).

Bowel Management

Mr. Smith is dependent on his bowel program. His program is done every other day and consists of a suppository and digital stimulation. His personal care attendant transfers him to the shower/commode chair, the nurse performs the program, then his attendant positions the chair over the commode (Total Assist).

Transfers (Bed, Chair, Wheelchair, Toilet, Tub, Shower)

Because of problems with skin breakdown and his hip condition, he uses a lift in his home. The lift is also used to transfer him to and from the shower/commode chair. Mr. Smith uses an air bed at this time. He notes the lift is used to bring him from a lying to sitting position and his attendant moves his feet and legs off the bed. He uses a slide board for transfers but needs assistance with moving his legs and feet (Total Assist/Moderate Assist).

Mobility

Mr. Smith uses a manual wheelchair with adaptive equipment for mobility in the home and community setting. He is able to maneuver the manual wheelchair on hard surfaces, such as concrete or pavement, but has difficulties in wet or snowy conditions and on uneven terrain. He has not been on long community outings (such as shopping) so his abilities in this area unknown. He notes he primarily has used his power wheelchair when outside in his yard (Modified Independence).

At the time of this report he was limited to use of a power wheelchair or total assistance with his manual wheelchair, because his right hand will be casted for approximately one month.

Transportation

Mr. Smith has done very limited driving since his injury; however, he did undergo a driver's evaluation while at Craig Hospital. As a result of this evaluation driver's training, vehicle modifications, and adaptive equipment were recommended (Modified Independence).

He has a current Montana driver's license with no restrictions other than glasses. At this time he has a Ford Econoline van which has a raised roof (not including the driver's place), lift, and electric door. It does not have any adaptive equipment for driving.

Household Activities

The client has not done household chores such as cleaning, cooking, or laundering since his injury. Mr. Smith relates he "used to do a lot of cooking" and helped with the housework, including cleaning and laundering. He states he would like to be able to do some of the housework but adds that "it's just hard to do."

Mr. Smith relates that his new home is barrier free and does not need any additional modifications other than possibly a stairway lift to allow him access to the basement where he hopes to eventually locate his exercise equipment. The client is unable to perform any home maintenance/repair activities and will need assistance with maintaining this property (snow removal, lawn mowing, etc.).

He would require assistance and/or adaptive equipment to do shopping, cooking, cleaning, and household chores.

Social Activities

Mr. Smith does not participate in any church or community activities at this time nor does he belong to any community groups or clubs. As noted previously, he belongs to the Faith Lutheran Church but no longer attends on a regular basis.

He did not belong to any community groups prior to his injury. Mr. Smith did belong to the spinal cord injury support group in Whitefish in the past, but this group is no longer active.

Health Maintenance/Recreational Activities

Immediately prior to tendon transfer surgery Mr. Smith was going to a health club approximately three days a week. His physical therapist supervised his exercise program, a trainer worked with him one day a week, and his wife assisted him during the other days. Mr. Smith also expresses an interest in obtaining exercise equipment to use at home to work on physical conditioning. He relates he has explored the possibility of home exercise equipment and provided information to his case manager but has not heard back regarding purchasing such equipment.

In terms of present recreational activities, Mr. Smith relates he typically reads, watches television, and "looks at stuff in my room." He adds that he is working with a loaner computer which is very outdated and has a regular keyboard with no modifications (including no mouse) and he has problems using the keyboard.

Mr. Smith expresses an interest in learning to use computers, especially in such areas as word processing, spreadsheets, and the Internet. He is also interested in a voice activated computer system, because he relates he is very slow at using a keyboard and it bothers his neck to look down for long periods of time.

Mr. Smith reports that prior to the injury his hobbies included hunting, fishing, reloading, boating/rafting, and hiking and he was "real active" in pursuing these interests, especially hunting. He notes he tried hunting once since his injury but it was "difficult." He relates he tried using his power wheelchair but became stuck and had to wait for someone to come to assist him. He notes the power wheelchair is extremely rough, describing it as "it beats you to death." He adds that he had a rest built for his wheelchair to support his rifle but it did not work very well. Mr. Smith relates he ended up hunting in a "very controlled environment." He continues to be interested in pursuing adaptive hunting.

The only time he has been fishing since the injury was on 6/11/99 when he went on a chartered boat outing for persons with disabilities called Crossing the Barriers, in conjunction with the Montana Department of Fish, Wildlife & Parks. He notes there was no adaptive equipment on the boat and someone held the fishing rod for him and the only part he could do in fishing was to use his palm to reel. Mr. Smith relates that the experience has sparked an interest in returning to fishing and boating on a modified basis. He states, "It was really fun but takes a lot of doing." He also is interested in doing reloading but is concerned about the degree of manual dexterity required for this activity.

CURRENT MANAGEMENT AND CARE

The client's treating physiatrist continues to be Dr. Stone in Kalispell and he reports he last saw Dr. Stone on 5/19/99. Mr. Smith reports that at this time he sees Dr. Stone on an as-needed basis and will probably be seeing him again some time in September.

He reports his treating "medical doctor" continues to be Dr. Jones, who provides follow-along services, draws blood for protimes, and prescribes and monitors medication. The client relates that he sees Dr. Jones on an at least monthly basis at this time and he last saw her on 8/28/99. He is scheduled to have his protimes checked again on 9/7/99 and will see Dr. Jones again on 9/27/99.

Mr. Smith notes that, because of the Coumadin he is prescribed, he has a blood test done on a monthly basis at Dr. Jones's office to check his protimes levels to determine if the Coumadin dosage needs to be changed. If problems with his protimes level occur, then blood tests are taken on a more frequent basis by the registered nurse who comes to his home. He continues to be on a 7.5 mg dosage at this time but Mr. Smith notes this could change based on the results of the test on 9/7/99.

Mr. Smith saw Perry C. Howard, M.D., a neurosurgeon, on 6/11/99 regarding recent neck pain. The client relates he had cervical x-rays at that time which showed his neck continues to be stable. Mr. Smith is now doing a home neck exercise program and taking pain medication as needed. He will not continue seeing Dr. Howard for neck pain at this time, because this condition will be monitored by Drs. Stone and Jones.

In 6/99 the client was having problems with hematuria (blood in the urine) and saw Dennis R. Scopes, M.D., a urologist, who did an IVP and cystogram. No kidney stones were present. Mr. Smith does not see a urologist on a regular basis but will probably be seen every six months to one year for a cystogram. This treatment may vary depending on whether he can return to an external catheter bladder program. At this time he has urine tests done only when a urinary tract infection is suspected.

The client is being seen by Dr. Cook for individual counseling; Dr. Cook has also seen the Smiths on three occasions for marital counseling. Mr. Smith reports he was seeing him one time a week but at this time is seeing him one time every two weeks. He last saw Dr. Cook on 8/11/99; although another appointment is not scheduled at this time, Dr. Cook anticipates seeing him again soon.

Ms. Smith was also being seen for psychological services on an ongoing basis by Linda Logan, MA, LPC. Ms. Smith last saw Ms. Logan on 6/28/99.

Mr. Smith underwent the first part of a two-part tendon transfer surgery on his right hand on 8/22/99 by Chad Henry, M.D., at Swedish Hospital (Craig Hospital) in Denver, Colorado. The procedure required hospitalization for two days; his right hand will be casted for four weeks, followed by several weeks of occupational therapy. Bert James, M.D., in Kalispell and his current occupational therapist, Troy Terrell, OTR/L, will provide local follow-up care. It is not yet known when the second part of the procedure will be done, but Dr. Henry notes the second procedure is typically performed two months after the first. The recovery period for the second part of the tendon transfer procedure will be approximately the same time as the first part. Mr. Smith relates at this time that he is uncertain whether he will eventually have a tendon transfer procedure performed on his left hand because this will depend on the outcome of the procedure done to his right hand.

Dr. Olson has noted a medialization laryngoplasty procedure would allow better vocalization with more strength and clarity. Mr. Smith relates he would like a stronger voice, particularly because he has difficulty being heard if he is calling someone in another room; however, he is leaving consideration for vocal cord surgery until the future, when he has recovered from the tendon transfer surgery.

Current medications (as of 8/25/99) include:

- Baclofen (Lioresal), 10 mg, four times a day for muscle spasm control
- Ditropan, 5 mg, two times a day for bladder spasm control
- Florinef, 0.1 mg, two times a day for blood pressure
- Coumadin, 7.5 mg, one time a day for anticoagulation
- Magic Bullet, one time every other day for bowel management (suppository)
- Senokot-S, as needed for stool softener
- Endocet, mg unknown, as needed for pain (one time per day while in therapy)
- Lodine, 400 mg, as needed for neck pain
- Vicodin, 500 mg, one time every three to four hours (as of 8/25/99) or as needed for post-surgical pain
- Prozac, 20 mg, two times a day for depression
- Temazepan, 30 mg, one time a night for sleep aid
- Centrum multivitamin, mg unknown, one time a day as a dietary supplement
- Vitamin C, 500 mg, two times a day for bladder program
- Niferex Forte, 150 mg, one time a day as iron supplement;
- Vitamin E, 400 units, one time a day as a dietary supplement/skin aid.
- Tylenol 500 mg, as needed for fever reduction

Mr. Smith reports he had stopped taking Coumadin in preparation for surgery and was taking Lovenox as an anticoagulant for two weeks. He notes he began taking Coumadin again on 8/25/99.

Mr. Smith relates the only adverse side affects he notices from the medication is drowsiness.

Mr. Smith currently has a personal care attendant from Whitefish Home Medical Services come in twice a day for approximately three hours in the morning and one hour in the evening to help with activities of daily living such as showering, dressing, grooming, emptying the leg bag, and transfers. The attendant also provides range of motion exercises. He was receiving personal care attendant services from NorthMont until 8/14/99, at which time he switched service providers so that he would be able to self-direct his care. A registered nurse from Glacier County Home Health Agency comes in once every other day for an average of one to one and one-half hours per visit to do his bladder and bowel programs, take his vital signs, and monitor his skin condition.

The client's wife periodically helps the attendant with transfers, empties the leg bag, and provides range of motion exercises.

Medical case management services are being provided by Robin Quinnell, RN, CCM, of Community Wellness. Mr. Smith reports at this time that she calls on the average of once a week and he occasionally stops in to see her when he is exercising at the Summit.

Until recently Mr. Smith was receiving physical therapy one time per week from Kent Smyth, PT, at the Summit. However, physical therapy is on hold at this time because of the recent tendon transfer surgery Mr. Smith underwent. Mr. Smyth relates he will be seeing him again in the future to complete the transition to an independent exercise program. Prior to surgery, the client was participating in a supervised exercise program (clinical membership) at the Summit three days a week. A trainer was providing supervision one day a week and his wife assisted him the other two days. Mr. Smith reports he needs assistance to set up the machines and pull the pulleys down to his level. Although this exercise program is currently on hold pending recovery from surgery, he is scheduled to resume it on 9/12/99.

Mr. Smith's occupational therapy program is currently on hold while his right arm is casted. His occupational therapist, Troy Terrell, OTR/L, at Kalispell Regional Hospital Outpatient Therapy, will provide follow-up treatment after the cast is removed from Mr. Smith's right hand. In addition, future therapy will involve adaptive driving, van modifications, and community outings. Mr. Terrell has also been working on modifications for some of the exercise equipment Mr. Smith uses at the Summit.

Initially following the injury, limited vocational rehabilitation services were provided regarding possible evaluations, possible computer use/modification, and transportation issues. Mr. Smith has been receiving private vocational rehabilitation services from Michael Simms, MS, CRC, of Vocational Rehabilitation Counseling in Kalispell. In 9/98 Mr. Simms prepared a job analysis of an alternate position—data entry clerk—with Mr. Smith's employer at injury (Rocky Mountain Manufacturing) and job site modification needs were determined. Dr. Stone approved the data entry clerk job but noted concerns regarding the need for prolonged sitting, bending, stooping, and gradual increase in sitting and work tolerance. A vocational rehabilitation plan outlining the specifics of an on-the-job training agreement with Rocky Mountain Manufacturing has been developed. He will initially work one hour per day and attempt to increase his work hours as appropriate. Mr. Smith was initially scheduled to begin this on-the-job training program on 8/14/99 but construction delays occurred because of inclement weather conditions. As of 8/28/99 the client relates that the work site accommodations and modifications have not yet been completed and he is not aware of another starting date having been set.

The client relates he has been working with Veronica Sands, rehabilitation counselor, at the state Rehabilitative Service Division regarding van modification.

CURRENT FINANCIAL STATUS

Mr. Smith currently receives workers compensation benefits and Social Security Disability Income benefits. He was found eligible for SSDI benefits in 1/98 and therefore will not be eligible for Medicare benefits until 1/2000.

The client describes his overall financial status by stating, "I guess it's all right. There's a lot of stuff we have to do yet that depends on finances."

CONCLUSIONS

Careful consideration has been given to all of the medical, psychosocial, rehabilitation, and evaluation data contained within the client's file and my report. Clearly, Mr. Smith has incurred significant disability and handicapping conditions secondary to complete C6 tetraplegia (ASIA A). His history of post-injury complications suggests the need for close monitoring and follow-up strategies of Mr. Smith's physical, psychological, functional, and social needs, particularly as he ages with spinal cord injury.

Given Mr. Smith's level of injury, even the most minor functional loss can create significant secondary disability, requiring substantially greater personal care assistance and costly interventions. Consequently, extra vigilance will be needed to ensure that appropriate alternatives and interventions are implemented at times critical to the long-term preservation of function. A key to addressing Mr. Smith's long-term health care needs will be a primary care physician at the local level, such as Dr. Stone, who can oversee the big picture and effectively address his changing physical, psychosocial, environmental, equipment, and attendant care needs. In addition, I would also see the need for Mr. Smith to have contact with the Craig Hospital Spinal Cord Injury Care System every one to three years, or more frequently if problems develop or as generalized decline becomes more apparent, to provide comprehensive medical, equipment, psychological, and social assessments and updated recommendations relevant to the increasing needs he will experience from aging with spinal cord injury.

In terms of Mr. Smith's vocational rehabilitation potential, I would question if the income levels associated with his current vocational objective of return to work with his employer at injury as a data entry clerk would be sufficient to provide a meaningful wage beyond the additional health care and transportation needs he has, particularly as these increase in the future. Further, given his age, education, work experience, and the fact that people with spinal cord injury show a significant decrease in their vocational activities at a relatively earlier age than the general population, I would not see further retraining or additional education as substantially enhancing Mr. Smith's re-employment potential.

Consequently, for all practical purposes, I see Mr. Smith as totally disabled from substantial, competitive employment at this stage in his work life cycle given the factors of age, education, and disability. This is not to say he should not be encouraged to continue to pursue the highly modified job option his employer at injury is willing to provide. However, it must be kept in mind that this option will likely be on a part-time basis at best and require significant adaptive equipment and work site modification. And the success of this option will further depend on Mr. Smith's ability to establish and maintain a program of care that will allow him to sustain employment on a consistent basis so that he does not have a record of missed days or repetitive tardiness for work because of a range of physical and psychological factors that tend to prevent job stabilization in the open labor market.

Although competitive employment may not be a realistic goal at this stage in Mr. Smith's work life cycle given the combination of factors previously described, I do, however, think it will be important to continue to encourage and support other forms of productivity through community involvement and recreation and health maintenance activities to maintain his quality of life.

After you have had an opportunity to review this report and the attached appendix, please contact me should you have further questions.

Respectfully submitted,

Terry L. Blackwell, Ed.D.
Certified Case Manager
Certified Life Care Planner
Certified Rehabilitation Counselor
Associate Professor of Rehabilitation Counseling

Attachment: Life Care Plan

C: Brett and Sandy Smith

Terry L. Blackwell, Ed.D.
Louisiana State University
Health Sciences Center
1900 Gravier Street
New Orleans, LA 70112
(504) 568-2420

LIFE CARE PLAN
Brett E. Smith
Projected Evaluations

	Date of Birth:	5/3/56
	Date of Injury:	7/3/97
	Date Prepared:	9/1/99
	Primary Disability:	Tetraplegia

Item/Service	Age / Year	Frequency/ Replacement	Purpose	Cost	Comment	Provider
Physical therapy	Beginning: 42 1/99; Ending: Life expectancy	1 × /1–3 years*	Maintain strength and reduce complications	Per Unit: $0 Per Year: $0	Cost included in periodic inpatient/outpatient spinal cord injury re-evaluation	Spinal Cord Injury Care System (Craig Hospital)
Occupational therapy	Beginning: 42 1/99; Ending: Life expectancy	1 × /1–3 years*	Assess equipment and aids for independence which can be used as age and disability combine to create greater dependence	Per Unit: $0 Per Year: $0	Cost included in periodic inpatient/outpatient spinal cord injury re-evaluation	Spinal Cord Injury Care System (Craig Hospital)
Nursing	Beginning: 42 1/99; Ending: Life expectancy	1 × /1–3 years*	Assess bowel/bladder management, skin care	Per Unit: $0 Per Year: $0	Cost included in periodic inpatient/outpatient spinal cord injury re-evaluation	Spinal Cord Injury Care System (Craig Hospital)
Psychological/ Social	Beginning: 42 1/99; Ending: Life expectancy	1 × /1–3 years*	Assess psychosocial adjustment	Per Unit: $0 Per Year: $0	Cost included in periodic inpatient/outpatient spinal cord injury re-evaluation	Spinal Cord Injury Care System (Craig Hospital)
Recreational therapy	Beginning: 42 1/99; Ending: Life expectancy	1 × /1–3 years*	Assess leisure interests and recommend adaptive equipment	Per Unit: $0 Per Year: $0	Cost included in periodic inpatient/outpatient spinal cord injury re-evaluation	Spinal Cord Injury Care System (Craig Hospital)
Disabled driver	Beginning: 42 1/99; Ending: 42 1/99	1 × only	Assess driving and recommend adaptive equipment	Per Unit: $0 Per Year: $0	Already accomplished as of 1/23/99 evaluation	Craig Hospital

Format Adapted from Paul M. Deutsch, Ph. D, CRC, Copyright 1994.
Growth Trend to be Determined by Economist
*See Routine Future Medical Care chart re: periodic inpatient/outpatient spinal cord injury care system evaluation. Frequency of periodic evaluation may increase if problems develop or as generalized decline becomes more apparent.

Terry L. Blackwell, Ed.D.
Louisiana State University
Health Sciences Center
1900 Gravier Street
New Orleans, LA 70112
(504) 568-2420

LIFE CARE PLAN
Brett E. Smith
Future Medical
Care—Routine (1)

Date of Birth:	5/3/56
Date of Injury:	7/3/97
Date Prepared:	9/1/99
Primary Disability:	Tetraplegia

Item/Service	Age	Year	Frequency/ Replacement	Purpose	Cost	Comment	Provider
Periodic inpatient/ outpatient spinal cord injury care system evaluation[a]	Beginning: 42 Ending: Life expectancy	1/99	1 × /1–3 years or more frequently if problems develop or as generalized decline becomes more apparent	Provide comprehensive evaluation to include medical, equipment, psychological, and social assessments, and updated recommendations to preserve function or reduce complications through the aging process	Per Unit: $2,500– $6,500/periodic evaluation Per Year:	Initial evaluation has already been provided. Per unit cost is a range for subsequent 5-day evaluation on an inpatient/outpatient basis	Spinal Cord Injury Care System (Craig Hospital)
General medical	Beginning: 43 Ending: Life expectancy	9/99	2 × /year	Routine assessment	Per Unit: $45–$65/visit Per Year: $90–$130		Mary Jones, M.D.
Physical medicine and rehabilitation	Beginning: 43 Ending: Life expectancy	9/99	3–4 × /year	Routine assessment	Per Unit: $73/visit Per Year: $219–$292		James Stone, M.D.
Orthopedic	Beginning: 43 Ending: 44	8/99 8/00	5–7 × /post-surgery	Routine follow-up after tendon transfer procedures performed by Dr. Henry	Per Unit: $45/visit Per Year: $225–$315		Bert James, M.D.
Otolaryngology	Beginning: 43 Ending: 45	9/99 9/01	2–3 × /post-surgery	Routine follow-up after medialization laryngoplasty	Per Unit: $0 Per Year: $0	Cost included in procedure cost	Cory Olson, M.D.

Format Adapted from Paul M. Deutsch, Ph. D., CRC, Copyright 1994.
Growth Trend to be Determined by Economist

Terry L. Blackwell, Ed.D.
Louisiana State University
Health Sciences Center
1900 Gravier Street
New Orleans, LA 70112
(504) 568-2420

Date of Birth: 5/3/56
Date of Injury: 7/3/97
Date Prepared: 9/1/99
Primary Disability: Tetraplegia

LIFE CARE PLAN
Brett E. Smith
Future Medical
Care—Routine (2)

Item/Service	Age	Year	Frequency/Replacement	Purpose	Cost		Comment	Provider
Urology	Beginning: 43	9/99	1 × / year	Routine assessment	Per Unit:			D. Scopes, M.D.
	Ending:	Life expectancy			Per Year: $29			
Miscellaneous laboratory work[b]	Beginning: 43	9/99	See below for specific recommendations	Routine assessment	Per Unit:		See below for breakdown of costs	Kalispell Regional Hospital
	Ending:	Life expectancy			Per Year:			

Format Adapted from Paul M. Deutsch, Ph. D., CRC, Copyright 1994.
Growth Trend to be Determined by Economist

[a] Additional costs for periodic inpatient/outpatient spinal cord injury care system evaluation would include airline travel for two people, ground transportation, and apartment accommodations for 5 nights at a cost of $911–$2,037. Attendant care is already covered (see Home Care/Facility Care chart).

[b] Laboratory work to include: CBC/SMAC (including lipid profile) 1 × / year @ $21.85/each; U/A 3–4 × / year @ $3.00–$23.85 (if positive)/each; renogram 1 × every other year @ $648.25/each; cystoscopy 1 × / year or less @ $1,500–$1,800/each; AP pelvis 3–5 × during lifetime @ $83.75/each; IVP 1–2 × during lifetime @ $278/each; voiding cystourethrogram 1–2 × / year @ $109; EKG 1 × / 1–3 years @ $172.50/each. Other studies may include fecal occult blood @ $16.85/each and flexible sigmoidoscopy @ $170/each (noted "recommended per general medical needs but not related to accident"). Such studies are typically performed at 1 × / 1–5 years.

Terry L. Blackwell, Ed.D.
Louisiana State University
Health Sciences Center
1900 Gravier Street
New Orleans, LA 70112
(504) 568-2420

**LIFE CARE PLAN
Brett E. Smith
Future Medical
Care—Aggressive
Treatment**

Date of Birth: 5/3/56
Date of Injury: 7/3/97
Date Prepared: 9/1/99
Primary Disability: Tetraplegia

Item/Service	Age	Year	Frequency/Replacement	Purpose	Cost	Comment	Provider
Tendon transfers (two-part procedure)*	Beginning: 43 Ending: 43	Beginning: 8/99 Ending: 10/99	1 × only (involves two separate procedures)	Improved hand function	Per Unit: $23,122–$26,174 for 2 procedures Per Year:	Cost includes physicians' fees, hospital charges, transportation, and attendant care housing	Chad Henry M.D., Craig Hand Clinic/Swedish Hospital
Medialization laryngoplasty	Beginning: 43 Ending: 45	Beginning: 9/99 Ending: 10/01	1 × only	Improved vocalization	Per Unit: $7,730–$7,830 Per Year:	Cost includes physician's fees, follow-up with Dr. Olson, and hospital charges	Cory Olson, M.D., Kalispell Regional Hospital

Format Adapted from Paul M. Deutsch, Ph. D., CRC, Copyright 1994.
Growth Trend to be Determined by Economist

*First part of tendon transfer procedure was performed on 3/22/99; Dr. Henry reports second part of procedure is typically performed within 2 months after the first. Cost does not include follow-up with Dr. Jones and outpatient occupational therapy (see Routine Medical Care and Projected Therapeutic Modality charts).

The need for a surgical procedure pertaining to cervical stabilization (plate removal) may be likely in the future but is not indicated at this time.

Terry L. Blackwell, Ed.D.
Louisiana State University
Health Sciences Center
1900 Gravier Street
New Orleans, LA 70112
(504) 568-2420

LIFE CARE PLAN
Brett E. Smith
Projected Therapeutic Modalities

Date of Birth: 5/3/56
Date of Injury: 7/3/97
Date Prepared: 9/1/99
Primary Disability: Tetraplegia

Item/Service	Age	Year	Frequency/ Replacement	Purpose	Cost	Comment	Provider
Individual/family counseling and education	Beginning: 43 Ending: Life expectancy	9/99	1 × /every other week for 2–3 months; followed by 1 × /3–4 weeks for 2–3 months; as-needed basis thereafter	Aid in psychosocial/ disability adjustment	Per Unit: $540–$900 Per Year:	Cost based on $90 per session	Local provider
Sexuality counseling	Beginning: 43 Ending: 44	9/99 9/00	10–20 sessions	Aid in sexual adjustment to disability	Per Unit: $900–$1,800 Per Year:	Cost based on $90 per session	Local provider
Spousal counseling (wife)	Beginning: 39 Ending: 40	9/99 9/00	1 × /week for 1 year	Spousal support and adjustment	Per Unit: Per Year: $3,120–$3,600	Cost based on $65–$75 per session	Local provider
SCI support group/peer counseling	Beginning: 43 Ending: Life expectancy	9/99	As needed	Peer support in disability adjustment	Per Unit: $0 Per Year: $0	No cost services available	Local support group as available
Physical therapy	Beginning: 43 Ending: 43	9/99 10/99	1 × /week for 1 month	Monitor independent exercise program	Per Unit: $256–$432 Per Year:	Unit cost based on $64–$108/hour	Local provider
Occupational therapy	Beginning: 43 Ending: 44	9/99 9/00	16–28 times	Disabled driver training, adaptive equipment training, independent community reintegration/training, post-tendon transfer follow-up	Per Unit: $1,408–$3,803 Per Year:	Unit cost based on $88–$136/hour	Local provider

Format Adapted from Paul M. Deutsch, Ph. D., CRC, Copyright 1994.
Growth Trend to be Determined by Economist

Terry L. Blackwell, Ed.D.
Louisiana State University
Health Sciences Center
1900 Gravier Street
New Orleans, LA 70112
(504) 568-2420

LIFE CARE PLAN
Brett E. Smith
Medication/Supply Needs

	Date of Birth:	5/3/56
	Date of Injury:	7/3/97
	Date Prepared:	9/1/99
	Primary Disability:	Tetraplegia

Item/Service	Age	Year	Frequency/ Replacement	Purpose	Cost	Comment	Vendor
Catheter/miscellaneous supplies[a]	Beginning: 43 Ending: Life expectancy	9/99	1 × /year allowance	Miscellaneous supplies	Per Unit: Per Year: $1,652	See below for breakdown of individual supply costs	Local supplier
Prescribed pharmaceuticals[b]	Beginning: 43 Ending: Life expectancy	9/99	1 × /year allowance	Routine pharmaceuticals as prescribed	Per Unit: Per Year: $3,523– $4,752	See below for breakdown of individual pharmaceutical costs	Local supplier

Format Adapted from Paul M. Deutsch, Ph. D., CRC, Copyright 1994.
Growth Trend to be Determined by Economist

[a]Miscellaneous supplies include: abdominal binder $14.25; thigh-high Ted hose $46.32; #16 French Foley catheter $22.32; drainage leg bag $317.72; overnight bag $546.00; leg tubing $178.36; underpads $176.90; disposal washcloths $152.60; disposal gloves $53.29; Betadyne $13.80; cotton tip applicators $9.52; KY jelly $13.20. Costs represent yearly usage. If intermittent catheter program becomes feasible in the future, associated costs must be adjusted accordingly.

[b]Prescribed pharmaceuticals include: Lioresal $74.70 (Baclofen $37.20); Ditropan $32.10 (Oxybutnin $14.49); Florinef $28.94 (none); Coumadin $26.26 (none); Percocet $5.91 (Endocet $1.90); Lodine $46.65 (Etodolac $23.52); Restoril $25.83 (Temazepam $7.16); Niferex Forte $9.97 (none); Prozac $133.09 (none). Over-the-counter pharmaceuticals include: Tylenol $0.27 (0.10); (Vitamin C $1.54); (Vitamin E $1.17); Centrum multivitamin $2.70 ($1.36); Senokot S $0.31 (none); Magic Bullet suppository $6.59 (none). Costs represent monthly usage; brand is listed first with generic noted in parenthesis.

Terry L. Blackwell, Ed.D.
Louisiana State University
Health Sciences Center
1900 Gravier Street
New Orleans, LA 70112
(504) 568-2420

LIFE CARE PLAN
Brett E. Smith
Orthotics

Date of Birth: 5/3/56
Date of Injury: 7/3/97
Date Prepared: 9/1/99
Primary Disability: Tetraplegia

Item/Service	Age	Year	Frequency/ Replacement	Purpose	Cost	Comment	Vendor
Tenodesis splint	Beginning: Already purchased (1997) Ending: 41	1997	1 × only	Enhance independence	Per Unit: Per Year:	Cost not available	St. Jude's Institute of Rehabilitation
Bilateral AFO boots	Beginning: Already purchased (7/98) Ending: 42	7/98	1 × only	Rehabilitation/ medical management	Per Unit: $1,200 Per Year:	Unit cost incurred one time only	Northwestern Care
Splinting after tendon transfer surgery	Beginning: 43 Ending: 43	8/99 11/99	1 × after each part of two-part procedure	Medical management	Per Unit: $400 Per Year:	Cost for fabricating each splint is approximately $200	Kalispell Regional Hospital Outpatient Occupational Therapy

Format Adapted from Paul M. Deutsch, Ph. D., CRC, Copyright 1994.
Growth Trend to be Determined by Economist

LIFE CARE PLAN
Brett E. Smith
Wheelchair Needs

Terry L. Blackwell, Ed.D.
Louisiana State University
Health Sciences Center
1900 Gravier Street
New Orleans, LA 70112
(504) 568-2420

		Date of Birth:	5/3/56
		Date of Injury:	7/3/97
		Date Prepared:	9/1/99
		Primary Disability:	Tetraplegia

Item/Service	Age	Year	Frequency/ Replacement	Purpose	Cost	Comment	Vendor
Quickie Revolution ultralite manual wheelchair (anti-tip, laterals, Jay back, Applewood board, seat belt)	Beginning: Ending: Life expectancy	Already purchased (1997)	1 × /4–6 years to age 50; than 1 × /6–8 years as a back-up	Mobility	Per Unit: $3,060 Per Year:	Per unit cost based on 1999 dollars because original purchase price not available; includes accessories added to wheelchair at Craig Hospital	North Medical
Quickie P200 power wheelchair	Beginning: Ending: 41	Already purchased (1997) 1997	1 × only	Mobility	Not available	Power wheelchair recommended as age and disabiliy combine to create greater dependence	North Medical
Quickie P300 power wheelchair (detachable leg rests, padded adjustable arm rests, chest strap, tilt back)*	Beginning: 46–48 Ending: Life expectancy	2002–2004	1 × /5–7 years	Mobility	Per Unit: $13,595 Per Year:	Per unit cost based on 1999 price	Local supplier
Activeaid roll-in shower/commode chair	Beginning: Already purchased (2/98) Ending: Life expectancy		1 × /3–5 years	Aid in bathing/ toileting	Per Unit: $613 Per Year:	Per unit cost based on purchase price	Whitefish Medical Equipment

Format Adapted from Paul M. Deutsch, Ph. D., CRC, Copyright 1994.
Growth Trend to be Determined by Economist

*Tilt back for power wheelchair has been recommended. P300 model would replace P200 model, because it would cost approximately $6,000 to add tilt to current power wheelchair.

Terry L. Blackwell, Ed.D.
Louisiana State University
Health Sciences Center
1900 Gravier Street
New Orleans, LA 70112
(504) 568-2420

LIFE CARE PLAN
Brett E. Smith
Wheelchair Accessories

Date of Birth: 5/3/56
Date of Injury: 7/3/97
Date Prepared: 9/1/99
Primary Disability: Tetraplegia

Item/Service	Age	Year	Frequency/ Replacement	Purpose	Cost	Comment	Vendor
High profile Roho cushion (1)	Beginning: Already purchased (4/98) Ending: Life expectancy		1 × /2–3 years	Pressure reduction while seated in wheelchair	Per Unit: $425 Per Year:	Per unit cost based on purchase price	Local supplier
High profile Roho cushion (extra)	Beginning: 43 Ending: Life expectancy	9/99	1 × /2–3 years	Pressure reduction while seated in wheelchair	Per Unit: $448 Per Year:	Per unit cost based on 1999 cost	Local supplier
Roho cushion cover (extra)	Beginning: 43 Ending: Life expectancy	6/99	1 × /1–2 years	Maintain cushion	Per Unit: $40 Per Year:	Per unit cost based on purchase price	Local supplier
Bean bag lapboard	Beginning: 43 Ending: Life expectancy	1/99	1 × year	Work and activity site	Per Unit: $10 Per Year:	Per unit cost based on purchase price	Local supplier
Quad wheelchair gloves	Beginning: 43 Ending: 46–48	5/99 2002–2004	1 × /3–6 months	Safety aid	Per Unit: $30–$40 Per Year: $120–$240	Per unit cost based on 1999 price	Local supplier
Transfer board	Beginning: Already purchased (8/97) Ending: Life expectancy		1 × 10 years	Transfer aid	Per Unit: $45–$55 Per Year:	Per unit cost based on 1999 price	Local supplier
Wheelchair backpack	Beginning: Already purchased (3/99) Ending: Life expectancy		1 × 2–3 years	Enhance independence	Per Unit: $40–$55 Per Year:	Per unit cost based on 1999 price	Local supplier

Format Adapted from Paul M. Deutsch, Ph. D., CRC, Copyright 1994.
Growth Trend to be Determined by Economist

LIFE CARE PLAN
Brett E. Smith
Wheelchair Maintenance

Terry L. Blackwell, Ed.D.
Louisiana State University
Health Sciences Center
1900 Gravier Street
New Orleans, LA 70112
(504) 568-2420

Date of Birth: 5/3/56
Date of Injury: 7/3/97
Date Prepared: 9/1/99
Primary Disability: Tetraplegia

Item/Service	Age	Year	Frequency/ Replacement	Purpose	Cost	Comment	Vendor
Manual wheelchair	Beginning: 43 Ending: Life expectancy	Beginning: 9/99 Ending: Life expectancy	1×/year to age 50; 1×/every other year when used as back-up	Maintain equipment	Per Unit: Per Year: $45	Unit cost not incurred on year new wheelchair purchased	Local supplier
Shower/commode wheelchair	Beginning: 43 Ending: Life expectancy	Beginning: 9/99 Ending: Life expectancy	1×/year	Maintain equipment	Per Unit Per Year: $45	Unit cost not incurred on year new wheelchair purchased	Local supplier
Power wheelchair	Beginning: 43 Ending: Life expectancy	Beginning: 9/99 Ending: Life expectancy	1×/2–3 years until age 45–47; 1×/year thereafter	Maintain equipment	Per Unit: Per Year: $45–$90	Maintenance scheduled based on increased use after age 50	Local supplier
Replacement tires and tubes*	Beginning: 43 Ending: Life expectancy	Beginning: 9/99 Ending: Life expectancy	1–2×/year—tires and tubes; 1×/every other year—upholstery	Replace/ maintain equipment	Per Unit: Per Year: $124–$158	Per year cost based tires $25/each, tubes $9/each, upholstery replacement $180	Local supplier
Power wheelchair batteries (2)	Beginning: 43 Ending: Life expectancy	Beginning: 9/99 Ending: Life expectancy	1×/year	Equipment power supply	Per Unit: $100–$180 Per Year: $200–$360:		Local supplier

Format Adapted from Paul M. Deutsch, Ph.D., CRC, Copyright 1994.
Growth Trend to be Determined by Economist

*Has extra set of wheels for manual wheelchair at this time

Terry L. Blackwell, Ed.D.
Louisiana State University
Health Sciences Center
1900 Gravier Street
New Orleans, LA 70112
(504) 568-2420

LIFE CARE PLAN
Brett E. Smith
Home Care/Facility Care

Date of Birth: 5/3/56
Date of Injury: 7/3/97
Date Prepared: 9/1/99
Primary Disability: Tetraplegia

Item/Service	Age/Year	Frequency/Replacement	Purpose	Cost	Comment	Provider
Interior/exterior maintenance allowance	Beginning: 43 9/99 Ending: Life expectancy	Yearly allowance	Assistance in household activities, lawn care, snow removal	Per Unit: $60 Per Year: $720	Per unit allowance based on $60 per month	Local vendor
Attendant care services	Beginning: 43 9/99 Ending: 60 2016	10–12 hrs/day	Provide care/assistance with activities of daily living	Per Unit: Per Year: $40,150–$52,560	Per year cost based on $11–$12/hour for 10–12 hours per day to age 60, at which time 24-hour care begins	Local provider/ agency
24-hour attendant care	Beginning: 60 2016 Ending: Life expectancy	24 hrs/day	Provide care/ assistance as age and disability combine to create greater dependence	Per Unit: Per Year: $51,100–$92,710	Per year cost based on $140–$254 per day	Local provider/ agency
Skilled nursing care services	Beginning: 43 9/99 Ending: Life expectancy	1–2 hrs/every other day	Provide care planning and monitoring services in addition to regular nursing services	Per Unit: Per Year: $9,125–$13,870	Per year cost based on $50–76/visit	Local provider/ agency

Format Adapted from Paul M. Deutsch, Ph. D., CRC, Copyright 1994.
Growth Trend to be Determined by Economist

Terry L. Blackwell, Ed.D.
Louisiana State University
Health Sciences Center
1900 Gravier Street
New Orleans, LA 70112
(504) 568-2420

	Date of Birth:	5/3/56
	Date of Injury:	7/3/97
	Date Prepared:	9/1/99
	Primary Disability:	Tetraplegia

LIFE CARE PLAN
Brett E. Smith
Aids for Independent Function

Item/Service	Age	Year	Frequency/ Replacement	Purpose	Cost	Comment	Vendor
Adaptive clothing allowance	43	Beginning: 9/99 Ending: Life expectancy	Yearly allowance	Enhance independence	Per Unit: Per Year: $518	Per year allowance based on Department of Veterans Affairs guidelines	Local supplier
Long-handled reacher (wrist driven)	43	Beginning: 9/99 Ending: Life expectancy	1 × /3–5 years	Enhance independence	Per Unit: $95–$140 Per Year:	Unable to use regular reachers because of hand function	Local supplier
Cellular phone service	43	Beginning: 9/99 Ending: Life expectancy	Monthly service	Safety aid	Per Unit: $18/month Per Year: $216	Safety aid, especially during travel	Local supplier
Environmental control unit (ECU)	43	Beginning: 9/99 Ending: Life expectancy	1 × /10 years	To enhance independence in activities of daily living	Per Unit: $2,000–$6,500 Per Year:	Cost depends on number and type of items included on ECU	Local supplier
Adaptive equipment allowance*	43	Beginning: 9/99 Ending: Life expectancy	Yearly allowance	Enhance independence	Per Unit: Per Year: $100		Local supplier

Format Adapted from Paul M. Deutsch, Ph. D., CRC, Copyright 1994.
Growth Trend to be Determined by Economist

*Yearly allowance includes adaptive equipment used now or used in the past, such as bath mitt, shower sponge, fingernail clipper, dysem, universal cuffs, knife, fork, cupholder, keyholder, typing stick, pen/pencil holder, zipper pull, reading board, transfer belt. An adaptive knife, plate guard, adjustable arm for computer monitor, and document holder have also been recommended.

Terry L. Blackwell, Ed.D.
Louisiana State University
Health Sciences Center
1900 Gravier Street
New Orleans, LA 70112
(504) 568-2420

**LIFE CARE PLAN
Brett E. Smith
Home Furnishings and
Accessories**

Date of Birth: 5/3/56
Date of Injury: 7/3/97
Date Prepared: 9/1/99
Primary Disability: Tetraplegia

Item/Service	Age	Year	Frequency/Replacement	Purpose	Cost	Comment	Vendor
Invacare micro air bed*	Beginning: Already purchased (10/98) Ending: 42	10/98	1 × only	Prevention of pressure sores	Per Unit: $12,000 Per Year:	For informational purposes	Norco
Air bed replacement components: Filter Overlay pad Blower Mattress	Beginning: 43 Ending: Life expectancy	9/99	Filter—1×/month Pad—1×/2–3 years Blower—1×/5 years Mattress—1×/8 years	Prevention of pressure sores	Per Unit: Filter—$25 Pad—$191 Blower—$11,000 Mattress—$3,563 Per Year:		Local supplier
Overbed table	Beginning: 43 Ending: 43	9/99	1 × only	Enhance independent functioning	Per Unit: $105–$115		Local supplier
Invacare lift	Beginning: Already purchased (7/98) Ending: Life expectancy		1×/10–15 years	Transfer aid	Per Unit: $889 Per Year:	Per unit cost based on purchase price	Norco
Sling for lift	Beginning: Already purchased (10/98) Ending: Life expectancy		1×/3–5 years	Transfer aid	Per Unit: $107 Per Year:	Per unit cost based on purchase price	Norco

Format Adapted from Paul M. Deutsch, Ph. D., CRC, Copyright 1994.
Growth Trend to be Determined by Economist

*When sleeping in regular bed with wife, an egg crate ($40–$60) mattress pad is needed to prevent pressure sores during that time.

Terry L. Blackwell, Ed.D.
Louisiana State University
Health Sciences Center
1900 Gravier Street
New Orleans, LA 70112
(504) 568-2420

Date of Birth: 5/3/56
Date of Injury: 7/3/97
Date Prepared: 9/1/99
Primary Disability: Tetraplegia

LIFE CARE PLAN
Brett E. Smith
Architectural Renovations

Accessibility/Accommodations		Comment
Front Ramping		Many of these accommodations have already been provided in the barrier-free home which Mr. Smith and his family moved into in 11/98.
Emergency Exit Ramping	X	
Light Controls		
Floor Coverings		
Hallways		Accommodations which still need to be made include emergency ramping (cost $337–$695) and an intercom system (cost $41–$91). An elevator/stairway lift would allow access to the basement, where the client wishes to eventually locate home exercise equipment. Cost for these accommodations would be $15,000–$18,000. Annual service contract would be $300/yr.
Doorways		
Parking		
Kitchen:		
Sinks/Fixtures		
Cabinets		
Appliances		
Side-by-side Refrigerator		
Bathroom:		
Sink		
Cabinets		
Roll-in-Shower		
Hand Held Shower		
Temperature Control Guards		
Heater		
Fixtures		
Door Handles		
Additional Electrical Outlets		
Central Heat/Air		
Therapy/Equipment Room	X	
Elevator/Stairway Lift to Basement	X	
Bedroom Windows		Note: Kitchen accommodations were not included because the kitchen was designed for Ms. Smith and was not built to be completely accessible for Mr. Smith. It is projected he will not be cooking independently.
Other Windows		
Fire Alarm		
Smoke Detectors		
Intercom System	X	

Format Adapted from Paul M. Deutsch, Ph. D., CRC, 1994

Terry L. Blackwell, Ed.D.
Louisiana State University
Health Sciences Center
1900 Gravier Street
New Orleans, LA 70112
(504) 568-2420

LIFE CARE PLAN
Brett E. Smith
Transportation

	Date of Birth:	5/3/56
	Date of Injury:	7/3/97
	Date Prepared:	9/1/99
	Primary Disability:	Tetraplegia

Item/Service	Age	Year	Frequency/Replacement	Purpose	Cost	Comment	Vendor
1998 Ford club wagon van with 4-wheel drive, Braun swing away lift, raised roof	Beginning: Already purchased (1998) Ending: 42	7/98	1 × only	Transportation	Per Unit: $23,000 Per Year:	Per unit cost based on purchase price (unknown if includes modifications)	Rugg Ford
Adaptive van (at time of replacement of current van)	Beginning: 46–48 Ending: Life expectancy	2002–2004	1 × /5–7 years	Transportation	Per Unit: $14,171 Per Year:	Driver evaluation at Craig Hospital indicated driving from wheelchair would be preferred method.	Freewheel Vans
Adaptive equipment maintenance	Beginning: 43 Ending: Life expectancy	9/99	1 × /3 months	Maintain equipment	Per Unit: $41–$134 Per Year: $162–$536	Per unit cost based on $27–$67/hour per servicing	Local supplier

Format Adapted from Paul M. Deutsch, Ph. D, CRC, Copyright 1994.
Growth Trend to be Determined by Economist

Currently has a 1998 van with above listed modifications. Further adaptations (6-way power seat, shelf for feet, quad hand controls) will be undertaken in the future. However, full adaptations as recommended by Craig Hospital cannot be made on present vehicle because 4-wheel drive control is located on floor. When current van is replaced, should be with an adapted van that will allow for wheelchair driver. Specific recommendations for wheelchair driver include: lift; outside magnetic lift switch; front dash switches for lift and door; drop floor (Ford only); remove shelf over driver; MPS quad hand controls; 3-inch steering column; tri-pin steering device; alternate driver seat with front plate; seat base expansion; EZ Lock electric lockdown for wheelchair with 6-point shoulder and lap belt; adapt shoulder strap for independent access; Grandmar chest strap; dash extension on wash, wipe, headlights, and temperature controls as needed; electric parking brake.

Note: Average cost of a family vehicle is $18,300. This amount should be deducted from the cost of the van. Trade-in value to be determined by economist.

Terry L. Blackwell, Ed.D.
Louisiana State University
Health Sciences Center
1900 Gravier Street
New Orleans, LA 70112
(504) 568-2420

LIFE CARE PLAN
Brett E. Smith
Health
Maintenance/Recreational Needs (1)

Date of Birth: 5/3/56
Date of Injury: 7/3/97
Date Prepared: 9/1/99
Primary Disability: Tetraplegia

Item/Service	Age	Year	Frequency/ Replacement	Purpose	Cost	Comment	Vendor
Health club membership	Beginning: 43 Ending: 60	9/99 9/16	3 ×/week	Health maintenance	Per Unit: $49 Per Year: $588	Unit cost based on $49 month membership fee, includes trainer at no additional cost	Summit
Health club initiation fee	Beginning: 43 Ending: 43	9/99 9/99	1 × only	Health maintenance	Per Unit: $90	one-time initiation fee	Summit
Uppertone (home based exercise equipment)	Beginning: 43 Ending: 43	9/99 9/99	1 × only	Health maintenance	Per Unit: $2,609 Per Year:		G.P.K., Inc.
Adaptive recreational equipment: Gun mount, receiver and trigger activator; reel with joystick, EZ cast Lift with sling for boat	Beginning: 43 Ending: 60	9/99 9/16	1 × only	Recreational activities	Per Unit: Gun mount, etc., $640 Reel, etc. $498 Lift $1,140 Per Year:	Costs represent equipment needed for start-up only	Access to Recreation
Computer hardware	Beginning: 43 Ending: 60	9/99 9/16	1 ×/5–7 years	Enhance independence in avocational pursuits, home budget maintenance, educational/leisure endeavors	Per Unit: $1,700–$2,000 Per Year:	Cost includes monitor, hard drive, printer	Local supplier

Format Adapted from Paul M. Deutsch, Ph. D., CRC, Copyright 1994.
Growth Trend to be Determined by Economist

LIFE CARE PLAN
Brett E. Smith
Health Maintenance/Recreational Needs (2)

Terry L. Blackwell, Ed.D.
Louisiana State University
Health Sciences Center
1900 Gravier Street
New Orleans, LA 70112
(504) 568-2420

Date of Birth: 5/3/56
Date of Injury: 7/3/97
Date Prepared: 9/1/99
Primary Disability: Tetraplegia

Item/Service	Age	Year	Frequency/Replacement	Purpose	Cost	Comment	Vendor
Voice-activated computer system hardware	Beginning: 43 Ending: 43	9/99 9/99	1 × only	Enhance independent use of computer and lessen energy requirements	Per Unit: $395–$695 Per Year:		Dragon Systems
Computer software	Beginning: 43 Ending: 43	9/99 9/99	1 × /2–3 years	Enhance independence in avocational pursuits, home budget maintenance, educational/leisure endeavors	Per Unit: $60–$300 Per Year:	Includes software for word processing, spreadsheets, database, Internet	Local supplier

Format Adapted from Paul M. Deutsch, Ph. D., CRC, Copyright 1994.
Growth Trend to be Determined by Economist

LIFE CARE PLAN
Brett E. Smith
Potential Complications

Terry L. Blackwell, Ed.D.
Louisiana State University
Health Sciences Center
1900 Gravier Street
New Orleans, LA 70112
(504) 568-2420

Date of Birth: 5/3/56
Date of Injury: 7/3/97
Date Prepared: 9/1/99
Primary Disability: Tetraplegia

Complication/Risk Factor(s)	Complication/Risk Factor(s)	Comment
Pressure sores — immobility; shearing; moisture; inadequate nutrition; lack of pressure relief in bed/wheelchair	**Respiratory complications** — loss of physical fitness; obesity; respiratory infections; progressive kyphosis	Cost varies according to extent of complication
Contractures — inappropriate or lack of range of motion; complications from fractures; severe spasticity; improper positioning	**Renal complications** — chronic infections; incomplete voiding; urinary reflux; inadequate fluid intake; hypertension	The frequency and duration, as well as the type of complication, cannot be accurately predicted. This page is for informational purposes only.
Upper extremity impairments — overuse and aging; inadequate equipment	**Autonomic dysreflexia** — lack of proper skin, bowel, and/or bladder management; tight clothing, shoes, leg bag strapping, etc.	
Deep venous thrombosis — lack of movement, range of motion; inadequate fluid intake	**Cardiovascular complications** — physical inactivity; hypertension; obesity; emotional stress and depression; lack of access to appropriate health care services and appropriate equipment modification	
Urinary tract infections — lack of proper bladder management; indwelling catheter; inactivity; inadequate fluid intake		
Gastrointestinal complications — lack of proper dietary, bowel management		
Spasticity		
Depression — inactivity; decreased functioning; shrinking support systems; lack of access to appropriate health care services and effective personal care assistance; lack of recreational activities		

Format Adapted from Paul M. Deutsch, Ph. D., CRC, 1994

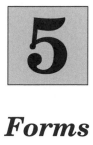

Forms

LIFE CARE PLAN INTERVIEW & HISTORY QUESTIONNAIRE

Date _____

Location _____

Referral Source _____

File # _____

IDENTIFYING INFORMATION

Client's Name _____

Date of Birth _____ Age _____ Social Security # _____

Address _____

City/State/Zip _____

Home Telephone _____ Work Telephone _____

Message Telephone _____ Name _____

Own Home _____ Rent _____

Accessible to Public Transportation: Yes _____ No _____

Race: White _____ Black _____ Asian _____ Hispanic _____ Other _____

Bilingual _____ Glasses _____ Dominant Hand _____

Height _____ Weight (present) _____ Weight (pre-injury) _____ Sex _____

Appearance _____
_____

Assistive Devices and Equipment _____
_____

Marital Status:
Married ____ Single ____ Divorced ____ Never Married ____ Number of Marriages ____

FAMILY HISTORY

Spouse's Name _____ Age _____

Number of Dependent Children _____

Children(s) Name   Age   By Marriage Number

_____   _____   _____
_____   _____   _____
_____   _____   _____
_____   _____   _____
_____   _____   _____

Client's Place of Birth _____

Previous Residences: 1. _____
                        2. _____
                        3. _____
                        4. _____

Number of Siblings _____

Brother(s)/Sister(s)   Age   Current/Past   Health
                                    Occupation   (good/fair/poor)

_____   _____   _____   _____
_____   _____   _____   _____
_____   _____   _____   _____
_____   _____   _____   _____
_____   _____   _____   _____
_____   _____   _____   _____
_____   _____   _____   _____

If any of above siblings are disabled, include name and disability:

Brother(s)/Sister(s)   Disability

_____   _____
_____   _____
_____   _____
_____   _____

Parents' Names   Current Residence   Current/Past Occupation

_____   _____   _____
_____   _____   _____

Comments _____
_____
_____
_____

EDUCATION/TRAINING

Highest Grade Completed _____ School _____

Special Classes/Assistance _____ GPA _____

Grades While Attending School _____

Transcripts Available: Yes _____ No _____

Degree/Certification _____ Year _____

Honors/Scholarships _____ Year _____

Special Training _____

Location _____ Year _____

Previous License/Certification/Registration _____

Present License/Certification/Registration _____

Did you like attending school? Yes _____ No _____ Explain why/why not? _____
_____
_____

Other Schools Attended:

Name of School	Location	Program/Subjects	GPA	Dates

School Subjects:

Liked Most _____

Like Least _____

Best Grades _____

Worst Grades _____

Other School Activities Participated In: _____
_____
_____

Do you now wish to attend school? Yes _____ No _____

How long are you willing to attend?

6 months _____ 1 year _____ 2 years _____ 4 years _____

Which of the following would you prefer?

1. College/University _____
2. Vocational/Technical School _____
3. On-The-Job Training _____
4. Direct Job Placement _____
5. Obtain GED _____
6. Academic Skill Building _____

Comments _____
_____
_____

MILITARY SERVICE

Branch _____ Dates of Service _____ Rank at Discharge _____

Occupation and Duties _____
_____
_____

Special Training _____

Service Connected Disability _____ Disability %Rating _____

Service Connected Disability Conditions:

1. _____
2. _____
3. _____
4. _____
5. _____

Comments _____
_____
_____
_____
_____
_____
_____

EMPLOYMENT HISTORY (Starting with most recent job)

Employer _____ Job Title _____ Salary _____

Address _____ City _____ State _____

Date Began _____ Date Ended _____ Length _____

Full-time _____ Part-time _____ Reason for Leaving _____

Union Member: Yes _____ No _____ Name of Union _____

Specific Duties _____
_____

Supervisory Responsibilities: Yes _____ No _____ Describe _____
_____

Job Skills _____
_____

What did you like best about the job? _____
_____

What did you like least about the job? _____
_____

Would you like to do this type of work again? Yes _____ No _____ Explain why/why not? _____

Did your disability interfere with your ability to do this job? Yes _____ No _____

If yes, explain how: _____
_____

Employer _____ Job Title _____ Salary _____

Address _____ City _____ State _____

Date Began _____ Date Ended _____ Length _____

Full-time _____ Part-time _____ Reason for Leaving _____

Union Member: Yes _____ No _____ Name of Union _____

Specific Duties _____
_____

Supervisory Responsibilities: Yes _____ No _____ Describe: _____
_____

Job Skills _____
_____

What did you like best about the job? _____
_____

What did you like least about the job? _____
_____

Would you like to do this type of work again? Yes _____ No _____ Explain
why/why not? _____

Did your disability interfere with your ability to do this job? Yes _____ No _____

If yes, explain how: _____
_____

Employer _____ Job Title _____ Salary _____

Address _____ City _____ State _____

Date Began _____ Date Ended _____ Length _____

Full-time _____ Part-time _____ Reason for Leaving _____

Union Member: Yes _____ No _____ Name of Union _____

Specific Duties _____
_____

Supervisory Responsibilities: Yes _____ No _____ Describe: _____
_____

Job Skills _____

What did you like best about the job? _____
_____

What did you like least about the job? _____
_____

Would you like to do this type of work again? Yes _____ No _____ Explain
why/why not? _____

Did your disability interfere with your ability to do this job? Yes _____ No _____

If yes, explain how: _____
_____

Have you ever lost a job or been denied employment due to your disability?

Yes _____ No _____ If yes, explain how: _____
_____
_____

Do you have skills and experience in the following areas (check all skill areas)?

Skill Area	Yes	No	Extent of Skill/Experience
Office Machines	___	___	_____
Computers	___	___	_____
Word Processors	___	___	_____
Keyboarding	___	___	_____
Bookkeeping	___	___	_____
Communications Equipment	___	___	_____
Construction Equipment	___	___	_____
Transport Equipment	___	___	_____
Farm Equipment	___	___	_____
Mechanical/Machines	___	___	_____
Machine Shop Tools	___	___	_____
Shipping/Receiving	___	___	_____
Inventory Control	___	___	_____
Scheduling	___	___	_____
Instructing/Teaching	___	___	_____
Supervising	___	___	_____
Sales	___	___	_____

Other _____

Comments _____

_____

_____

_____

DISABILITY CONDITIONS

Date of SCI _____ Level of SCI _____

Complete or Incomplete Injury _____

Sensory _____ Motor _____

How Injured _____

_____

Initial Treatment _____

_____

Summary of Treatment to Date _____

_____

_____

Bowel Program (Include bowel care procedure, frequency, and time required) ___

_____

Type of Bladder Management _____

_____

Current Nursing/Attendant Care Needs _____

_____

Have you worked since injury? (If worked, for whom? Part- or full-time? Any problems doing? Any modifications/accommodations made, etc.?) _____

_____

_____

Other Medical Conditions _____
_____

Significant Injuries/Accidents/Illnesses Prior to SCI (Include type and age/date)? __
_____
_____

Surgeries prior to SCI (include type and date)? _____
_____

Surgeries after SCI (include type and date)? _____
_____

Secondary Problem(s) _____
_____
_____

Client's perceptions of disability condition(s) and how these impact on ability to perform activities of daily living (ADLs) and work-related activities: _____
_____
_____
_____

Comments _____
_____
_____
_____

HISTORY OF COMPLICATIONS

Skin:
   (pressure sores) _____

Musculoskeletal System:
   (joint contractures, heterotopic _____
   ossification, osteoporosis, _____
   degenerative joint disease, _____
   fractures, etc.) _____

Cardiovascular System:
   (deep venous thrombosis, _____
   pulmonary embolism, _____
   autonomic dysreflexia, etc.) _____

Respiratory System:
   (atelectasis, pneumonia, etc.) _____

Genitourinary System:
   (genitourinary bleeding, _____
   urinary tract infections, _____
   bladder/kidney stones, _____
   bladder cancer, etc.) _____

Gastrointestinal System:
   (neurogenic bowel, _____
   cholelithiasis, diverticulitis, _____
   fecal impactions, colorectal _____
   cancer, hemorrhoids, etc.)

Nervous System:
   (spasticity, neurogenic pain, _____
   carpal tunnel syndrome, _____
   cystic myelopathy, _____
   noncystic myelopathy, etc.) _____

Endocrine System:
   (diabetes, etc.)   _____

Psychosocial Complications:
   (suicide attempt(s), self-neglect, _____
   depression, substance
   abuse, etc.)   _____

Fatigue: _____
Other: _____
                                      _____
                                      _____
                                      _____

Comments _____
_____

PHYSICAL LIMITATIONS

Activity	Yes	No	Extent
Sitting			
Standing			
Walking			
Lifting			
Carrying			
Pushing			
Pulling			
Climbing			
Balancing			
Stooping			
Kneeling			
Crouching			
Crawling			
Reaching			
Handling			
Fingering			
Feeling			
Talking			
Hearing			
Tasting/Smelling			
Seeing			
Hand/Arm Controls			
Foot/Leg Controls			
Bowel			
Bladder			
Driving			
Physical Stamina			
Other			

Comments _____
_____
_____
_____

NEUROBEHAVIORAL LIMITATIONS

Behavioral Symptom	Yes	No	Extent
Inattention/Reduced Alertness	_____	_____	_____
Somatic Concerns	_____	_____	_____
Disorientation	_____	_____	_____
Anxiety	_____	_____	_____
Expressive Deficit	_____	_____	_____
Emotional Withdrawal	_____	_____	_____
Conceptual Disorganization	_____	_____	_____
Disinhibition	_____	_____	_____
Guilt Feelings	_____	_____	_____
Memory Deficit	_____	_____	_____
Agitation	_____	_____	_____
Depressive Mood	_____	_____	_____
Hostility/ Uncooperativeness	_____	_____	_____
Decreased Initiative/Motivation	_____	_____	_____
Suspiciousness	_____	_____	_____
Fatigability	_____	_____	_____
Hallucinatory Behavior	_____	_____	_____
Motor Retardation	_____	_____	_____
Unusual Thought Content	_____	_____	_____
Blunted Affect	_____	_____	_____
Excitement	_____	_____	_____
Poor Planning	_____	_____	_____
Lability of Mood	_____	_____	_____
Tension	_____	_____	_____
Comprehension Deficit	_____	_____	_____
Speech Articulation Deficit	_____	_____	_____
Other	_____		

Comments _____
_____
_____
_____

ENVIRONMENTAL LIMITATIONS

Condition	Yes	No	Extent
Inside	_____	_____	_____
Outside	_____	_____	_____
Cold	_____	_____	_____
Heat	_____	_____	_____
Wet/Humidity	_____	_____	_____

Noise   _____ _____ _____
Vibration   _____ _____ _____
Fumes/Odors   _____ _____ _____
Other   _____ _____

_____

Comments _____
_____
_____

WORK SITUATIONS/LIMITATIONS

Work Situation/ Limitation	Yes	No	Extent
Variety of Duties	_____	_____	_____
Shift Work	_____	_____	_____
Repetitive Work	_____	_____	_____
Fast Paced Work	_____	_____	_____
Following Instructions	_____	_____	_____
Exacting Performance	_____	_____	_____
Meeting Emergencies	_____	_____	_____
Competitive Work	_____	_____	_____
Working Alone	_____	_____	_____
Working Around Others	_____	_____	_____
Working With Others	_____	_____	_____
Other _____			

Comments _____

PRESENT MEDICAL TREATMENT

Physician(s)	Speciality	Telephone Number	Frequency of Visits	Date of Last/Next Appointment
_____	_____	_____	_____	_____
_____	_____	_____	_____	_____
_____	_____	_____	_____	_____
_____	_____	_____	_____	_____
_____	_____	_____	_____	_____

Therapist(s)	Name	Telephone Number	Facility	Frequency
Occupational Therapy	_____	_____	_____	_____
Physical Therapy	_____	_____	_____	_____
Speech/Language	_____	_____	_____	_____
Other _____				

Medication	Dosage	Purpose	Frequency	Side Effects
_____	_____	_____	_____	_____
_____	_____	_____	_____	_____
_____	_____	_____	_____	_____
_____	_____	_____	_____	_____
_____	_____	_____	_____	_____

Over-the-counter medication(s) _____

_____

_____

Laboratory work, counseling, etc. _____

_____

Comments _____

_____

ADAPTIVE EQUIPMENT

Item/Model	Date of Purchase	Purchase Price	Dealer Supplier	Present Condition
Physical Mobility (e.g., wheelchair, wheelchair accessories):				
_____	_____	_____	_____	_____
_____	_____	_____	_____	_____
_____	_____	_____	_____	_____
Transfer Mobility (e.g., bed lift, bathtub trapeze):				
_____	_____	_____	_____	_____
_____	_____	_____	_____	_____
_____	_____	_____	_____	_____
Support/Positioning (e.g., standing frame, lift, hospital bed, special mattress):				
_____	_____	_____	_____	_____
_____	_____	_____	_____	_____
_____	_____	_____	_____	_____
Self-Care:				
_____	_____	_____	_____	_____
_____	_____	_____	_____	_____
Eating:				
_____	_____	_____	_____	_____
_____	_____	_____	_____	_____
_____	_____	_____	_____	_____
Grooming:				
_____	_____	_____	_____	_____
_____	_____	_____	_____	_____
Bathing:				
_____	_____	_____	_____	_____
_____	_____	_____	_____	_____
Dressing — Upper Body:				
_____	_____	_____	_____	_____
_____	_____	_____	_____	_____
_____	_____	_____	_____	_____

Dressing — Lower Body:

_____   _____ _____ _____ _____
_____   _____ _____ _____ _____
_____   _____ _____ _____ _____

Toileting:

_____   _____ _____ _____ _____
_____   _____ _____ _____ _____
_____   _____ _____ _____ _____

Bowel/Bladder
   Management:

_____   _____ _____ _____ _____
_____   _____ _____ _____ _____
_____   _____ _____ _____ _____

Communication:

_____   _____ _____ _____ _____
_____   _____ _____ _____ _____
_____   _____ _____ _____ _____

Household Maintenance:

_____   _____ _____ _____ _____
_____   _____ _____ _____ _____
_____   _____ _____ _____ _____

Transportation:

_____   _____ _____ _____ _____
_____   _____ _____ _____ _____
_____   _____ _____ _____ _____

Recreation/Health
   Maintenance:

_____   _____ _____ _____ _____
_____   _____ _____ _____ _____
_____   _____ _____ _____ _____

Vocational:

_____   _____ _____ _____ _____
_____   _____ _____ _____ _____
_____   _____ _____ _____ _____

Comments _____
_____
_____
_____
_____
_____
_____
_____
_____

SUPPLIES

Item/Type	Size	Replacement Frequency	Supplier	Cost
_____	____	_____	_____	____
_____	____	_____	_____	____
_____	____	_____	_____	____
_____	____	_____	_____	____
_____	____	_____	_____	____

_____ _____ _____ _____ _____
_____ _____ _____ _____ _____
_____ _____ _____ _____ _____
_____ _____ _____ _____ _____
_____ _____ _____ _____ _____
_____ _____ _____ _____ _____
_____ _____ _____ _____ _____
_____ _____ _____ _____ _____
_____ _____ _____ _____ _____

Comments _____
_____
_____

ACTIVITIES OF DAILY LIVING

Usually Arise _____ A.M. Usually Retire _____ P.M.

Average Hours Sleep/24 Hours _____

Sleep Difficulties _____
_____

Nap During the Day? Yes _____ No _____ If Yes, how long and how many times per day? _____

Activity	Independent	Require Assistance
Self Care:		
Eating	_____	_____
Grooming	_____	_____
Bathing	_____	_____
Dressing—Upper Body	_____	_____
Dressing—Lower Body	_____	_____
Toileting	_____	_____
Sphincter Control:		
Bladder Management	_____	_____
Bowel Management	_____	_____
Transfer/Mobility:		
Bed	_____	_____
Chair, Toilet	_____	_____
Wheelchair	_____	_____
Tub/Shower	_____	_____
Vehicle/Physical Mobility:		
Walk	_____	_____
Wheelchair Propulsion	_____	_____
Support/Positioning	_____	_____
Communication:		
Comprehension		
Auditory	_____	_____
Visual	_____	_____
Both	_____	_____
Expression		
Vocal	_____	_____
Non-Vocal	_____	_____
Both	_____	_____

Other _____
_____

Current Driver's License: Yes _____ No _____ Restrictions _____

Current Transportation/Vehicle Available: Yes _____ No _____ Type _____

Is transportation a problem? Yes _____ No _____ If Yes, explain: _____
_____
_____

Any DUI arrests? Yes _____ No _____

If Yes, when and in which city and state? _____

Comments _____
_____
_____
_____
_____
_____

SOCIAL ACTIVITIES

Organizations _____

Church _____ Work Volunteer _____

Hobbies/Recreational Interests — Preinjury: _____
_____

Hobbies/Recreational Interests — Present (tried preinjury hobbies since SCI? If not, why? If so, to what extent, what accommodations needed?) _____
_____
_____
_____

Comments _____
_____

PERSONAL HABITS

Cigarette Smoking   Yes _____ No _____ _____

Alcohol Drinking   Yes _____ No _____ _____

Non-Prescribed Drugs   Yes _____ No _____ _____

History of Substance Abuse/Treatment _____
_____

Comments _____
_____

FINANCIAL STATUS

	Income			Expenses	
Employment	$ _____ month	Rent/Mortgage	$ _____ month
VA Disability Compensation	$ _____ month	Food	$ _____ month
SSI/SSDI	$ _____ month	Utilities	$ _____ month
Spouse's Employment	$ _____ month	Auto	$ _____ month
Retirement	$ _____ month	Phone	$ _____ month
Pension (VA)	$ _____ month	Insurance	$ _____ month
Public Assistance	$ _____ month	Medical	$ _____ month
Relatives	$ _____ month	Personal	$ _____ month
Food Stamps	$ _____ month	Other	$ _____ month
Other	$ _____ month		
Total Income	$ _____ month	Total Expenses	$ _____ month

Current Financial Situation _____

Comments _____
_____
_____

OTHER INDIVIDUAL/AGENCY INVOLVEMENT

State Vocational Rehabilitation   Yes _____ No _____ _____
    State Job Service   Yes _____ No _____ _____
Rehabilitation Nurse(s)   Yes _____ No _____ _____

Other _____

Previous Arrest(s)/Conviction(s) _____
_____

Comments _____
_____

AVAILABLE SUPPORT TO CLIENT

Will your family be of help to you in your rehabilitation program? Yes _____
No _____
Explain in what capacity: _____
_____

Does your spouse support your goals? Yes _____ No _____
If No, explain why not: _____
_____

Is your spouse employed? Yes _____ No _____ Where? _____

How will your spouse's employment affect your rehabilitation program? _____
_____

Will other family members be able to offer you financial support while you train?
Yes _____ No _____ If yes, explain: _____
_____

Will you be willing or able to relocate? Yes _____ No _____ Explain: _____
_____
_____

Describe any current family problems, including other family members with medical
or other problems, which should be considered in developing your life care plan: ___
_____
_____
_____
_____

BEHAVIORAL OBSERVATIONS

Orientation _____ Approach to Evaluation: +   −

Stream of Thought _____ Concentration _____

Attitude/Motivation _____

Insight _____

Memory: Remote _____ Recent _____

Present Personal/Vocational Goals _____
_____
_____

TENTATIVE PLAN IMPLICATIONS/CONSIDERATIONS _____
_____
_____
_____
_____

IMPRESSIONS/COMMENTS _____
_____
_____
_____

REVIEWED/SIGNED RELEASE OF INFORMATION

Yes _____ No _____

(Adpated from *Life Care Planning for Spinal Cord Injury: A Resource Manual for
case Managers* by T.L. Blackwell, R.O. Weed & A.S. Powers. Elliott & Fitzpatrick,
Inc., 1994. Reprinted by permission.)

QUESTIONS FOR PRIMARY CARE PHYSICIAN/PHYSIATRIST RE: LIFE CARE PLANNING NEEDS FOR (Patient) _____

CLASSIFICATION OF SPINAL CORD INJURY:

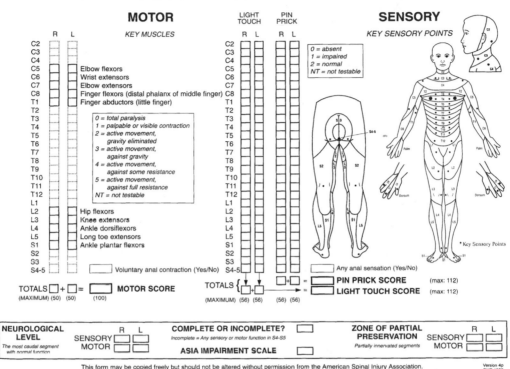

Figure 5-3. (American Spinal Injury Association; Version 4p, GHC 1996.)

OTHER DIAGNOSES/COMPLICATIONS/COMORBIDITY: _____

_____

_____

_____

_____

FUNCTIONAL INDEPENDENCE ASSESSMENT:

Please rate _____ on present levels of functional independence for the following areas:

Levels
NO HELPER
7   Complete Independence (Timely, Safely)
6   Modified Independence (Device)

HELPER
Modified Dependence

5   Supervision
4   Minimal Assistance
     (Subject=75%+)
3   Moderate Assistance
     (Subject=50%+)

Complete Dependence

2   Maximal Assistance
     (Subject=25%+)
1   Total Assistance
     (Subject=0%+)

	Level			Level
Self Care		**Communication**		
Eating	_____	Comprehension		
Grooming	_____	Auditory		_____
Bathing	_____	Visual		_____
Dressing — upper body	_____	Both		_____
Dressing — lower body	_____	Expression		
Toileting	_____	Vocal		_____
Sphincter Control		Non-vocal		_____
Bladder management	_____	Both		_____
Bowel management	_____			
Transfer		**Social Cognition**		
Bed, chair, wheelchair	_____	Social interaction		_____
Toilet	_____	Problem solving		_____
Tub/shower	_____	Memory		_____
Locomotion				
Walk/Wheelchair	_____			
Walk				
Wheelchair	_____			
Both	_____			
Stairs	_____			

HEALTH CARE NEEDS:

What are your recommendations regarding _____ future health care needs:

Physician	Yes	No	Frequency	Duration	Purpose	Necessary vs Desirable
Physiatry	____	____	_____	_____	_____	_____
Pediatrics	____	____	_____	_____	_____	_____
Neurology	____	____	_____	_____	_____	_____
Orthopedics	____	____	_____	_____	_____	_____
Otolaryngology	____	____	_____	_____	_____	_____
Urology	____	____	_____	_____	_____	_____

Ophthalmology   ____ ____ _____ _____ _____ _____ _____
Dermatology   ____ ____ _____ _____ _____ _____ _____
Obstetrics/
    Gynecology   ____ ____ _____ _____ _____ _____ _____
Rheumatology   ____ ____ _____ _____ _____ _____ _____
Cardiology   ____ ____ _____ _____ _____ _____ _____
Gastroenterology   ____ ____ _____ _____ _____ _____ _____
Internal Medicine   ____ ____ _____ _____ _____ _____ _____
Psychiatry   ____ ____ _____ _____ _____ _____ _____
Other   _____

Non-Physician

Physical Therapy   ____ ____ _____ _____ _____ _____ _____
Occupational
    Therapy   ____ ____ _____ _____ _____ _____ _____
Respiratory Therapy   ____ ____ _____ _____ _____ _____ _____
Speech/
    Communication
    Therapy   ____ ____ _____ _____ _____ _____ _____
Rehabilitation
    Nursing   ____ ____ _____ _____ _____ _____ _____
Dietetics   ____ ____ _____ _____ _____ _____ _____
Rehabilitation
    Counseling   ____ ____ _____ _____ _____ _____ _____
Psychology/
    Social Work   ____ ____ _____ _____ _____ _____ _____
Neuropsychology   ____ ____ _____ _____ _____ _____ _____
Rehabilitation
    Engineering   ____ ____ _____ _____ _____ _____ _____
Other   _____

What do you see as _____ sexual health care needs? _____
_____

What do you project as ____   long-term health care needs through aging
with spinal cord injury? _____
_____

REHABILITATION MANAGEMENT:

What are your recommendations regarding future evaluations for _____:

	Yes	No	Frequency	Purpose
Physical Therapy Evaluation	____	____	_____	_____
Occupational Therapy Evaluation	____	____	_____	_____
Home Evaluation	____	____	_____	_____
Speech/Communication Therapy Evaluation	____	____	_____	_____

Respiratory Therapy
   Evaluation   ____ ____ _____ _____

Sexual Function/Fertility
   Evaluation   ____ ____ _____ _____

Dietary Assessment   ____ ____ _____ _____

Driving Evaluation   ____ ____ _____ _____

Educational Evaluation   ____ ____ _____ _____

Functional Capacities
   Evaluation   ____ ____ _____ _____

Inpatient/Outpatient
   Spinal Cord Injury
   Center Evaluation   ____ ____ _____ _____

Leisure
   Activity/Recreational
   Therapy Evaluation   ____ ____ _____ _____

Nursing Evaluation   ____ ____ _____ _____

Orthopedic Evaluation   ____ ____ _____ _____

Neuropsychological
   Evaluation   ____ ____ _____ _____

Psychological/Social
   Assessment   ____ ____ _____ _____

Vocational Evaluation   ____ ____ _____ _____

Do you see the need for any additional evaluations such as visual, hearing, dental (please include frequency and purpose, as appropriate)? _____

_____

_____

_____

_____

_____

_____

Along with the previous medical care, do you see the need for any additional tests or lab work, such as CBC, SMAC, Protime, x-rays, urinary tract functioning, bone scans, vital capacity assessment, arterial blood gases, sleep studies, diagnostic ECG, fecal occult blood test, sigmoidoscopy, etc.?

Test/Lab	Frequency	Purpose
_____	_____	_____
_____	_____	_____
_____	_____	_____
_____	_____	_____
_____	_____	_____
_____	_____	_____
_____	_____	_____
_____	_____	_____

MEDICATIONS:

What are _____ current medication needs?

Medication	Purpose	Dosage	Schedule	Common Side Effects
_____	_____	_____	_____	_____
_____	_____	_____	_____	_____
_____	_____	_____	_____	_____
_____	_____	_____	_____	_____
_____	_____	_____	_____	_____
_____	_____	_____	_____	_____
_____	_____	_____	_____	_____
_____	_____	_____	_____	_____

What do you project as future medication needs?

Medication	Purpose	Dosage	Schedule	Common Side Effects
_____	_____	_____	_____	_____
_____	_____	_____	_____	_____
_____	_____	_____	_____	_____
_____	_____	_____	_____	_____

BOWEL/BLADDER MANAGEMENT:

What is _____ current bowel care routine and what level of assistance is needed with this?

_____

_____

_____

What is _____ current bladder program and what level of assistance is needed with this?

_____

_____

_____

What changes in bladder/bowel programs and level of assistance would you project for the future as _____ ages with spinal cord injury (please indicate estimated age of initiation, as appropriate)?

_____

_____

_____

HOME/FACILITY CARE NEEDS:

What level of home/facility care do you see as most appropriate for _____ at this time?

Facility Care
  Intermediate living   _____
  Transitional living   _____
  Skilled nursing facility   _____

Home Care

   Full-time home attendant care   _____

   Part-time home attendant care   _____

      Level of attendant care, i.e., RN, LPN, home care attendant, etc. (Please specify amount of skilled and unskilled care needed): _____

_____

_____

_____

What level of household assistance (help required for cleaning, cooking, laundering, shopping, etc.) do you see as most appropriate for _____ at this time? _____

_____

_____

_____

Do you foresee a change in the future in the level of attendant care and household assistance _____ will need?

   No _____

   Yes _____ If yes, after what time period or age would you project this change might occur and what level of care would be needed then? _____

      _____

      _____

SPINAL CORD INJURY COMPLICATIONS:

What do you see as potential complications both as a consequence of injury and from aging with spinal cord injury?

	Condition/Complication	Expected	Possible
Skin (e.g., pressure sores)	_____	_____	_____
Musculoskeletal system (e.g., joint contractures, heterotopic ossification, osteoporosis, degenerative joint disease, fractures)	_____	_____	_____
Cardiovascular system (e.g., deep venous thrombosis, pulmonary embolism, autonomic dysreflexia)	_____	_____	_____
Respiratory system (e.g., atelectasis, pneumonia)	_____	_____	_____
Genitourinary system (e.g., genitourinary bleeding, urinary tract infections, bladder/kidney stones, bladder cancer)	_____	_____	_____
Gastrointestinal system (e.g., neurogenic bowel, cholelithiasis, diverticulitis, fecal impactions, colorectal cancer, hemorrhoids)	_____	_____	_____

Nervous system
   (e.g., spasticity, neurogenic
   pain, carpal tunnel syndrome,
   cystic myelopathy, noncystic
   myelopathy)
Endocrine system
   (e.g., diabetes)
Psychosocial complications
   (e.g., suicide, self-neglect,
   depression, drug and alcohol
   abuse)
Fatigue
Other _____

_____

Do you see the need for any surgical intervention for _____ now or in the
future?
   No _____
   Yes _____   Type of procedures and at what ages: _____
                    _____
                    _____
                    _____
                    _____
                    _____

ADAPTIVE EQUIPMENT:

What are your recommendations regarding _____ equipment needs in the
following areas? (Include both present and future needs and age of initiation you
anticipate equipment needs change):

   Physical mobility (e.g., wheelchair, include type, seating requirements, accessories) _____
   _____
   _____

   Transfer mobility (e.g., bed lift, bathtub trapeze, etc.) _____
   _____
   _____

   Support/positioning (e.g., standing frame, lift, hospital bed, special mattress,
   etc.) _____
   _____
   _____

   Self care _____
   _____
   _____

   Eating _____
   _____
   _____

   Grooming _____
   _____
   _____
   _____

Bathing _____

_____

_____

Dressing — upper body _____

_____

Dressing — lower body _____

_____

_____

Toileting _____

_____

_____

Bowel/bladder management _____

_____

_____

Communication _____

_____

_____

Household maintenance _____

_____

_____

Transportation _____

_____

_____

Recreation/health maintenance _____

_____

_____

_____

Vocational _____

_____

_____

_____

EDUCATIONAL/VOCATIONAL IMPLICATIONS:

In an eight-hour time period, what would _____ capacity be in each of the following:

Total at one time uninterrupted (in hours)   Total during entire eight-hour time period (in hours)

Sit	0	1/2	1	2	3	4	5	6	7	8	Sit	0	1/2	1	2	3	4	5	6	7	8
Stand	0	1/2	1	2	3	4	5	6	7	8	Stand	0	1/2	1	2	3	4	5	6	7	8
Walk	0	1/2	1	2	3	4	5	6	7	8	Walk	0	1/2	1	2	3	4	5	6	7	8

Note: In terms of an eight-hour time period, "Occasionally" equals 1% to 33%; "Frequently" equals 34% to 66%, "Constantly" equals 67% to 100%.

	Never	Occasionally	Frequently	Constantly
Lift:				
Up to 10 pounds	_____	_____	_____	_____
11–20 pounds	_____	_____	_____	_____

	Never	Occasionally	Frequently	Constantly
21–50 pounds	_____	_____	_____	_____
51–100 pounds	_____	_____	_____	_____
100+ pounds	_____	_____	_____	_____

	Never	Occasionally	Frequently	Constantly
Carry:				
Up to 10 pounds	_____	_____	_____	_____
11–20 pounds	_____	_____	_____	_____
21–50 pounds	_____	_____	_____	_____
51–100 pounds	_____	_____	_____	_____
100+ pounds	_____	_____	_____	_____
Push/Pull:				
Up to 10 pounds	_____	_____	_____	_____
11–20 pounds	_____	_____	_____	_____
21–50 pounds	_____	_____	_____	_____
51–100 pounds	_____	_____	_____	_____
100+ pounds	_____	_____	_____	_____

Can _____ do repetitive movements as in operating controls?

	Yes	No
Right Hand/Arm	_____	_____
Right Foot/Leg	_____	_____
Left Hand/Arm	_____	_____
Left Foot/Leg	_____	_____

	Never	Occasionally	Frequently	Constantly
Can _____:				
Climb	_____	_____	_____	_____
Stoop	_____	_____	_____	_____
Balance	_____	_____	_____	_____
Kneel	_____	_____	_____	_____
Crouch	_____	_____	_____	_____
Crawl	_____	_____	_____	_____
Reach (all directions)	_____	_____	_____	_____
Handle (gross manipulation)	_____	_____	_____	_____
Finger (fine manipulation)	_____	_____	_____	_____
Feel	_____	_____	_____	_____

	None	Mild	Moderate	Severe
Would _____ have difficulties involving:				
Talking	_____	_____	_____	_____
Hearing	_____	_____	_____	_____
Tasting/Smelling	_____	_____	_____	_____
Seeing (near, far depth, color, accommodation, or field of vision)?	_____	_____	_____	_____

	None	Mild	Moderate	Severe
Any restriction of activities involving:				
Exposure to cold, heat, wet, or humidity	_____	_____	_____	_____
Noise	_____	_____	_____	_____

Vibration   ____   ____   ____   ____
Exposure to fumes, odors,
   dusts, mists, gases, or
   chemicals   ____   ____   ____   ____
Moving mechanical parts   ____   ____   ____   ____
Unprotected heights   ____   ____   ____   ____
Operating automotive
   equipment?   ____   ____   ____   ____

Is _____ involved with treatment and/or medication that might affect ability to work?

   No _____

   Yes _____   Describe: _____

   _____

   _____

   _____

Has _____ reached maximum medical improvement (MMI)?

   Yes _____   As of?   _____

   No _____   Projected MMI date? _____

Can _____ return to work according to the restrictions defined above?

   Yes _____

   No _____   If not, give estimated date for return to work: _____

Is _____ able to work full-time?

   Yes _____

   No _____

Is _____ able to work part-time?

   Yes _____   How many hours/days? _____

   No _____

What neurobehavioral limitations are reasonable to expect? _____

_____

_____

_____

How will these limitations impact _____ future life adjustment and ability to work? _____

_____

_____

_____

OTHER:

Do you have any additional comments about anything not covered in the previous questions and which we should be aware of when addressing _____ long-term health care or safety-related needs?

_____

_____

_____

_____

_____

_____

_____

Signature   Date

(Adapted from *Life Care Planning for Spinal Cord Injury: A Resource Manual for Case Managers* by T.L. Blackwell, R.O. Weed & A.S. Powers. Elliott & Fitzpatrick, Inc., 1994. Reprinted by permission.)

**QUESTIONS FOR NURSE RE: LIFE CARE PLANNING NEEDS FOR
(Patient) _____**

Please complete the following table regarding _____ current medications:

Medication	Purpose	Dosage	Schedule	Side Effects

What is _____ current bowel program and what level of assistance is needed with this? (Please indicate bowel program frequency, average length of program and how often incontinence occurs.) _____
_____
_____
_____

What supplies does _____ need for this bowel program? List specific amount used if possible. _____
_____
_____

What is _____ current bladder program and what level of assistance is needed with this? (Please specify bladder program frequency, as appropriate, and how often incontinence occurs.) _____
_____
_____
_____

What supplies does _____ need for this bladder program? If a catheter is used, please give the brand or item number and replacement schedule. _____
_____
_____

What changes in bowel/bladder program and level of assistance would you project for the future as _____ ages with spinal cord injury? (Please indicate estimated age of initiation, as appropriate). _____
_____
_____
_____

Does _____ typically experience sleep difficulties at this time?
      No _____
      Yes _____
      If Yes, describe: _____
_____
_____
_____

How long is _____ able to remain up during the day? _____
_____
_____
_____

Does _____ nap or rest during the day? _____
_____
_____

Do you see the need for routine nursing care and follow-up?
    No _____
    Yes _____
    If Yes, please estimate how often you would recommend _____ receive
    nursing care and how long this care should continue. Please include purpose,
    frequency, and duration of nursing care recommendations:
    Purpose _____
    _____
    _____

    Frequency _____
    _____
    _____

    Duration _____
    _____
    _____

Do you project the need for nursing evaluation in the future as _____ ages
with spinal cord injury?
    No _____
    Yes _____
    If Yes, at what time periods would you recommend an evaluation be performed
    (e.g., 1 time every 12 months)? _____
    _____
    _____

Does _____ need to be reminded of safety directions? _____
_____
_____

Is _____ able to turn, transfer, and perform weight shifts independently?
    Yes _____
    No _____
    If no, describe: _____
    _____
    _____
    _____

What level of assistance does _____ require for turning, transfers, and weight
shifts? _____
_____
_____
_____

Is _____ independent in basic activities of daily living?
    Yes _____
    No _____
    If no, describe: _____
    _____
    _____
    _____

What activities of daily living does _____ require assistance with to perform?

_____
_____
_____
_____

What changes would you anticipate in the future as age and disability combine to create an increased need for assistance with activities of daily living? (Please include at what age you would anticipate this change might occur and what level of care would be needed then.) _____

_____
_____
_____

Any cognitive impairments observed?

No _____
Yes _____
If Yes, describe: _____
_____
_____

What other supplies does _____ currently require?

Type/Item	Size	Frequency of Replacement	Supplier
_____	_____	_____	_____
_____	_____	_____	_____
_____	_____	_____	_____
_____	_____	_____	_____
_____	_____	_____	_____
_____	_____	_____	_____

Do you have any additional comments about anything not covered in the previous questions and which we should be aware in addressing _____ long-term health care or safety-related needs? _____

_____
_____
_____
_____
_____
_____
_____
_____
_____
_____
_____
_____
_____

_____   _____
Signature   Date

(Adapted from *Life Care Planning for Spinal Cord Injury: A Resource Manual for Case Managers* by T.L. Blackwell, R.O. Weed & A.S. Powers. Inc., 1994 Elliott & Fitzpatrick. Reprinted by permission.)

QUESTIONS FOR OCCUPATIONAL THERAPIST RE: LIFE CARE PLANNING NEEDS FOR (Patient) _____

Do you see the need for occupational therapy?

No _____

Yes _____

If yes, please estimate how often you would recommend _____ receive therapy and how many months such therapy should continue. If possible, also list what general areas such therapy should encompass.

Frequency _____
_____
_____

Duration _____
_____
_____

Goals _____
_____
_____

Do you project the need for occupational therapy evaluation in the future as _____ ages with spinal cord injury?

No _____

Yes _____ If Yes, at what time periods would you recommend an evaluation be performed (e.g., 1 time only or 1 time every 6 months of therapy, etc.)? _____
_____
_____
_____

What type of adaptive equipment does _____ require (please include maintenance and replacement schedules and age of initiation and suspension)?

Self Care:

Eating _____
_____
_____
_____

Grooming _____
_____
_____
_____

Bathing _____
_____
_____

Dressing — upper body _____
_____
_____

Dressing — lower body _____
_____
_____

Toileting _____
_____
_____
_____

Sphincter Control:
   Bladder management _____
_____
_____
_____

   Bowel management _____
_____
_____
_____

Transfer/Mobility:
   Bed/Chair/Wheelchair _____
_____
_____
_____

   Toilet _____
_____
_____
_____

   Tub/shower _____
_____
_____
_____

   Vehicle _____
_____
_____
_____

Physical Mobility:
   Wheelchair propulsion _____
_____
_____
_____

   Support/positioning _____
_____
_____
_____

   Wheelchair accessories _____
_____
_____
_____

   Other _____
_____
_____
_____

Communication:
   Receptive _____
_____
_____
_____

   Expressive _____
_____
_____
_____

Sexual functioning _____
_____
_____
_____

Environment:

Home _____

_____

_____

_____

School/Worksite _____

_____

_____

_____

Recreation/Avocational _____

_____

_____

_____

Other _____

_____

_____

_____

What level of home/facility care do you see as most appropriate for _____ at this time?

Facility Care

Intermediate living   _____
Transitional living   _____
Skilled nursing facility   _____

Home Care:

Full-time home attendant care   _____
Part-time home attendant care   _____
Level of attendant care, i.e., RN, LPN, home care attendant, etc. Please specify amount of skilled and unskilled care needed: _____

_____

_____

_____

What level of household assistance (help required for cleaning, cooking, laundering, shopping, etc.) do you see as most appropriate for _____ at this time? _____

_____

_____

_____

_____

Do you foresee a change in the future in the level of attendant care and household assistance _____ will need?

No _____

Yes _____   If yes, after what time period or age would you project this change might occur and what level of care would be needed then? _____

_____

_____

_____

_____

Please rate _____ on present level of functional independence for the following areas:

Levels
NO HELPER
7 Complete Independence (Timely, Safely)
6 Modified Independence (Device)
HELPER
Modified Dependence
5 Supervision
4 Minimal Assistance (Subject = 75%+)
3 Moderate Assistance (Subject = 50%+)
Complete Dependence
2 Maximal Assistance (Subject = 25%+)
1 Total Assistance (Subject = 0%+)

	Level			Level
Self Care		**Communication**		
Eating	_____	Comprehension		
Grooming	_____	Auditory	_____	
Bathing	_____	Visual	_____	
Dressing—upper body	_____	Both	_____	
Dressing—lower body	_____	Expression		
Toileting	_____	Vocal	_____	
Sphincter Control		Non-vocal	_____	
Bladder management	_____	Both	_____	
Bowel management	_____	**Social Cognition**		
Transfer		Social interaction	_____	
Bed, chair, wheelchair	_____	Problem solving	_____	
Toilet	_____	Memory	_____	
Tub/shower	_____			
Locomotion				
Walk/Wheelchair	_____			
Walk				
Wheelchair	_____			
Both	_____			
Stairs	_____			

Do you project _____ will eventually be able to drive with adaptive equipment? What type of adaptive equipment would be required (please include maintenance and replacement schedules and age of initiation and suspension)? Would a driving evaluation be beneficial?

_____

_____

_____

_____

_____

_____

_____

Should a home visit be performed?

     Yes _____

     No _____

Any recommendations regarding architectural renovations needed such as additional room(s), kitchen/bathroom counters, electrical work, ramps, widened doors, grab bars, door handles, alarms, etc.? _____

_____

_____

_____

_____

Any cognitive deficits observed?

     No _____

     Yes _____   If yes, describe: _____

_____

_____

_____

_____

_____

Any behavioral deficits observed?

     No _____

     Yes _____   If yes, describe: _____

_____

_____

_____

_____

_____

What is _____ current level of stamina/endurance? What changes do you anticipate in the future as _____ ages with spinal cord injury? _____

_____

_____

_____

_____

Do you have any recommendations regarding future recreational services? _____

_____

_____

_____

_____

_____

_____

Do you have any additional comments about anything not covered in the previous questions which we should be aware of when working with ＿＿＿＿＿, which address long-term health care needs? ＿＿＿＿＿＿＿＿＿＿＿＿＿＿＿＿＿＿＿＿＿

_____
_____
_____
_____
_____
_____
_____
_____
_____
_____
_____
_____
_____
_____
_____
_____
_____
_____
_____
_____
_____
_____
_____
_____
_____
_____
_____
_____
_____
_____
_____
_____
_____
_____
_____
_____
_____
_____
_____
_____
_____
_____

Signature   Date

(Adapted from *Life Care Planning for Spinal Cord Injury: A Resource Manual for Case Managers* by T.L. Blackwell, R.O. Weed & A.S. Powers. Elliott & Fitzpatrick, Inc., 1994. Reprinted by permission.)

QUESTIONS FOR PHYSICAL THERAPIST RE: LIFE CARE PLANNING NEEDS FOR (Patient) _____

Do you see the need for physical therapy?

      No _____

      Yes _____   If yes, please estimate how often you would recommend _____ receive therapy and how many months such therapy should continue. If possible, also list what general areas such therapy should encompass.

    Frequency _____

_____

_____

_____

    Duration _____

_____

_____

_____

    Goals _____

_____

_____

_____

Do you project the need for physical therapy evaluation in the future as _____ ages with spinal cord injury?

      No _____

      Yes _____   If yes, at what time periods would you recommend an evaluation be performed (e.g., 1 time only or 1 time every 6 months of therapy, etc.)? _____

_____

_____

_____

_____

Would you recommend a home exercise program for _____?

      No _____

      Yes _____   If yes, what does the program involve, what level of assistance would be needed to perform the exercises as recommended, and what equipment is required?

_____

_____

_____

_____

_____

What brand and model of wheelchair/ambulation aids and accessories does _____ need at this time (please include type of accessories, age of initiation, and replacement and maintenance schedules)? _____

_____

_____

_____

_____

What would you identify as _____ future wheelchair needs as aging with spinal cord injury occurs (please include type of accessories, age of initiation, and replacement and maintenance schedules)? _____

_____

_____

_____

_____

What type of adaptive equipment does _____ require (please include maintenance and replacement schedules and age of initiation and suspension)?
Transfer Mobility:

    Bed _____

_____

_____

_____

    Chair _____

_____

_____

    Wheelchair _____

_____

_____

    Toilet _____

_____

_____

    Tub/shower _____

_____

_____

_____

    Vehicle _____

_____

_____

_____

Physical Mobility:

    Wheelchair propulsion _____

_____

_____

    Support/positioning _____

_____

_____

_____

    Wheelchair accessories _____

_____

_____

    Other _____

_____

_____

What is _____ current level of stamina/endurance? Do you anticipate changes as aging with spinal cord injury occurs (please comment on changing needs as these relate to preservation of function)?

_____

_____

_____

Do you have any additional comments about anything not covered in the previous questions which we should be aware of when working with _____, which address long-term health care needs? _____

_____
_____
_____
_____
_____
_____
_____
_____
_____
_____
_____
_____
_____
_____
_____
_____
_____
_____
_____
_____
_____
_____
_____
_____
_____
_____
_____
_____
_____
_____
_____
_____
_____
_____
_____
_____
_____
_____
_____
_____
_____

_____   _____
Signature   Date

(Adapted from *Life Care Planning for Spinal Cord Injury: A Resource Manual for Case Managers* by T.L. Blackwell, R.O. Weed & A.S. Powers. Elliott & Fitzpatrick, Inc., 1994. Reprinted by permission.)

QUESTIONS FOR PSYCHOLOGIST/NEUROPSYCHOLOGIST RE: LIFE CARE PLANNING NEEDS FOR (Patient) _____

Current DSM-IV Diagnosis:

Axis I _____

_____

Axis II _____

_____

Axis III _____

_____

Axis IV _____

_____

Axis V _____

_____

Do you see the need for mental health services at this time?

No _____

Yes _____

If yes, please describe what type of services, frequency, duration, and age of initiation and suspension: _____

_____

_____

_____

Do you see the need for mental health services as _____ ages with spinal cord injury?

No _____

Yes _____

If yes, please describe what type of services, frequency, duration, and age of initiation and suspension: _____

_____

_____

_____

Please summarize _____ cognitive and behavioral strengths and weaknesses and psychosocial adaptation to disability: _____

_____

_____

_____

_____

What implications do you see for _____ current and future adjustment to disability? _____

_____

_____

_____

_____

_____

_____

What do you see as mental health needs (including type of service, frequency and duration) for _____ family members/significant others? _____

_____

_____

_____

_____

What do you project as _____ future treatment needs?

	No	Yes	Frequency	Duration
Case Management Services	_____	_____	_____	_____
Cognitive/Behavioral Management	_____	_____	_____	_____
Individual Counseling	_____	_____	_____	_____
Family Counseling/Education	_____	_____	_____	_____
Group Counseling	_____	_____	_____	_____
Pain Management	_____	_____	_____	_____
Social Skills/Assertiveness Training	_____	_____	_____	_____
Stress Management, Biofeedback, and Relaxation Techniques	_____	_____	_____	_____
Behavior Management	_____	_____	_____	_____
Substance Abuse Prevention	_____	_____	_____	_____
Resource Referrals	_____	_____	_____	_____
Sexuality Counseling	_____	_____	_____	_____
Referral to specialized services	_____	_____	_____	_____

such as: peer counseling,
psychiatric consultations,
vocational counseling,
psychological consultations,
spiritual support (circle
which)

Other _____
_____

Along with the previous treatment(s), what do you see as needs regarding any additional evaluations, such as educational, vocational, neuropsychological/psychological, etc. at the present time and as _____ ages with spinal cord injury?

Evaluation	Purpose	Frequency/Duration
_____	_____	_____
_____	_____	_____
_____	_____	_____
_____	_____	_____
_____	_____	_____

Please give current test findings, observations, and/or your opinion regarding _____ functional levels:

Intelligence level _____
_____
_____
_____

Personality style with regard to the school/work and home _____
_____
_____
_____

Stamina _____
_____
_____

Functional limitations and assets _____
_____
_____
_____

Ability for education and/or training _____

_____

_____

_____

Vocational implications _____

_____

_____

_____

_____

_____

_____

_____

_____

_____

_____

_____

_____

_____

_____

_____

_____

_____

Do you have any additional comments about anything not covered in the previous
questions and which we should be aware of in addressing _____ long-term
psychosocial adaptation needs? _____

_____

_____

_____

_____

_____

_____

_____

_____

_____

_____

_____

_____

_____

_____

_____

_____

_____

_____

_____

_____

_____

_____

Signature	Date

(Adapted from *Life Care Planning for Spinal Cord Injury: A Resource Manual for Case Managers* by
T.L. Blackwell, R.O. Weed & A.S. Powers. Elliott & Fitzpatrick, Inc., 1994. Reprinted by permission.)

SUPPLEMENTAL QUESTIONS FOR INDIVIDUALS WITH TRAUMATIC BRAIN INJURY IN ADDITION TO SPINAL CORD INJURY

As _____ has also incurred a traumatic brain injury, please give current test findings, observations, and/or your opinion regarding functional levels in the following:

Level of insight into present functioning _____
_____
_____
_____

Ability to compensate for deficits _____
_____
_____
_____

Ability to initiate action _____
_____
_____

Ability to maintain attention/concentration _____
_____
_____
_____

Ability to handle stress/tension _____
_____
_____
_____

Ability to problem solve _____
_____
_____
_____

Ability to identify and correct errors _____
_____
_____
_____

Presence of depressive symptoms _____
_____
_____
_____

Memory impairments (short term, long term, auditory, visual, etc.) _
_____
_____
_____

Lowered frustration tolerance _____
_____
_____

Recommendations for compensation strategies/aids _____
_____
_____

Please complete the following with respect to _____ ability to perform school/work related activities:

	Not Significantly Limited[a]	Moderately Limited[b]	Markedly Limited[c]	No Evidence of Limitation in This Category
A. Understanding and Memory				
• The ability to remember locations and work-like procedures	_____	_____	_____	_____
• The ability to understand and remember very short and simple instructions	_____	_____	_____	_____
• The ability to understand and remember detailed instructions	_____	_____	_____	_____
B. Sustained Concentration and Persistence				
• The ability to carry out very short and simple instructions	_____	_____	_____	_____
• The ability to carry out detailed instructions	_____	_____	_____	_____
• The ability to maintain attention and concentration for extended periods	_____	_____	_____	_____
• The ability to sustain an ordinary routine without special supervision	_____	_____	_____	_____
• The ability to perform activities within a schedule, maintain regular attendance, and be punctual within customary tolerances	_____	_____	_____	_____
• The ability to work in coordination with or proximity to others without being distracted by them	_____	_____	_____	_____
• The ability to make simple decisions	_____	_____	_____	_____
• The ability to complete a normal school/work day and week without interruptions from psychologically based symptoms and to perform at a consistent pace without an unreasonable number and length of rest periods	_____	_____	_____	_____
C. Social Interaction				
• The ability to interact appropriately with peers	_____	_____	_____	_____
• The ability to ask simple questions or request assistance	_____	_____	_____	_____

---

[a]Not Significantly Limited: No significant limitation in this area.

[b]Moderate: An impairment which seriously limits but does not preclude the individual's ability to function in the designated area.

[c]Marked: An impairment which seriously interferes with the individual's ability to function independently, appropriately, and effectively in the designated area.

	Not Significantly Limited[a]	Moderately Limited[b]	Markedly Limited[c]	No Evidence of Limitation in This Category
• The ability to accept instructions and respond appropriately to criticism from authority figures	_____	_____	_____	_____
• The ability to get along with peers without distracting them or exhibiting behavioral extremes	_____	_____	_____	_____
• The ability to maintain socially appropriate behavior and to adhere to basic standards of neatness and cleanliness	_____	_____	_____	_____

D. Adaptation

• The ability to respond appropriately to changes in school/home settings	_____	_____	_____	_____
• The ability to be aware of normal hazards and take appropriate precautions	_____	_____	_____	_____
• The ability to travel in unfamiliar places or use public transportation	_____	_____	_____	_____
• The ability to set realistic goals or make plans independently of others	_____	_____	_____	_____

---

[a]Not Significantly Limited: No significant limitation in this area.

[b]Moderate: An impairment which seriously limits but does not preclude the individual's ability to function in the designated area.

[c]Marked: An impairment which seriously interferes with the individual's ability to function independently, appropriately, and effectively in the designated area.

What are your recommendations for specific cognitive/behavioral treatment needs and suggestions regarding treatment approaches? (Identify abilities that may be used to circumvent or compensate for deficit skills; identify kinds of cues or modifications that are likely to enhance performance; and, identify components of cognitive processes on which alternative functional approaches to deal with cognitive impairment can be built.) _____

_____

_____

_____

_____

Do you see the need for follow-up by a neurologist?

No _____

Yes _____ Frequency _____ Duration _____

Does _____ need companion or attendant care? If so, what level? (Please include details relevant to the level of care required, hours that care is needed, etc.)

_____

_____

_____

_____

Do you project a change in the future in the level of companion or attendant care _____ will need?

No _____

Yes _____   If Yes, at approximately what age would this occur and what would needs be then (including recommendations regarding possible group home setting, if appropriate)? _____

_____

_____

_____

Do you project _____ would be able to successfully function in academic training or in the work setting? Would accommodations need to be provided? _____

_____
_____
_____
_____
_____
_____
_____
_____
_____
_____
_____
_____
_____
_____
_____
_____
_____
_____
_____
_____
_____
_____
_____
_____
_____
_____
_____
_____
_____
_____
_____
_____
_____

_____   _____

Signature   Date

(Adapted from *Life Care Planning for Traumatic Brain Injury: A Resource Manual for Case Managers* by T.L. Blackwell, A.S. Powers & R.O. Weed. Elliott & Fitzpatrick, Inc., 1994. Reprinted by permission.)

APPENDIX A

Demographic Characteristics of Spinal Cord Injury

Incidence

The reported incidence (number of new cases of SCI occurring in the U.S. each year) of SCI varies according to source (Go, DeVivo, & Richards, 1995; Stover & Fine, 1986). Based on an earlier study of SCI incidence conducted in northern California during 1970 and 1971, Kraus, Franti, Riggins, Richards, and Borhani (1975) estimated that SCI occurs at the rate of 53 cases per million population, but only 32 per million survive 24 hours after the injury. In their study of national incidence of hospitalized SCI, Bracken, Freeman, and Hellenbrand (1981) found an increased annual incidence rate of 40 cases per million population. Several subsequent studies, derived from state-mandated SCI central registries, revealed annual hospitalized SCI incidence rates ranging from 26 to 76 cases per million population (Acton et al., 1993; Colorado Department of Health and Environment, 1997; Ergas, 1985; Georgia Central Registry, 1993; Hickman, 1993; Lawrence, Bayakly, & Mathison, 1992; Louisiana Office of Public Health, 1999; Oklahoma State Department of Health, 1998; Utah Department of Health, 1993). Given the findings from various studies, Go et al. (1995) summarized the national annual incidence of SCI for people who survive the initial trauma at between 30 and 40 cases per million population. This corresponds to approximately 7,000 to 10,000 new cases of traumatic SCI per year in the U.S. (DeVivo et al., 1999; Hall et al., 1999; NSCISC, 2000).

Prevalence

Because SCI is relatively rare, attempts to determine prevalence (number of existing cases of SCI in the U.S. at a given point in time) by actually counting individuals with disability are not practical because of the time and resources that would be required (Go et al., 1995). Survey-based studies have produced a variety of prevalence rates for persons with SCI, with estimates ranging from 525 per million population to 1,124 per million population (Collins, 1986; Ergas, 1985; Harvey, Rothschild, Asmann, & Stripling, 1990; Kurtzke, 1975). Probably the most widely cited SCI prevalence rates however (based on probability sampling techniques and mathematical relationships with incidence and mortality) are estimated at between 721 and 906 per million (Berkowitz, Harvey, Greene, & Wilson, 1992; DeVivo, Fine, Maetz, & Stover, 1980). Based on 1999 U.S. Census population estimates, these rates correspond to an estimated SCI population total of approximately 183,000 to 230,000 people (NSCISC, 2000).

Age

Population-based studies reveal that SCI occurs primarily among individuals between 16 and 30 years of age, with approximately 80 percent of the injuries occurring between 16 and 45 years of age (Acton et al., 1993; Bayakly & Lawrence, 1992; Colorado Department of Public Health and Environment, 1997; Go et al., 1995; Kraus et al., 1975; Lawrence et al., 1992; Nobunaga, Go, & Karunas, 1999; Oklahoma State Department of Health, 1998). Model Systems data show that 54.1 percent of SCI occur in the age group 16 to 30 with the average age at injury being 31.7 years. Since 1973, there has been an increase in the mean age at time of injury. Individuals who were injured in 1973 to 1977 had a mean age of 28.5; those injured in 1994 to 1998 had a mean age of 36 years.

Another trend shown in these Model Systems data is an increase in the proportion of those who were at least 61 years of age at injury. In 1973 to 1977, persons older than 60 years of age at injury comprised 4.5 percent of the database. From 1994 to 1998, this increased to 11.5 percent (Nobunaga et al., 1999). This trend has important health care and management implications, because older persons who incur SCI have more pre-existing major medical conditions (e.g., diabetes, obesity, heart disease, and arthritis), are more likely to have higher level injuries, develop secondary medical complications during initial hospitalization and rehabilitation, have lower levels of independence in care, and have more frequent rehospitalizations than their younger counterparts at SCI onset (DeVivo, Shewchuk, Stover, Black, & Go, 1992; Go et al., 1995; Menter & Hudson, 1995; Roth, Lovell, Heinemann, Lee, & Yarkony, 1992; Yarkony, Roth, Heinemann, & Lovell, 1988).

Gender

Findings from various demographic studies have consistently shown a greater occurrence of SCI in males compared to females (Berkowitz et al., 1992; Fine, Kuhlemeier, DeVivo, & Stover, 1979; Stover & Fine, 1986; Young, Burns, Bowen, & McCutchen, 1982). Overall, 81.5 percent of all persons enrolled in the National SCI Database are male. This greater than four-to-one male-to-female ratio has varied little throughout the 25 years of Model Systems data collection. However, Nobunaga et al. (1999) noted the National SCI Database appears to be slightly biased toward the inclusion of males compared to findings from population-based samples, which range from 69.1 percent to 80.6 percent male (Bayakly & Lawrence, 1992; Colorado Department of Public Health and Environment, 1997; Georgia Central Registry, 1993; Hickman, 1993; Kraus et al., 1975; Louisiana Office of Public Health, 1999; Oklahoma State Department of Health, 1998; Utah Department of Health, 1993).

Race/Ethnicity

Demographic studies continue to show that the majority of new SCIs are white (Berkowitz, O'Leary, Kruse, & Harvey, 1998). However, a significant trend over time has been observed in the racial distribution of persons in the Model Systems database. Among persons injured between 1973 and 1977, 76.9 percent were white, 14.0 percent were African-American, 6.2 percent were Hispanic, 2.1 percent were Native American, and 0.8 percent were Asian. However, between 1994 and 1998, only 67.2 percent of persons enrolled in the National SCI Database were white, while 21.5 percent were African-American, 8.0 percent were Hispanic, 1.1 percent were Native American, 1.4 percent were Asian, and 0.8 percent were classified as "other"(Nobunaga et al., 1999). It is important to note that most Model Systems are located in large urban areas that may not be representative of the country at large. Further, because the Model Systems designation is based on five-year federal funding cycles, the composition of the centers changes over time. Therefore, it is also possible that the changing racial/ethnic composition reflects a change in the number or composition of the Model Systems (possibly the inclusion of more urban-based centers). Although Go et al. (1995) surmise that it is reasonable to assume a slight bias exists in the National SCI Database toward the disproportionate inclusion of minorities, Berkowitz et al. (1998) concluded from their studies that the Model Systems data may reflect the national SCI demographics more closely than previously thought.

Marital Status

Although earlier studies of veterans with SCI suggested there was little if any impact of SCI on marital status (Abrams, 1981; Deyoe, 1972; El Ghatit & Hanson, 1976), a later study by Berkowitz et al. (1992) found that persons with SCI have a rate of divorce nearly twice that of the general U.S. population. Data on marriage and divorce rates of persons enrolled in the National SCI Database also demonstrate that the proportions of single (never married) and divorced individuals with SCI was substantially higher than those of the general U.S. population of comparable age and gender (DeVivo, Hawkins, Richards, & Go, 1995; DeVivo & Richards, 1996). Age (younger persons are more likely to divorce), gender and race (females and African-Americans more frequently get divorced), prior divorce, having no children, and a more severe injury were factors found to be associated with divorce (Brown & Giesy, 1986; Crewe, Athelstan, & Krumberger, 1979; DeVivo & Fine, 1985; El Ghatit & Hanson, 1975). However, the influence of age, race, prior divorce, and childlessness on divorce rates was similar to the effects these factors have for the general population (Dijkers, Abela, Gans, & Gordon, 1995).

Post-injury outcome studies have found that the likelihood of getting married after SCI is also reduced. Although research on marriage rates post-injury have been limited, findings from the National SCI Database suggest that people with SCI have significantly fewer marriages in the first several years post-injury than would be expected based on age and gender-specific first-marriage rates for the general population (DeVivo & Fine, 1985). Further, these data found that post-injury marriages of persons with SCI were no more stable than pre-injury marriages, as previously thought (DeVivo et al., 1995).

A number of factors associated with onset of SCI produce stressors for both spouses that in turn may result in increased likelihood of separation and divorce (Brown & Giesy, 1986; Crewe et al., 1979; Crewe & Krause, 1988; DeLoach & Greer, 1981; El Ghatit & Hanson, 1975; El Ghatit & Hanson, 1976; Kerr & Thompson, 1972; Trieschmann, 1988). Dijkers et al. (1995) summarize these factors to include the injured partner's limited capacity to fulfill household and child care tasks; his or her care needs; reduced mobility, resulting in reduction of outings and social contacts; loss of social supports; financial pressures and lowered standard of living; changes in sexual function; job loss and resulting loss of social status; assumption of the stigmatized disabled status; and problems with psychological adjustment.

Education

Studies that look at individual educational level at the time of injury reveal on average that persons with SCI have educational levels somewhat below that of persons in the U.S. general population, whereas individuals who have been injured for a number of years have educational levels somewhat higher than that of the general population (Go et al., 1995). Findings from the National SCI Database demonstrated that 66 percent of persons with SCI admitted between the ages of 18 and 21 years of age were at least high school graduates, compared to 86 percent for the U.S. general population (Go et al., 1995; U.S. Bureau of the Census, 1992).

Several population-based studies have subsequently reported distribution of educational levels for persons who incur SCIs to be similar to that reported by the Model Systems (Colorado Department of Public Health and Environment, 1997; Georgia Central Registry, 1993; Hickman, 1993). Berkowitz et al. (1992, 1998) found the overall education of persons with SCI aged 25 years or more to be somewhat higher than the general population. However, the authors were measuring education at the time of the survey study and not at the time of injury. These findings would tend to support the trends found in Model Systems follow-up data, which demonstrates a gradual increase of average educational level attained at each anniversary year post-injury. Dijkers et al. (1995) found that at five years post-injury the educational level of persons enrolled in the National SCI Database was still somewhat less than that of the general U.S. population. However, at 10 years post-injury the educational level was somewhat higher, suggesting a delay and prolongation of the education process. This is probable evidence of successful adaptation to injury. As discussed in the section on employment, the level of educational attainment is a very significant factor for predicting the likelihood of a person's return to work after SCI (DeVivo, Rutt, Stover, & Fine, 1987; El Ghatit & Hanson, 1978, 1979; Krause, 1992; Krause & Anson, 1996; Krause, Sternberg, Maides, & Lottes, 1998).

Etiology

The National SCI Database documents 37 causes of injury, which for convenience are often grouped into five categories: motor vehicle accidents; falls; acts of violence; recreational sporting activities; and, other causes that do not fit into any of these categories (Go et al., 1995; Stover & Fine, 1986). Causes of SCI vary considerably by age, gender, and race.

Population-based studies have shown motor vehicle accidents to be the leading cause of SCI among whites and Native Americans; motor vehicle accidents account for nearly half of all injuries among whites and approximately two-thirds among Native Americans (Acton et al., 1993; Berkowitz et al., 1998; Colorado Department of Public Health and Environment, 1997; Kraus et al., 1975; Louisiana Office of Public Health, 1999; Nobunaga et al., 1999). Falls usually rank second, accounting for between 13 and 23 percent of SCIs, with recreational sporting activities and acts of violence each accounting for approximately 3 to 17 percent of injuries (Go et al., 1995).

Acts of violence are the leading cause of SCI for African-Americans and Hispanics. Population-based studies have shown the incidence rate of SCI caused by acts of violence to be between six and twelve times higher among African-Americans than among whites (Acton et al., 1993; Bayakly & Lawrence, 1992; Go et al., 1995; Louisiana Office of Public Health, 1999). Motor vehicle accidents, falls, and recreational sporting activities are the next most important injury categories in descending order of incidence among non-white racial/ethnic groups (Stover & Fine, 1986; Trieschmann, 1988; University of Alabama, 1998).

The difference in distribution of SCI etiologies by gender is most pronounced in the proportion of motor vehicle accident-related injuries and recreational sporting activities. Motor vehicle accidents account for a larger proportion of SCI in women than men, whereas the reverse is evident in the proportion of recreational sporting related injuries. Falls and acts of violence are fairly evenly distributed across genders (Acton et al., 1993; Bayakly & Lawrence, 1992; Berkowitz et al., 1998; Go et al., 1995; Kraus et al., 1995; Nobunaga et al., 1999; Trieschmann, 1988).

Both population-based studies and hospital-based studies reveal that the cause of SCI also differs substantially by age (Go et al., 1995; Stover & Fine, 1986). Motor vehicle accidents are the leading cause of SCI before age 45, while falls are the leading cause after age 45. The proportion of SCIs resulting from recreational sporting activities and acts of violence steadily declines with advancing age at injury (Acton et al., 1993; Berkowitz et al., 1992, 1998; Go et al., 1995; Kraus et al., 1975; Nobunaga et al., 1999; Stover & Fine, 1986).

Injury Characteristics

The relative proportion of persons with tetraplegia and paraplegia enrolled in the National SCI Database has varied little over the years (Nobunaga et al., 1999; Stover & Fine, 1986). Slightly more than half of these individuals are classified as having tetraplegia. The most common area of injury is the C4, C5, and C6 levels; the second most common area is between T12 and L1 (Go et al., 1995). Since 1994 the most frequent neurologic category for persons enrolled in the National SCI Database has been incomplete tetraplegia (30 percent) followed by complete paraplegia (26 percent), complete tetraplegia (23 percent), and incomplete paraplegia (20 percent) (Go et al., 1995; Nobunaga et al., 1999; Stover & Fine, 1986). Population-based studies from several statewide registries suggest that the National SCI Database may be somewhat biased toward over-representation of persons with more severe injuries (Acton et al., 1993; Bayakly & Lawrence, 1992).

Findings from studies of etiologic categories report motor vehicle accident-related SCIs are likely to result in neurologically incomplete tetraplegia (32.0 percent) and complete paraplegia (25.7 percent). By comparison, complete paraplegia (42.2 percent) and incomplete paraplegia (26.4 percent), are the usual outcomes of SCI resulting from acts of violence. Recreational sporting related accidents are most likely to result in tetraplegia, with an almost equal outcome probability of complete tetraplegia (44.0 percent) and incomplete tetraplegia (45.1 percent). Falls are more likely to result in incomplete tetraplegia (36.3 percent), followed by incomplete paraplegia (22.9 percent), up to age 45. After age 45 the incidence of tetraplegia rapidly increases with advancing age at time of injury (Go et al., 1995; Nobunaga et al., 1999).

National Spinal Cord Injury Database

The National SCI Database has been in existence since 1973 and captures data from an estimated 13 percent of new SCI cases in the United States each year (DeVivo, Jackson, Dijkers, & Becker, 1999; Stover, DeVivo, & Go, 1999). Since its inception, 24 federally funded Model SCI Care Systems have contributed data to the National SCI Database. The National Spinal Cord Injury Statistical Center (NSCISC) was established in 1984, succeeding the National Spinal Cord Injury Data Research Center as the central facility to collect and analyze data reported by the Model Systems. Over the years, these data have been used to conduct longitudinal (cohort) studies of the long-term natural history of persons with SCI. In addition, this information has been analyzed to assess trends in demographic characteristics, health services provided, and treatment outcomes for people enrolled in the National SCI Database (Stover et al., 1999). As of September 1999, the database contained information on more than 19,648 persons who sustained traumatic SCI (NSCISC, 2000).

IMPLICATIONS FOR LIFE CARE PLANNING

Although the NSCISC is the best available source of data regarding the demographic characteristics of people with SCI, it must be pointed out that these data are not population-based (a primary requirement of epidemiology), and therefore have unknown generalizability to the SCI population as a whole. Specifically, the database includes only persons who have been treated at a Model Systems within the first year following SCI. Further, most Model Systems that contribute data to the NSCISC come from large urban hospitals in high-population states (e.g., Boston, Chicago, Detroit, Houston, New York). Consequently, there may be an underrepresentation of individuals from rural areas, where health care delivery systems may be quite different. Furthermore, the Model Systems have changed over the years, because these federally designated centers recompete for funding in five-year cycles, with the number and locations of the centers changing to some degree between cycles.

Even the type of individuals who are treated at a center in a particular area may vary as a function of socioeconomic status (SES) or economic resources and whether the center is part of a county funded, university affiliated, or private setting. As a result, changes in overall demographics in Model Systems cases over time will not only reflect the changing trends in demographics among people with SCI, but also differences in the characteristics of the patient populations being treated by the hospitals that have been added over the five-year cycle (once funded, few centers lose their Model Systems designation). Lastly, it must be pointed out that the Model Systems were not implemented until 1971 and then only on a limited scale. Therefore, there is an underrepresentation of individuals whose SCIs occurred prior to the past two decades, with no participants who have been injured 30 years or more. These limitations must be considered when evaluating data reported by NSCISC, particularly as related to demographics, etiology, costs, and mortality.

APPENDIX B

Costs Associated with Spinal Cord Injury

Although SCI is proportionally rare compared to the prevalence of other types of injuries, its costs are high to the individual and society. According to a report by the Agency for Health Care Policy and Research (1996), SCI was the most expensive condition or principle diagnosis treated in U.S. hospitals. Further, given that the majority of SCIs involve younger adults and demand a high volume of medical and rehabilitation services over the person's lifetime, the direct costs (costs that result from treatment, rehabilitation, and other expenditures caused directly by the SCI) often exceed $1 million (Berkowitz et al., 1992; Berkowitz et al., 1998; DeVivo, Whiteneck, & Charles, 1995a; Harvey, Wilson, Greene, Berkowitz, & Stripling, 1992; Johnson, Brooks, & Whiteneck, 1996; NSCISC, 2000). The costs are highly correlated with the severity of injury.

The following is a summary of three studies that describe the direct costs associated with SCI. These figures represent costs for goods and services that have been provided and do not represent the costs of goods and services that may be needed for care. There may be very significant discrepancies between the level of care needed and that which is provided using available resources. Because life care plans should always be based on an assessment of *needs*, rather than any compromise between needs and resources, studies of costs for services delivered will typically underestimate resources needed based on a comprehensive LCP. Consequently, average figures from cost studies cannot be used to estimate costs for individual cases. However, cost studies can be helpful as a guide to determine the relative distribution of costs for some of the various needs categories. These studies may also help to identify the frequency of events (e.g., rehospitalizations) that may be projected for a given individual when there is no basis for a different individual projection (except perhaps cost of the item in the particular geographic location where the individual with SCI may live).

PSA-DIS STUDY

Berkowitz et al. (1992) evaluated the economic consequences of SCI under a project with the Paralysis Society of America (PSA), a unit of the Paralyzed Veterans of America, which funded the study, and Disability Income Systems, Inc. (DIS), a group of Rutgers University researchers responsible for carrying out this study. After interviewing 758 individuals with SCI, the authors provided a comprehensive analysis of the direct costs resulting from SCI, then averaged these costs over the entire SCI population to develop an estimated average cost profile (adjusted to 1988 dollars). Included in the study was information about individuals who survived initial treatment. Costs for items such as emergency medical services, post-rehabilitation laboratory tests and procedures, specific physician services (e.g., physician fees for surgery), vocational rehabilitation, and transportation were excluded.

The study was designed to examine the various costs associated with SCI, including acute care, rehabilitation, and annual treatment/maintenance. Survey respondents were asked questions regarding the costs associated with the following areas:

- Hospitalization
- Medical practitioner services
- Personal assistance services
- Prescription/non-prescription drugs and supplies
- Adaptive equipment
- Home modifications

Given the inability of some respondents to provide accurate information on SCI-related expenses, the authors also collected survey data on the quantities of medical goods and services used. This information was used to price the incremental demand for items and services attributable to SCI using the market prices for these items in 1988.

In this study, Berkowitz et al. (1992) utilized a prevalence-based sample augmented by individuals who were members of various organizations that represent people with disabilities, individuals residing in long-term care facilities as well as in the community, and individuals from referrals by persons already included in the study. The participants included both veterans (25.4 percent) and nonveterans (74.6 percent). They were further divided into people who were tetraplegic (43.7 percent) and those who were paraplegic (55.5 percent). Of the study sample 0.8 percent were classified as unknown relevant to level/extent of injury.

Hospitalization

In this study the authors estimated the overall average costs for initial hospitalization and rehabilitation during the first two years post-injury to be $95,203 (the average costs were $118,785 for persons with tetraplegia and $73,319 for those with paraplegia). Factors that may impact the length of stay post-injury include severity of injury, age, injury complications or comorbidity of preexisting conditions, and source of payment for treatment.

Following initial hospitalization and rehabilitation, people with SCI had a higher rate of rehospitalization than non-SCI persons. On average, the study found that individuals with SCI spend almost six days more each year in the hospital than non-SCI individuals. This increase in hospitalization time results in an incremental (i.e., attributed to SCI) average cost of $2,958 per year.

Medical Practitioner Services

Individuals with SCI may consult a variety of health care practitioners during their post-injury lives. Included in the treatment team of health care practitioners are physicians (e.g., physiatrists, urologists, etc.) and nonphysicians such as physical therapists, nurses, psychologists, and others. Survey respondents were asked to identify the types of health care practitioners they had seen outside of the hospital setting in the previous year, the number of times they were consulted, the reasons for consultation, and the sources of payment for these appointments. Overall, more than 90 percent of respondents had seen a physician or other health care practitioner during the previous year.

The estimated average cost of practitioner visits for individuals with SCI was $2,334 per year compared with the $86 per year predicted for non-SCI individuals. Consequently, the costs due to SCI for practitioner services were estimated at $2,248 per year.

Personal Assistance Services

Individuals with SCI often require some type of assistance with activities of daily living. Factors that may impact the need for personal assistance include level of injury, age, gender, and level of involvement in household activities. The study found that, on average, individuals with SCI received 25.1 hours per week of assistance.

Cost estimates for personal assistance averaged $6,080 per year. The costs were calculated for an assistant wage of $5 per hour based on data collected in a national survey of attendant care programs in the U.S. The survey was conducted by the World Institute on Disability and figures were adjusted to 1988 dollars. Fringe benefits and other agency fees were not included. Obviously, the $5 per hour figure significantly underestimates current attendant care wages, particularly in larger metropolitan areas.

Prescription/Nonprescription Drugs and Supplies

Although the study attempted to identify specific information regarding prescription medications, the information gathered from respondents was often incomplete relevant to quantities used. Nevertheless, the authors were able to gather information on the types of medications used frequently by individuals with SCI. Muscle relaxants were the most frequently used medication (33.3 percent used regularly, 7.4 percent as needed) followed by pain medication (19 percent used regularly, 15.6 percent as needed), urinary antiseptics (17.7 percent used regularly, 3.2 percent as needed), and antibiotics (15.7 percent used regularly, 18.5 percent as needed). Least commonly used drugs included cortisone, anti-muscle calcification drugs, gastric medications, and male hormones.

On average, the authors reported that individuals with SCI pay $113 more per year than their non-SCI counterparts for prescription medications. This figure may grossly underestimate what can be expected in terms of prescription medication costs. At today's cost, one treatment of an urinary tract infection with antibiotics can cost more than $113, excluding any other medications the individual may require. Factors such as age, severity of injury, SCI-related complications, or comorbid medical conditions may impact usage patterns. Medication costs were highest for individuals with complete tetraplegia, incomplete paraplegia, incomplete tetraplegia, and complete paraplegia, respectively.

In addition to prescription medications, nonprescription supplies and medications were also used by individuals with SCI each day. Typically, items necessary in bladder programs were the single largest expenditure within the category of supplies.

The authors calculated the costs for nonprescription items by pricing out the actual quantities of each type of item as reported by study respondents. On average, they estimated that persons with SCI pay $1,686 per year for nonprescription medications and supplies, varying with severity of injury. Although these data show a decrease in costs by age, the authors caution that these age comparisons are not adjusted for differences in severity of injury.

Adaptive Equipment

Berkowitz et al. (1992) attempted to assess the number and types of individuals with SCI who utilize adaptive equipment to complete 14 activities of daily living. Bed and hygiene aids and mobility aids were more heavily utilized by the SCI population than other types of adaptive equipment. The largest portions of SCI population surveyed relied on equipment for getting around outside of their residence (63.2 percent), getting around inside residence (59.0 percent), bladder care (40.3 percent), bowel care (32.4 percent), getting into and out of the bathtub (30.0 percent), bathing (27.1 percent), and getting into and out of bed (21.0 percent).

In creating the LCP, life care planners must remember that adaptive equipment must be maintained and serviced periodically and equipment costs may vary depending upon the gender of the person with SCI, his or her age, and the time that has elapsed since the injury.

Home Modifications

Approximately 60 percent of study respondents made some modification to their living quarters to accommodate their SCI. The most frequent addition was a ramp. More than 20 percent of the respondents reported modifications that included widening doorways, installing grab bars, and/or building a new home or an addition to an existing residence. People with complete tetraplegia were found to be more likely (82.4 percent) than individuals with paraplegia (59 percent) to make home modifications. These figures should not be taken to imply that the home was not in need of modification in cases where no modification was made, because many individuals with limited resources often live in housing with poor or virtually nonexistant accessibility.

Cost estimates for home modifications were $14,545 on average for individuals making modifications. People with tetraplegia had higher home modification expenses than those with paraplegia.

Institutional Care Costs

A very small percentage of the SCI population was found to live in nursing homes and other long-term care facilities (2.6 percent). Of these, 52 percent had incomplete tetraplegia and 27.4 percent had complete tetraplegia. Because of the low percentage of the total of individuals with SCI in institutionalized care facilities, the cost for these services over the general SCI population was low.

Summary of Costs

Berkowitz et al. (1992) concluded that following the high costs for initial treatment and rehabilitation, individuals with SCI can expect to incur ongoing costs of more than $14,000 per year throughout their post-rehabilitation lives. The authors note, however, that whenever possible they used conservative methodologies in calculating the average cost estimates. Further, they surmised that the cost estimates will likely rise as persons with SCI age. Table B-1 summarizes how the costs were distributed across the various areas of this study. These figures were based on estimates averaged over the entire SCI population.

Table B-1. Average Incremental SCI Direct Costs (1988 Dollars)

Type of Cost	Average Costs
Initial costs of:	
Hospitalization	$ 95,203
Home modifications	8,208
Total initial cost	103,411
Recurring annual expenses for:	
Post-rehabilitation hospitalization	2,958
Medical practitioner services	2,248
Personal assistance services	6,080
Prescription drugs	113
Nonprescription drugs and supplies	1,686
Adaptive equipment	861
Institutional care	189
Total recurring annual expenses	14,135

(From Direct Costs of Traumatic SCI in *The Economic Consequences of Traumatic Spinal Cord Injury* by Berkowitz, Harvey, Greene, & Wilson, p. 74. Paralyzed Veterans of America, 1992. Reprinted with permission.)

The most extensive source of data on the direct costs of SCI was collected by the Model Systems. However, it is important to note that these data describe the experiences of facility-specific systems and may not be representative for cost investigations of individuals with SCI who receive treatment in other settings. It is not known how costs may differ in non-Model Systems. It may be surmised that initial costs are higher in a Model System (because to more diverse treatment programs), but that follow-up costs are lower because of to fewer recurring problems. As with the Berkowitz et al. (1992) study, Model Systems-based research used estimates based on charges rather than needs.

DeVivo, Whiteneck, and Charles (1995a) provided an overview of the average first-year post-injury charges and subsequent average annual follow-up costs incurred as a consequence of injury. These data were based on a prospective one-year cost study between 1989 and 1990 and were subsequently adjusted to 1992 dollars. The study population represented a random sample of 508 persons initially treated at a Model System since 1973 and enrolled in the National SCI Database, in addition to 227 newly injured persons with SCI (DeVivo et al., 1995a).

Emergency Medical Services, Acute Care, and Rehabilitation

DeVivo et al. (1995a) found that 82.9 percent of the average first-year post-SCI charges were associated with emergency medical services (0.5 percent), acute care (34.1 percent), and initial rehabilitation (48.3 percent). These total charges from injury to completion of rehabilitation ranged from $339,906 for individuals with high tetraplegia (Frankel A, B, or C) to $107,365 for persons with incomplete motor function at any level (Frankel D). The average charge was $164,364 (1992 dollars).

Outpatient Services and Physician Visits

This category includes costs associated with physician visits, physical therapy, occupational therapy, speech therapy, psychology, laboratory, x-ray, and other miscellaneous charges associated with outpatient visits. Charges for physician visits and associated costs were calculated separately. The average charges for all individuals in the study was $2,758 for the remainder of the first-year post-injury and $1,032 annually thereafter. The average outpatient physician fees for the study population were $526 and $322 for the remainder of the first year and subsequent years post-injury, respectively.

Durable Medical Equipment

The average charges for durable medical equipment (DME) was $5,633 for the remainder of the first year post-injury and $1,361 annually for subsequent years post-injury. DME-included costs relate to the purchase, rental, or repair of equipment, such as hospital beds, special mattresses, commodes, wheelchairs, wheelchair cushions, wheelchair backpacks, cushion covers, caliper straps, crutches, braces, splints, orthoses, ventilators, ventilator parts, and environmental control units. The costs for DME were much higher during the first year post-injury.

The study excluded costs associated with the purchase or lease price of a new car or van, because individuals in the general population were presumed to purchase new cars at the same pace as persons with SCI. However, the accuracy of this assumption has never been determined.

Environmental Modifications

In looking at costs for environmental modifications the authors included charges incurred for modification of residences and work sites. Also included in this category were costs related to car or van modifications such as hand controls, lifts, and the like. The average first-year post-injury charges were $4,672. Subsequent year charges post-injury were calculated at $790 annually.

Medication and Supplies

Charges for both prescription and nonprescription drugs and supplies were included in this category. Medications for SCI typically include muscle relaxants, urine acidifiers, antacids, laxatives, analgesics, and antibiotics. Typical supplies included catheters, tubing, leg and bed bags, disposable gloves, adhesive tape, cement, detergent, skin lotions, powder, bed pads, bandages, and diapers. The authors found the costs of medications and supplies to increase with severity of injury. Average costs for medications was $875 for the remainder of the first year post-injury and $1,007 for each subsequent year. Average charges for supplies were $939 and $1,204, respectively.

Attendant Care and Household Assistance

Average annual charges for attendant care were $8,317 for the remainder of the first year post-injury and $11,448 per year thereafter. DeVivo et al. (1995a) noted that the costs varied substantially by severity of injury, as evidenced by the average charges for persons with high tetraplegia, which were $25,358 during the remainder of the first year post-injury and $47,563 per year thereafter. The study further found that many participants did not incur additional charges for paid household assistance other than that provided by their attendants. On average, charges for household assistance was $220 during the remainder of the first year and $398 annually for subsequent years post-injury.

Attendant care costs included charges for unskilled services provided by paid family members, friends, neighbors, aides, and orderlies, as well as skilled services by registered nurses or licensed practical nurses. Included in household assistance costs were charges for paid help needed for activities such as cleaning, cooking, laundering, shopping, and yard work. These figures included fringe benefits and agency fees.

Rehospitalizations and Nursing Home Care

Included in the rehospitalization charges were costs associated with SCI and secondary complications. Charges averaged $7,756 during the remainder of the first year post-injury for the study population and $5,255 annually thereafter. The charges varied by severity of injury.

Information from the National SCI Database indicated that, initially, persons with SCI were rehospitalized an average of once every two years. With the increase of time post-injury, rehospitalizations became less frequent and occurred about once every three years. The average length of stay per rehospitalization was approximately 17 days.

DeVivo et al. (1995a) noted that nursing home care charges were somewhat unstable, given that only 3.1 percent of the study participants required this level of care during the first year post-injury and only 2 percent required nursing home care during a subsequent study year. Among the few individuals with SCI who actually spent time in nursing home or extended care facilities, the average charges were $46,294 during the remainder of the first year post-injury and $38,018 in other post-injury years.

Vocational Rehabilitation

Because most people in this sample did not incur any charges for vocational rehabilitation, the costs figures from these data were consequently low. As a result, charges incurred by study participants averaged $375 for the remainder of the first year post-injury and only $249 annually for each subsequent year. Included in this category were charges for vocational and education preparation and vocational counseling as purchased either by the person with SCI or a third party (such as a vocational rehabilitation agency).

Miscellaneous Costs

The authors used a miscellaneous costs category to include items not identified in the other categories, such as transportation to and from health care providers, appropriate long distance phone calls, and care and maintenance of service animals (excluding pets). Average first year post-injury miscellaneous charges subsequent to rehabilitation were $472 and $342 for follow-up years.

Distribution of Charges Summary

Comparison of the various service utilization categories revealed that, on average, over 80 percent of all expenses incurred during the first year post-injury are accounted for by acute care (34.1 percent) and rehabilitation (48.3 percent) services. During the follow-up years those categories with the highest average annual charges were attendant care and household assistance (49.0 percent) and rehospitalizations (21.8 percent). Within these averages there was considerable variability in costs by neurologic level of injury, as shown in Tables B-2 and B-3.

BERKOWITZ, O'LEARY, KRUSE, & HARVEY STUDY

In an extension study to the earlier PSA-DIS work, Berkowitz et al. (1998) focused in greater detail on the costs associated with adaptation and accommodation to SCI.

Table B-2. Average First-Year Post-Injury Charges (1992 Dollars) Incurred by Service Category

Service Category	High Tetraplegia (C1–C4)	Low Tetraplegia (C5–C8)	Paraplegia (T1–S5)	Incomplete Motor Functional at Any Level	All Groups
Number	26	50	73	78	227
Emergency medical services	$ 1,229	$ 974	$ 992	$ 810	$ 953
Acute care	160,567	73,867	51,742	47,437	67,601
Rehabilitation	178,110	144,028	72,676	59,118	95,810
Rehospitalizations	21,895	5,653	7,459	4,669	7,756
Nursing home care	0	5,893	243	149	1,428
Outpatient services	3,462	2,887	2,559	2,626	2,758
Outpatient physician fees	627	462	548	512	526
Durable equipment	14,170	10,279	3,511	1,795	5,633
Environmental modifications	7,988	7,568	6,175	304	4,672
Medications	1,374	1,224	887	475	875
Supplies	1,183	1,220	1,310	330	939
Attendant care	25,358	14,622	2,879	3,686	8,317
Household assistance	0	157	41	501	220
Vocational rehabilitation	877	152	583	157	375
Miscellaneous charges	227	338	791	345	472
Total mean charges	417,067	269,324	152,396	122,914	198,335
Total median charges	404,033	249,264	137,756	116,694	161,110

Table B-3. Average Charges (1992 Dollars) Incurred Annually after First Year Post-Injury by Service Category

Service Category	High Tetraplegia (C1–C4)	Low Tetraplegia (C5–C8)	Paraplegia (T1–S5)	Incomplete Motor Functional at Any Level	All Groups
Number	55	131	200	122	508
Rehospitalizations	$ 14,296	$ 5,064	$ 4,828	$ 2,082	$ 5,255
Nursing home care	1,666	578	1,064	0	748
Outpatient services	2,027	1,168	909	640	1,032
Outpatient physician fees	368	401	332	200	322
Durable equipment	3,421	1,660	1,132	486	1,361
Environmental modifications	616	1,048	1,115	58	790
Medications	1,467	1,393	887	581	1,007
Supplies	1,556	1,508	1,309	547	1,204
Attendant care	47,563	16,527	3,106	3,390	11,448
Household assistance	655	364	368	369	398
Vocational rehabilitation	408	421	184	98	249
Miscellaneous charges	664	470	273	163	340
Total mean charges	74,707	30,602	15,507	8,614	24,154
Total median charges	36,794	21,967	7,235	2,281	10,417

(From The Economic Impact of Spinal Cord Injury by M.J. DeVivo, G.G. Whiteneck, and E.D. Charles, Jr. in *Spinal Cord Injury: Clinical Outcomes for the Model Systems* by S.L. Stover et al., pp. 237–238. Aspen Publishers, Inc., 1995. Adapted with permission.)

Specifically, the study looked at costs related to wheelchairs, home, and vehicle modifications. The authors completed telephone interviews of 500 people (past one year post-injury) who were selected from four Model Systems (Craig Hospital, Kessler Institute for Rehabilitation, Santa Clara Valley Medical Center, and Shepherd Center) lists and the Paralyzed Veterans of America (PVA) membership lists. Of the 500 respondents in this study, 137 were PVA members, while 363 were affiliated with one of the four Model Systems samples. The participants were evenly split between 50.2 percent with tetraplegia and 49.2 percent with paraplegia (0.6 percent were classified as unknown relevant to level or extent of injury). The following summarizes the key areas assessed in this study on the direct costs of SCI. By using a more diverse participant sample, this study has greater generalizability than the Berkowitz et al. (1992) earlier investigation on costs of SCI.

First Year Costs

In presenting first year costs for SCI, Berkowitz et al. (1998) relied upon data from the NSCISC and from Model Systems patients (DeVivo et al., 1995a). The authors found that 87.6 percent of first-year post-injury costs were associated with initial acute care and rehabilitation. Based on these existing data the total direct costs of SCI were estimated to be $223,261 (1996 dollars) during the first year post-injury. The study further identified that for subsequent years, recurring costs for routine medical care and treatment of secondary complications are much lower than the high costs associated with initial injury.

Annual Medical Care Costs

Annual medical care costs were based on utilization rather than actual costs. In this study the respondents were asked to recall medical experiences over the last year, when they were treated, at what type of facility, whether they were admitted (to critical care units), surgery, and number of follow-up appointments necessary. The authors then calculated the annual costs of medical care from *Healthcare Cost and Utilization Project* data from the *Nationwide Inpatient Sample (NIS) Release 1*, Mutual of Omaha Insurance Company, and data published by the Department of Veterans Affairs in the *Federal Register*. Hospital charges were estimated based upon surgical and nonsurgical diagnosis-related groups (DRGs). Physician charges for inpatient services were based on 50 percentile fees for such services from the Practice Management Information Corporation (PMIC) physician fees guide. Average annual medical care costs were estimated at $9,007 a year. Higher costs were found for older people and for those with more severe injuries.

Medications and Supplies

Because medications and supply names were difficult for study respondents to recall, the authors relied on data gathered from a random sample of 508 Model Systems patients (DeVivo et al., 1995a). The medications typically identified included muscle relaxants, urine acidifiers, antacids, laxatives, analgesics, and antibiotics. Supplies included items such as catheters and other bladder management supplies.

The total annual costs for medications and supplies were estimated at $2,489. Initial costs for first year post-injury were not included and prices were inflated to reflect 1996 costs. The annual costs were fairly evenly distributed between medications and supplies, with supplies receiving a slightly larger share of the costs. The costs for medications and supplies were found to increase with level of injury.

Home Modifications

The responsibility for making the environment accessible following SCI typically falls to the individual and family. In this study, the costs for home modifications were determined by collecting data on the type and extent of modifications. These modifications were then priced out based upon Americans with Disabilities Act (ADA) modification pricing guides and the estimates subsequently reviewed by contractors for the homes of relatives validity. Secondary homes and the homes of relatives were also included in cost estimates because these are often necessary to provide an accessible environment. The authors found that most home modifications are made during the first year post-injury. Wheelchair ramps and widened doors were the most common single modification.

Findings from this study indicate that the cost of home modifications tends to increase with the age of persons with SCI, until they reach their late sixties. The average cost of home modification was estimated at $20,904 in 1996 with an additional $376 per year spent on repairs and maintenance. The authors caution that these cost estimates are conservative.

Vehicle Modifications

The costs of vehicle modification were derived by collecting cost data on modifications from a survey of 13 modification vendors that were then averaged and applied to each modification reported. The authors found that 77.4 percent of survey respondents had vehicles that were modified for their use, and 72.4 percent were able to drive. The most popular vehicle to modify was a full size van (51.3 percent), followed by automobiles (28.2 percent), minivans (10.5 percent), and trucks (8.7 percent). The most common conversion for full-sized vans included a wheelchair lift with raised roof. The most common conversion for minivans included a ramp with a lowered floor and air-kneel system. Most people with SCI stay in their wheelchair in both vans and minivans and rely on tiedowns to secure the chair. Driving modifications fell into two major categories: acceleration and brake control, and steering.

Costs for vehicle modifications ranged from $149 to $65,000, with an average of $6,497. The lowest modification costs were for cars and trucks. The average lifespan for modified vehicles was estimated at 8.8 years (based on respondent reports of when modifications were made).

Wheelchairs

The study looked at the types of wheelchairs and related options and accessories used by respondents, then combined this information with vendor data to estimate the overall costs. A listing of options and accessories typically prescribed was obtained with input from occupational therapist at the four Model Systems included in this study. Berkowitz et al. (1998) determined cost estimates based upon reported wheelchair information (model, accessories, etc.) and with vendor cost data. On average, the cost for a wheelchair was estimated at $4,965 with a range from $983 to $20,732. These figures represent the cost of purchasing the primary wheelchair. Many of the respondents had more than one chair, either as a backup or for special purposes. The overall average cost figure for a wheelchair in this study tends to mask the large difference between power wheelchairs and manual wheelchairs (average estimated costs for a manual wheelchair was $2,476 compared to $10,987 for a power wheelchair) and does not account for a backup or speciality chair.

Based on findings from the survey, the average expected lifespan of wheelchairs was calculated at 9.0 years for primary manual wheelchairs, 7.1 years for primary power wheelchairs, and 7.0 years for scooters. The average lifespan of shower/commode chairs was estimated at 6 years, based on vendor information.

The overall average annual costs for wheelchair maintenance and repair was estimated at $235 (average annual costs of $159 for manual wheelchairs and $421 for power wheelchairs). These cost estimates were derived by: 1) using the midpoint of cost ranges provided by dealers; and, 2) using the repair costs reported by three-fourths of the study respondents and imputing repair costs to the other one-fourth based on the types of repairs done.

Personal Assistance

Of the sample respondents in the study, 56 percent reported needing help with activities of daily living (ADLs). Four-fifths of those with tetraplegia but less than one-third of those with paraplegia required help. Assistance with ADLs was most commonly needed by individuals with complete injuries (26 percent of individuals with incomplete paraplegia compared to 31 percent of those with complete paraplegia and 77 and 92 percent of persons with incomplete and complete tetraplegia, respectively). Reaching was the activity where people were most likely to need help (53 percent). Almost three-fourths of the people with tetraplegia required help bathing and getting in or out of their bed, wheelchair, or tub/shower.

Berkowitz et al. (1998) found that approximately 70 percent of the respondents who needed assistance said it was provided by immediate family members. Those who received paid assistance typically have this provided by home health aides and personal attendants. The number of hours of assistance varied by injury severity, ranging from 6.7 hours per week for individuals with incomplete paraplegia to 47.8 hours per week for those with complete tetraplegia. When restricted to people who need help with ADLs, the average number of hours of assistance per week was 51.4.

The cost for providing assistance for people who were more than one year post-injury was estimated using the national average hourly pay for home health aides, nursing aides, orderlies and attendants ($7.91 in 1996). The average yearly cost of personal assistance in this sample was estimated at $11,464 (with approximately 61 percent paid and 39 percent unpaid).

Summary of SCI Costs

Table B-4 summarizes the distribution of SCI direct cost estimates developed from this updated study by Berkowitz et al. (1998).

Table B-4. Average Direct Costs (1996 Dollars)

| Cost Category | Total SCI Population | Level/Extent of Injury | | |
		Tetraplegia A, B, C	Paraplegia A, B, C	All Cases D, E
Direct costs				
First year medical costs	$ 223,261	$ 339,965	$ 174,007	$ 144,294
Home modifications	21,000	22,329	20,566	12,549
Total first year recovery	244,261	362,294	194,573	156,843
Average annual post-recovery cost of:				
Hospital	7,665	7,518	8,688	1,951
Practitioner services	1,342	1,472	1,234	1,161
Medications	1,138	1,600	1,003	657
Supplies	1,351	1,708	1,468	613
Wheelchairs	1,306	1,785	846	638
Personal assistance	11,464	20,178	3,537	2,506
Home modifications	376	420	342	294
Vehicle modifications	571	902	297	122
Total annual recurring costs	25,213	35,583	17,415	7,942

(From Direct Costs of Spinal Cord Injury in *Spinal Cord Injury: An Analysis of Medical and Social Costs* by Berkowitz, O'Leary, Kruse & Harvey, p. 74. Demos Medical Publishing, 1998. Reprinted with permission.)

SPINAL CORD INJURY COSTS STUDIES SUMMARY

It is obvious that the direct costs and related expenses associated with SCI can be significant over the person's lifetime. Although the actual average costs identified in the studies by Berkowitz et al. (1992, 1998) and DeVivo et al. (1995a) often showed considerable variation in some of the categories identified, the overall distribution of expenses were fairly consistent between studies. Table B-5 provides a summary of the distribution of costs for the major expense categories identified in these investigations.

These findings are intended as a guide to better understand the relative distribution of resource needs in the various categories of the LCP and cannot be applied to the individual case for costs projections. At best, these data can be viewed as baseline estimates that must be adjusted to reflect the individual impact of SCI on a needs-driven (opposed to cost-driven), case-by-case basis.

Table B-5. Cost Studies Summary: Distribution of Annual Charges Incurred after First Year Post-SCI

Category	PSA-DIS Study	Model Systems Study	Berkowitz *et al.* Study
Health Care/Follow-up	15.9%	5.6%	14.6%
Durable Medical Equipment	6.1	5.6	8.0
Medications/Supplies	12.7	9.2	16.0
Attendant Care/ Household Assistance	43.1	49.0	31.6
Environmental Modifications	—	3.3	5.2
Rehospitalizations	20.9	21.8	24.6
Institutional Care	1.3	3.1	—
Other	—	2.4	—

IMPLICATIONS FOR LIFE CARE PLANNING

There is a good deal of consistency between these various costs studies in terms of the nature of expense categories associated with the highest costs. Clearly, acute care and initial rehabilitation takes the greatest portion of expended resources during the first year post-SCI. Home modifications and durable medical equipment are also substantial expenses during the first year after onset of injury. During subsequent years, attendant care and household assistance are associated with the highest portion of expenditures among those with cervical level injuries. Rehospitalizations, medications and supplies, and upgrade of durable medical equipment also account for substantial resources after year one.

There are several significant limitations in the studies of costs after SCI, both to the general SCI case and to individual cases that are the focus of a LCP. In terms of the general SCI case, the Berkowitz et al. (1992, 1998) and DeVivo et al. (1995a) studies deal solely with charges and do not account for cases where needs are not being met because of limited resources. Therefore, the only time that charges are an accurate reflection of a cost associated in the general SCI case is when they are independent of resources (i.e., in cases where cost is not taken into account when making treatment decisions). The degree to which charges reflect needs varies dramatically, with some individuals having only the most essential needs met. It is not unusual to see cases where there is no insurance and no family support. Often, people are not even able to get into their wheelchairs because they have no one to assist them. These cases are averaged into the estimates. This limits applicability to the general case.

The situation in any individual case is much more problematic. Average charges are never likely to be an accurate indicator of costs associated for a given individual (because of the problems cited above). In addition, there are regional differences in the costs of particular items, particularly attendant care, because of differences in the labor market. States may also differ in terms of regulations regarding who may provide certain types of services. For example, some states mandate that only licensed or registered nurses perform intermittent catheterizations. This obviously increases the costs dramatically for individuals who need this procedure. Other problems with average charges are equally problematic. For example, costs for vocational rehabilitation may vary from nothing to completion of education through the doctoral level for others. Whereas research on costs (charges) invariably reflects a compromise between needs-based and resource-based decisions, the LCP should reflect only an assessment of needs. Consequently, costs research should never be used as the basis for projecting the costs of goods and services for a LCP.

In summary, data from the foregoing studies are not intended to apply to the individual LCP case for injury outcome or cost projection purposes. However, these data may provide the life care planner with a better understanding of the long-term consequences of disability and of specific service utilization categories and needs. This may help to show how costs may be distributed across categories so that a more accurate planning of resources can be provided for in the subsequent life care planning process. It is important for the life care planner to be aware that the cost estimates described in the various studies presented may grossly underestimate certain service need categories, such as outpatient services, attendant care services, and vocational rehabilitation services, when projected for the specific geographic region in which the individual resides.

The life care planner also must remember that, as persons with SCI age categories such as durable medical equipment needs, attendant care needs, the rate of rehospitalizations, or the need for extended facility care services may change. When rehospitalizations are accounted for in the LCP, it is necessary to reduce nonhospitalization-related costs during that time period. For example, if an annual seven-day rehospitalization is projected, then attendant care may need to be projected over a 51 week period annually unless other special needs circumstances are indicated — continued need for some portion of attendant care or homemaker services while the individual is hospitalized. Further, these cost figures do not represent any indirect costs that the person with SCI might experience in terms of reduction or elimination of work or other activity. These costs can be quite substantial and are relevant to actual loss for both the individual as well as other family members (Berkowitz et al., 1992). Consequently, it is imperative that the LCP be an individualized, needs-driven plan dictated by the onset of disability, with the focus on optimizing functional potential and independence through the process of aging with disability.

APPENDIX C

FIM™ Instrument

To more fully describe the impact of SCI on the individual and to monitor/evaluate progress associated with treatment, a standard measure of daily life activities is necessary (ASIA, 1996). Although there are a number of measures of functional independence (Hamilton, Granger, Sherwin, Zielezny, & Tashman, 1987), the instrument selected for inclusion in the National SCI Database—the FIM™ instrument—is currently the most widely used disability measure within rehabilitation medicine (Consortium for Spinal Cord Medicine, 1999a; Dijkers & Yavuzer, 1999; Ditunno et al., 1995; Hall, Cohen, Wright, Call, & Werner, 1999).

The FIM instrument was developed by a task force appointed in 1983 by the American Congress of Rehabilitation Medicine and the American Academy of Physical Medicine and Rehabilitation to develop a uniform method of documenting the severity of an individual's disability and medical rehabilitation outcomes (Hamilton et al., 1987; Heinemann, Linacre, Wright, Hamilton, & Granger, 1993).

The FIM instrument is an outcome assessment tool designed to measure the extent of disability and the need for assistance. Because it measures objective tasks and focuses on the burden of care, it is also capable of detecting changes in function over time as individuals with SCI age and their independence decreases (Mentor & Hudson, 1995). The American Spinal Injury Association (ASIA) International Standards for Neurological and Functional Classification of Spinal Cord Injury (1996) incorporates the FIM instrument as the disability measure to complement the impairment measures.

The FIM instrument has proved to be a reliable, easily administered measure of a person's ability to perform 18 basic activities of daily living (see Table C-1). Each activity is evaluated in terms of independence functioning using a seven-point scale (see Table C-2). A score of 1 indicates complete dependence and a score of 7 indicates complete independence. Scores below 6 require another person for supervision or assistance.

The FIM total score (summed across all items) estimates the impact of disability in terms of safety and dependence on others and/or technological devices. The profile of area scores and item scores pinpoints the specific aspects of daily living that have been most affected by SCI.

A derivation of the FIM instrument, called the WeeFIM®, was developed to measure severity of disability in children six months to seven years of age. The WeeFIM instrument can be used to determine the amount of assistance that is required beyond that considered to be developmentally appropriate, according to the age of the child. It is now being implemented in inpatient and outpatient pediatric programs.

The FIM/WeeFIM instruments can be of assistance in the life care planning process. Through ratings by the individual's therapist(s) and other health care providers, the FIM instrument can be used to demonstrate a relationship between disability and impairment. It can also aid the life care planner/case manager in assisting the individual with SCI to monitor functional gains and predict outcomes, plan service and equipment needs, estimate level of care requirements, and indicate changes in functional status through the individual's lifetime. A FIM score of 5 or less in any one area requires the life care planner to address that functional

Table C-1. The 18 FIM™ Performance Items

Area	Item
Self-Care	A. Eating
	B. Grooming
	C. Bathing
	D. Dressing — Upper Body
	E. Dressing — Lower Body
	F. Toileting
Sphincter Control	G. Bladder Management
	H. Bowel Management
Transfers	I. Bed, Chair, Wheelchair
	J. Toilet
	K. Tub, Shower
Locomotion	L. Walk/WheelChair
	M. Stairs
Communication	N. Comprehension Auditory, Visual, Both
	O. Expression Vocal, Nonvocal, Both
Social Cognition	P. Social Interaction
	Q. Problem Solving
	R. Memory

(FIM™ instrument. Copyright© 1997 Uniform Data System for Medical Rehabilitation (UDS_{MR}), a division of UB Foundation Activities, Inc. All rights reserved. Used with permission of UDS_{MR}.)

Table C-2. The Seven FIM™ Rating Levels of Independence of Functioning

Degree of Independence	Level of Functioning
INDEPENDENT	Another person is not required for the activity (NO HELPER).
7	*Complete Independence* — All of the tasks described as making up the activity are typically performed safely, without modification, assistive devices, or aids, and within a reasonable amount of time.
6	*Modified Independence* — One or more of the following may be true: the activity requires an assistive device; the activity takes more than reasonable time; or there are safety (risk) considerations.
DEPENDENT	Individual requires another person for either supervision or physical assistance in order for the activity to be performed, or it is not performed (REQUIRES HELPER).

Modified Dependence — The individual expends half (50%) or more of the effort. The levels of assistance required are:

5	*Supervision or Set Up* — Individual requires no more help than standby, cuing, or coaxing, without physical contact, or helper sets up needed items or applies orthoses or assistive/adaptive devices.
4	Minimal Contact Assistance — Individual requires no more help than touching, and expends 75% or more of the effort.
3	Moderate Assistance — Individual requires more help than touching, or expends half (50%) or more (but less than 75%) of the effort.

Complete Dependence — The individual expends less than half (less than 50%) of the effort. Maximal or total assistance is required, or the activity is not performed. The levels of assistance required are:

2	*Maximal Assistance* — Individual expends less than 50% of the effort, but at least 25%.
1	*Total Assistance* — Individual expends less than 25% of the effort.

(FIM™ instrument. Copyright© 1997 Uniform Data System for Medical Rehabilitation (UDS_{MR}), a division of UB Foundation Activities, Inc. All rights reserved. Used with permission of UDS_{MR}.)

deficit with an appropriate level of attendant care services. Further, in spite of the severe disability that many people with tetraplegia have they should be educated and trained to effectively direct their care by an attendant, whom they will manage.

IMPLICATIONS FOR LIFE CARE PLANNING AND CASE MANAGEMENT

In using the FIM instrument with SCI individuals, it should be kept in mind that the instrument was developed for the disabled population in general, and samples those areas of activity that have been found to be related to impairment among diverse disability groups. Although basic issues of reliability and validity have been explored by its developers, FIM's validity as an instrument for precisely gauging changed function with all SCI subpopulations has yet to be demonstrated empirically. For example, it is not yet clear that the self-care items sensitively gauge changes in self-care function experienced by people with tetraplegia during the course of rehabilitation. Subtle changes in upper extremity function that may have a significant effect on task performance may not be detected. Further, the reliability estimates for the communication and social cognition areas are lower than for other areas assessed. In addition, there is a need for some technical refinements with respect to assessment criterion for bladder, bowel, locomotion, comprehension, expression, and stair climbing (Granger & Fiedler, 1997). Despite these caveats, the use of the FIM instrument is recommended because of its relative ease of use. The instrument reflects functional issues of importance to SCI, and guidelines for its use have been carefully developed (ASIA, 1996, pp. 22–23).

The FIM instrument must be completed by a trained clinician familiar with its definitions and use. Otherwise, the results may be inaccurate and consequently could be detrimental to the life care planning process. Specific instructions for use of the FIM/WeeFIM instruments may be obtained directly from the developers of these instruments. The *Guide for The Uniform Data Set for Medical Rehabilitation (including the FIM*™ *instrument), Version 5.1* (1997) and the *WeeFIM System*^{SM} *Clinical Guide: Version 5* (1998) may be requested from Uniform Data System for Medical Rehabilitation, 232 Parker Hall, 3435 Main Street, Buffalo, NY, 14214-3007; (716) 829-2076. fax (716) 829-2080.

APPENDIX D

Functional Outcomes of Spinal Cord Injury

The following table provides some general guidelines for the reasonable predicted levels in functional independence in activities of daily living skills with respective levels of SCI, given optimal circumstances. Although individual functional capabilities vary, the primary determinant of expected functional outcomes relate to motor function (Consortium for Spinal Cord Medicine, 1999a; Winkler & Weed, 1999; Yarkony et al., 1987; Yarkony, 1994a).

Table D-1. Functional Rehabilitation Outcomes for Individuals with Spinal Cord Injury

Level of Injury	Functional Abilities
C1–C3	*Self-Care* Eating: Complete dependence. Grooming: Complete dependence. Bathing: Complete dependence. Dressing: Complete dependence. Toileting: Complete dependence. *Pressure Relief* Dependence or switch-operated power recline or tilt in space system. *Orthotic Devices* Ventilator dependent *Sphincter Control* Bladder Management: Complete dependence. Bowel Management: Complete dependence. *Mobility* Bed Mobility: Complete dependence; switch-operated power hospital bed. Wheelchair Transfers: Complete dependence. Toilet/Tub/Shower Transfers: Complete dependence. *Locomotion* Walk/Wheelchair: Not applicable/Modified independence, assistance in power recline/tilt wheelchair with head, chin, or breath control. *Transportation* Dependent on others in accessible van with lift or accessible public transportation.
C4	*Self-Care* Eating: Modified independence. May be able to feed self. Use of balanced forearm orthosis (BFOs) with universal cuff and adapted utensils indicated; drinks with long straw after set up. Grooming: Complete dependence. Bathing: Complete dependence. Dressing: Complete dependence. Toileting: Complete dependence.

(continued overleaf)

Table D-1. (*continued*)

Level of Injury	Functional Abilities
	Pressure Relief Independent in power recline/tilt wheelchair; dependent in bed or manual wheelchair. *Orthotic Devices* May require ventilator; upper extremity; external powered orthosis, dorsal cockup splint; BFOs. *Sphincter Control* Bladder Management: Complete dependence. Bowel Management: Complete dependence. *Mobility* Bed Mobility: Complete dependence; power hospital bed. Wheelchair Transfers: Complete dependence. Toilet/Tub/Shower Transfers: Complete dependence. *Locomotion* Walk/Wheelchair: Not applicable/Modified independence in pneumatic or chin control-driven power wheelchair with powered reclining feature. *Transportation* Dependent on others in accessible van with lift; unable to drive.
C5	*Self-Care* Eating: Modified independence with specially adapted equipment for feeding after set up. Grooming: Modified independence with specially adapted equipment for grooming after set up. Bathing: Complete dependence. Dressing: Modified independence with upper extremity dressing; complete dependence for lower extremity dressing. Toileting: Complete dependence. *Pressure Relief* Modified independence, may require assistance. *Orthotic Devices* Upper extremity; external powered orthosis, dorsal cockup splint, BFOs. *Sphincter Control* Bladder Management: Complete dependence. Bowel Management: Complete dependence. *Mobility* Bed Mobility: Complete dependence with assistance by others and by equipment; power hospital bed. Wheelchair Transfers: Complete dependence with assistance of one person with or without transfer board. Toilet/Tub/Shower Transfers: Complete dependence with assistance by others and with equipment. *Locomotion* Walk/Wheelchair: Not Applicable/Modified independence in power wheelchair indoors and outdoors; short distances in manual wheelchair with modified rims indoors. *Transportation* Independent driving van with highly specialized equipment.
C6	*Self-Care* Eating: Modified independence with equipment; drinks from glass. Grooming: Modified independence with equipment. Bathing: Independent in upper and lower extremity bathing with equipment. Dressing: Modified independence with upper extremity dressing; modified dependence with assistance needed for lower extremity dressing. Toileting: Dependence/Modified independence.

Table D-1. (*continued*)

Level of Injury	Functional Abilities
	Pressure Relief Independent. *Orthotic Devices* Wrist-driven orthosis. *Sphincter Control* Bladder Management: Complete dependence. Bowel Management: Complete dependence. *Mobility* Bed Mobility: Dependence/ Modified independence with equipment; power bed may be needed. Wheelchair Transfers: Dependence/Modified independence with transfer board. Toilet/Tub/Shower Transfers: Dependence/Modified independence with equipment. *Locomotion* Walk/Wheelchair: Not applicable/Modified independence with manual wheelchair with modified rims indoors; assistance needed outdoors. Much more functional with power wheelchair. *Transportation* Independent driving in specially adapted van with lift.
C7–C8	*Self-Care* Eating: Modified independence/Independent. Grooming: Modified independence with equipment. Bathing: Modified independence with equipment. Dressing: Modified independence in upper and lower extremity dressing with equipment. Toileting: Modified independence/Independent. *Pressure Relief* Independent. *Orthotic Devices* None. *Sphincter Control* Bladder Management: Modified independence. Bowel Management: Modified independence. *Mobility* Bed Mobility: Independent. Wheelchair Transfers: Modified independence with or without transfer board including car except to/from floor with assistance. Toilet/Tub/Shower Transfers: Independent. *Locomotion* Walk/Wheelchair: Not applicable/Independent manual wheelchair indoors. Much more functional with power wheelchair. *Transportation* Independent driving in car with hand controls or specially adapted van.
T1–T9	*Self-Care* Eating: Independent. Grooming: Independent. Bathing: Independent. Dressing: Independent. Toileting: Independent. *Pressure Relief* Independent. *Orthotic Devices* Knee-ankle-foot orthoses (KAFO) with forearm crutches or walker. *Sphincter Control* Bladder Management: Independent. Bowel Management: Independent. *Mobility* Bed Mobility: Independent.

(*continued overleaf*)

Table D-1. (*continued*)

Level of Injury	Functional Abilities
	Wheelchair Transfers: Independent. Toilet/Tub/Shower Transfers: Independent. *Locomotion* Walk/Wheelchair: Exercise only not functional with orthoses; modified independence requires physical assist or guarding. *Transportation* Independent driving in car with hand controls or specially adapted van.
T10–L1	*Self-Care* Eating: Independent. Grooming: Independent. Bathing: Independent. Dressing: Independent. Toileting: Independent. *Pressure Relief* Independent. *Orthotic Devices* KAFO or ankle-foot orthoses (AFO) with forearm crutches. *Sphincter Control* Bladder Management: Independent. Bowel Management: Independent. *Mobility* Bed Mobility: Independent. Wheelchair Transfers: Independent. Toilet/Tub/Shower Transfers: Independent. *Locomotion* Walk/Wheelchair: Modified independence, potential for independent functional ambulation indoors with orthoses; some individuals have potential for stairs using railing. *Transportation* Independent in driving car with hand controls or specially adapted van.
L2–S5	*Self-Care* Eating: Independent. Grooming: Independent. Bathing: Independent. Dressing: Independent. Toileting: Independent. *Pressure Relief* Independent. *Orthotic Devices* KAFO or AFO with forearm crutches or canes. *Sphincter Control* Bladder Management: Independent. Bowel Management: Independent. *Mobility* Bed Mobility: Independent. Wheelchair Transfers: Independent. Toilet/Tub/Shower Transfers: Independent. *Locomotion* Walk/Wheelchair: Community ambulation; modified independence indoors and outdoors with orthoses; AFO with forearm crutches or canes. *Transportation* Independent driving car with hand controls.

Assumptions:
(1) The SCI is motor complete, i.e., there is no useful movement below the level of injury.
(2) There are no significant constraining factors, e.g., obesity, extreme age, pre-existing disabilities, or other medical conditions.
(3) Appropriate attendant care is available.
(Adapted from Rehabilitation of the Spinal Cord Injured Patient by W.E. Staas, et al., in J.A. DeLisa (Ed.) *Rehabilitation Medicine: Principles and Practice* (2nd ed., pp. 898–899). J.B. Lippincott, 1993. Adapted with permission.)

IMPLICATIONS FOR LIFE CARE PLANNING

The above table represents a rather optimistic view of what may be accomplished by individuals with a given level of injury. As with nearly all aspects of SCI, there is tremendous individual variation in the extent to which any given individual may achieve these goals. Factors that may relate to lowered expectations include age, associated injuries, comorbidities, pre-injury fitness level, weight, adequacy of training, and value placed on physical independence. The last factor has often been equated to client "motivation," but it must be noted any given individual may have "competing motivations," such as attending school or work, that may place additional demands on him or her. It also must be noted that as individuals reach 15 or more years post-injury they experience many physiologic changes related to aging, including diminished physical independence (Menter & Hudson, 1995). Therefore, the ultimate degree of physical independence achieved depends on a number of individual factors, other than injury level, and will change over time. These factors must to be evaluated and addressed in the LCP.

APPENDIX E

Aging with Spinal Cord Injury

Long-term follow-up data suggests that people with SCI tend to "age faster," and that they experience some of the changes commonly associated with the normal aging process at an earlier age (Gerhart, Bergstrom, Charlifue, Menter, & Whiteneck, 1993; Gerhart, Charlifue, Menter, Weitzenkamp, & Whiteneck, 1997; Pentland, McColl, & Rosenthal, 1995; Winkler & Weed, 1999). Menter (1990) has developed a model of how aging may affect or impact the total function of individuals with SCI. Conceptually, this model identifies three phases that follow the onset of SCI: acute restoration, maintenance, and decline (see Figure E-1).

The acute restoration (acute rehabilitation) phase is described as the process by which an individual with SCI moves from having virtually no function immediately following injury to regaining the maximum amount of function consistent with the level of neurologic injury. Thus, a person with paraplegia will achieve modified independence in locomotion using a wheelchair and/or braces. An individual with low-level tetraplegia (C5–C8) may become largely independent in feeding, grooming, communication, and propelling a power wheelchair, but will likely still require assistance with transfers, dressing, and pushing a manual wheelchair outdoors. This phase is usually completed within two years following SCI and includes inpatient followed by outpatient and/or home-based rehabilitation (Menter, 1990; Menter, 1993).

The maintenance phase is identified as a variable but lengthy phase during which the person maintains the level of function that was established following injury and successful rehabilitation. In general, an individual's level of function will usually remain stable for 15 to 20 years. During this time the person with SCI typically completes education, begins or resumes his or her career, and returns to or begins a family (Menter, 1993).

The final phase, decline, occurs when the gradual onset of the physiologic aging process and the degenerative effects of an overuse syndrome combine and interfere with function (Stiens, Haselkorn, Peters, & Goldstein, 1996). A decline in

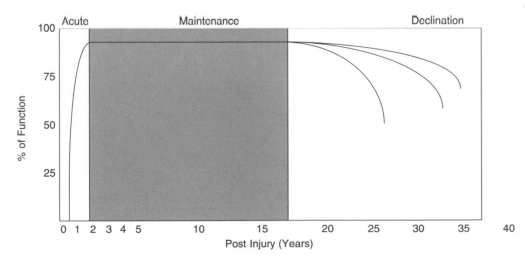

Figure E-1. Model of Aging and Spinal Cord Injury. (From Issues of Aging with Spinal Cord Injury by R.R. Menter in *Aging with Spinal Cord Injury* by G.G. Whiteneck, et al., p. 6. Demo Medical Publishing, 1993. Reprinted with permission.)

muscle strength, flexibility, joint range of motion, respiratory reserve, cardiovascular capacity (Stiens, Johnson, & Lyman, 1995), or an increase in skin breakdowns and/or other complications interfere with and decrease the overall function of the body. The rate of functional decline varies among individuals (Consortium for Spinal Cord Medicine, 1999a; Menter, 1990; Menter, 1993).

As individuals with SCI reach 20, 30, or 40 years post-injury, many face significant medical issues and complications, and functional declines as a consequence of disability. For individuals with tetraplegia, these changes can occur as early as in their 40s (Gerhart, Charlifue, Menter, Weitzenkamp, & Whiteneck, 1997; Pentland, McColl, & Rosenthal, 1995). For people with lower-level SCI, these changes might occur as early as in their 50s (Gerhart et al., 1993). It is important, however, to keep in mind that not everyone with SCI ages in the same way or have the same experiences.

Factors relating to the aging process include: 1) genetics; 2) trauma; 3) lifestyle; 4) adaptation to stress; and, 5) sociologic role (Menter, 1993). These factors must be taken into consideration when attempting to address the aging-related issues of a given individual with SCI. A person's family health history, lifestyle, and how well he or she deals with stress affects his or her health in old age. The strength or weakness of relationships with spouses and significant others, children, parents, and friends also affects the individual's later years, as well how much physical and emotional trauma he or she experienced at injury.

Other factors to consider for how individuals age depend on the level and severity of the neurologic defect and age at onset of injury. Injury at a particular stage in life creates a different set of demands, expectations, and resource needs. When the onset of SCI occurs late in life, the challenges typically are more difficult (Alander, Parke, & Stauffer, 1997; RTC/IL, 1994). In general, the older an individual is at onset of injury, the lower the level of functional independence he or she can be expected to achieve. In addition, the maintenance phase is correspondingly shorter the older the individual is at onset of SCI.

These aging-related changes have definite implications in life care planning for the individual's long-term needs. The further decline in levels of independence may substantially increase the need for attendant care and assistive aids, household assistance, and rehospitalizations as a result of increased SCI-related complications (DeVivo, et al., 1992). In addressing aging-related health care needs, the life care planner must focus on a broader primary and geriatric care orientation. This will involve an interdisciplinary team approach that may include various medical specialities, such as nursing, psychology, physical therapy, occupational therapy, and social services.

A detailed discussion of topics related to aging and SCI from a multiplicity of perspectives may be found in the text from the Craig Hospital, Rehabilitation Research and Training Center (RRTC) project, *Aging with Spinal Cord Injury* (1993) by Demos Medical Publishing.

IMPACT OF AGING ON SPINAL CORD INJURY

The normal aging of body systems creates special concerns for individuals with SCI. The following section was excerpted in large part from *SCI & Aging* by the University of Kansas, Research and Training Center on Independent Living (1994) and provides a brief overview of how the various parts of the body age in the normal individual and how these age-related changes can affect people with SCI. Also included is how the aging process may impact a person's psychosocial adjustment and how these changes can affect people with SCI.

NERVOUS SYSTEM

Normal Aging Process

Response times increase with age, the peripheral nerves conduct messages more slowly, and individuals become less coordinated, offering one explanation as to why older people fall so frequently. The nervous system also controls temperature regulation, and many people may feel unusually cold or hot even when room temperature is at normal levels. Damage to the nervous system may affect the body's immune system, which protects the body from infections of the skin, lungs, and urinary tract. Stress and depression may also affect the immune system and make the body less able to resist infection.

SCI Concerns

Pain, which is transmitted by the nervous system, is common in many people with SCI and is reported to increase with age (Jackson & Groomes, 1994; Little, 1998). Older people with SCI also tire more easily, have increased loss of sensation, experience greater spasticity, and lose some of their available motor control (Gerhart et al., 1993; Lammertse, 1993). As they age, people who also sustained a brain injury at the time of their spinal injury may experience *dementia*, a deterioration in their mental abilities. Spinal cord cysts (syringomyelia) near the original injury site are also common, and may cause pain, spasticity, and decreased function (Bursell, Little, & Stiens, 1999; Michals & Ramsey, 1996; Umbach & Heilporn, 1991).

RESPIRATORY SYSTEM

Normal Aging Process

With age, the lungs lose some of their elasticity, and the muscles that help the chest cavity to fill with air become stiffer and weaker. Consequently, an older person has a harder time getting a full breath and, with reduced breathing, is less likely to fight off colds and other chest infections. Less oxygen in the bloodstream also lowers a person's energy level and makes it more difficult to get through a normal day. When people do not get enough oxygen they can become dizzy, mentally confused, and disoriented.

SCI Concerns

Respiratory problems are a concern in a wide range of people with SCI (Little, 1998; Ragnarsson, Hall, Wilmot, & Carter, 1995). Those with high-level SCIs have reduced lung capacity (McKinley et al., 1999), and as they age they need increased help with coughing and draining fluids from their lungs. Lungs that are not fully drained of fluids and mucous are more prone to infections. People with tetraplegia who are ventilator-dependent are also prone to infection at the air tube insertion site.

Many people with SCI have difficulty coughing and clearing their lungs; some have muscle spasms in their chest walls that keep them from taking a full breath. Those who are overweight may tend to wheeze and have shortness of breath when engaging in activities of daily living. Sleep apnea is also a common development in

SCI that increases with age (Wilmot & Hall, 1993). In some cases cysts that develop on the spinal cord may impair lung function. An infection anywhere in the body can potentially lead to respiratory failure, particularly in individuals with tetraplegia and high paraplegia. The development of kyphosis and increasing spasticity can also lead to decreased respiratory system functioning. Respiratory complications are one of the leading causes of death for people with SCI (DeVivo, Krause, & Lammertse, 1999).

MUSCULOSKELETAL SYSTEM

Normal Aging Process

The normal process of aging causes the body to stiffen, particularly in the muscles and joints. With age, the tough cartilage tissue that protects and cushions the bones thins and become less supple. Tendons and ligaments also stiffen and weaken with age. They tear or bruise more easily and take longer to heal. As people age, their muscles become smaller and painful arthritis can develop in the joints.

Osteoporosis, a disease that makes bones weak, brittle, and at higher risk for fractures, is also more common in older people. The bones weaken as they lose important minerals such as calcium.

These changes in the bones, muscles, and joints can reduce range of motion and can make a person feel stiff and move with greater difficulty. These changes also may lead to fractures, dislocations, and deteriorating function.

SCI Concerns

People with SCI already face many challenges from their bones, joints, and muscles, and the natural process of aging makes them more prone to fatigue, pain, and injury. People who use wheelchairs or crutches rely heavily on their shoulder, elbow, and wrist joints. Overuse of these joints will cause dislocations; tears in the ligaments, muscles, and tendons; or carpal tunnel syndrome, a compression of the nerves in the wrist (Blankstein, Shmueli, Weingarten, Engel, & Ohry, 1985; Bursell et al., 1999; Goldstein, 1998; Sie, Waters, Adkins, & Gellman, 1992). As people with SCI age, they must be careful not to overuse their joints and muscles. They may have to take more time to perform their tasks of daily living and to rest more during and after each task. Further, this decrease in function may significantly change their ability to be independent and care for themselves (Waters, Sie, & Adkins, 1993).

The joints of people with SCI may already be in pain or have decreased range of motion due to *heterotopic ossification*, calcium deposits in the tissues around the joints, or from contractures, caused by a shortening in the muscle tendons (Goldstein, 1998). This shortening causes the joints to tighten and pull in. The arthritis that comes naturally with aging will most likely add to their discomfort.

Most older people have some level of osteoporosis, a loss of bone mass. However, many people with SCI will develop osteoporosis within six months of sustaining a SCI, regardless of their age (Garland, Stewart, & Adkins, 1992; Ragnarsson & Sell, 1981). Osteoporosis in people with SCI results from an absence of weight-bearing stress on the bone and a lack of muscle pull on the bone that comes with movement and likely from extensive hormonal changes. Without the natural stress from this weight and muscle pull, the calcium leaves the bone. The dissolved calcium may irritate the kidneys and bladder and can increase the risk for infections in the urinary tract and renal calculi. The amount of bone loss can be high and the bone that is lost cannot be regained (Szollar, Martin, Parthemore, Sartoris, & Deftos, 1997). Anyone with osteoporosis is at high risk for broken bones. Fractures are common among people with SCI, particularly to the lower extremities (McKinley et al., 1999; Nance, Schryvers, Leslie, Ludwig, Krahn, & Uebelhart, 1999).

CARDIOVASCULAR SYSTEM

Normal Aging Process

Heart disease is the number one cause of death among individuals older than 65. With aging there is decreased cardiac output, increased arrthymias, and increasing coronary artery disease. Some heart troubles are genetic or common in families. Others are caused by such things as smoking, stress, high blood pressure, obesity, and lack of exercise, all of which may be changeable risk factors.

SCI Concerns

Cardiovascular problems are a leading cause of death in people with SCI (Bauman, Raza, Spungen, & Machac, 1994; DeVivo, Black, & Stover, 1993; DeVivo, Krause, & Lammertse, 1999; Geisler, Jousse, Wynne-Jones, & Breithaupt, 1983; Go, DeVivo, & Richards, 1995; Krum, Howe, & Brown, 1992; Ragnarsson, 1993; Ragnarsson et al., 1995; Samsa, Patrick, & Feussner, 1993; Stiens, 1998; Stiens et al., 1995; Whiteneck, 1992). Many people who have been injured lead inactive lives and this sedentary lifestyle can affect the heart. The risks for cardiovascular disease may be magnified in people with SCI. Contributing risk factors include physical inactivity, low high-density lipoprotein cholesterol levels (HDL-C), proportionally increased body fat, and an increased incidence of glucose intolerance (Bauman & Spungen, 1994; Bauman et al., 1992; Stiens, 1998a; Stampfer, Sacks, Salvini, Willett, & Hennekens, 1991).

People with SCI also are at risk for irregular heart beats or blockage in the arteries. Reduced blood flow and high or low normal blood pressure also are common. Low blood pressure and an irregular heart beat are more common in those with a T5 or higher injury. People with SCI at or above the level of T6 are also at risk for *autonomic dysreflexia*, characterized by a sudden onset of high blood pressure, slow heartbeat, sweating, and severe headache (Consortium for Spinal Cord Medicine, 1997a; Goetz, 1998). Another cardiovascular system problem seen in people with SCI is deep venous thrombosis, a clotting of blood in the deep veins of the legs (Ragnarsson et al., 1995).

GASTROINTESTINAL SYSTEM

Normal Aging Process

Many older people suffer from constipation that can lead to hemorrhoids or even a bowel obstruction. Their stomach produces less acid, so their digestion slows. They are prone to stones in their gall bladders, and weaker anal muscles may lead to incontinence. The risk of colon cancer also increases with age.

SCI Concerns

Aging adds to the GI problems people with SCI already have. About one-quarter of those with SCI already complain about lower bowel problems, and one-fifth have serious problems with evacuating their bowels (Stiens, Bierner-Bergman & Goetz, 1997; Stone, Nino-Murcia, Wolfe, & Perkash, 1990). Problems with the GI tract can be serious and can cause death.

The most common GI problems in people with SCI are stool impaction, distention or swelling of the colon, abdominal bloating, and prolonged or incomplete emptying of the bowel (Cardenas, Farrell-Roberts, Sipski, & Rubner, 1995; Cosman, Stone, &

Perkash, 1993; Stiens, 1998b; Stiens, Bierner-Bergman, & Goetz, 1997) . Gallstones and hemorrhoids also are common (Moonka, Stiens, Eubank, & Stelzner, 1999).

GENITOURINARY SYSTEM

Normal Aging Process

The bladder shrinks with age, so an older person may have to urinate more often. The bladder muscles also weaken; therefore it is harder for older people to hold their urine or, conversely, to completely empty their bladders. Bladders that never empty completely are prone to infection. Weaker bladder sphincter muscles also can lead to urine leakage or incontinence.

SCI Concerns

In the past, urinary tract infections and kidney failure were major causes of death for people with SCI (Goetz & Little, 1998; Lanig, 1993). Better health services, antibiotics, and more information about how to manage bladder control (McKinley et al., 1999) have reduced death from urinary problems during the first 15 years after injury to just 2.7 percent (Lanig, 1993). Recurring bladder infections may lead to renal failure and a need for dialysis. For unexplained reasons, people with SCI also have a higher incidence of bladder cancer than the general population (Gerhart & Lammertse, 1997). They also experience more bladder and kidney stones.

As the bladder ages, urine leakage may become more common. Older people with SCI must be cautious of leaking and wetness because moisture can easily lead to skin breakdown and infections. People also tend to drink less water as they age. Fewer fluids will cause the urine to become concentrated, which can lead to bladder infections and urinary stones.

SKIN

Normal Aging Process

Aging skin is not a health problem but it can be a health concern. As skin ages it becomes dryer and thinner. It loosens and sags in places where once it was smooth and taut. Dry, thin, and loose skin protects less, blisters and injures more easily, and heals more slowly.

SCI Concerns

All older people should take care of their skin, but people with SCI must take especially good care of theirs (Garber, Rintala, Rossi, Hart, & Fuhrer, 1996; McKinley et al., 1999). Older skin has less moisture and elasticity, causing it to be more prone to pressure sores, blisters, cracks, and tears. People with SCI already stress many areas of their skin. Those who sit for long periods in wheelchairs place prolonged pressure on the skin of the back and buttocks. This in turn may present increased difficulty in maintaining sitting time and tolerance. Those who push wheelchairs or who use crutches develop large calluses and sometimes abrasions on the palms of their hands. Skin may also become rubbed or injured during transfers. In older people, these areas will become even more sensitive to tears, blisters, and pressure sores. People with SCI may also experience some incontinence, and skin that is wet for any length of time may be more likely to develop skin breakdown (Yarkony, 1993). Further, scars from previous pressure sores or surgeries may increase the risk of future skin breakdowns as the person with SCI ages.

PSYCHOSOCIAL FUNCTIONING

Normal Aging Process

Depression affects many older people, and they are considered the group most at risk for suicide. Feelings of worthlessness, helplessness, and hopelessness in combination with the biology of aging and a person's medical history and treatments are major factors contributing to depression and suicide among older individuals.

As people age, their body's ability to absorb and dispose of alcohol and other drugs changes. Alcohol is often harmful if mixed with certain prescription or over-the-counter drugs. This can be a problem for people over 65, because they are often heavy users of prescription drugs and over-the-counter medications.

Older people may develop a drinking problem late in life, often because of situational factors, such as retirement, lowered income, failing health, loneliness, or the death of friends or loved ones.

SCI Concerns

SCI is a catastrophic event that affects every aspect of the person's life and requires an enormous adjustment by even the most stable individuals. SCI has been compared to the death of a loved one, or other situations of extreme loss, in terms of the individual's emotional reaction to the event (Krause, 1992a). The loss of movement, sexual function, bowel and bladder functions, and pain are very hard to deal with for many individuals (Widerstrom-Noga, Felipe-Cuervo, Broton, Duncan, & Yezierski, 1999). People with SCI are at risk for depression, substance abuse, and suicide or self-neglect, leading to premature death (Charlifue & Gerhart, 1991; DeVivo, Black, Richards, & Stover, 1991; DeVivo, Black, & Stover, 1993; Dijkers, Buda Abela, Gans, & Gordon, 1995; Elliott & Frank, 1996; Fuhrer, Rintala, Hart, Clearman, & Young, 1993; Heinemann, Doll, Armstrong, Schnoll, & Yarkony, 1991; Kewman & Tate, 1998; Young, Rintala, Rossi, Hart, & Fuhrer, 1995). However, little is currently known about how people with SCI psychologically cope as they grow older and are faced with the complexities of the aging process and disability (Butt & Fitting, 1993). The process of adaptation that is required for individuals with SCI to maintain maximal control of their life and success with their goals is complex and differs for each person (Stiens, Biener-Bergman, & Formal, 1997). Successful adaptation is facilitated by family and peer support, education, assistive devices for independence, and realistic opportunities for participation in relationships and roles in the community.

INCOMPLETE INJURIES

Although longitudinal data indicate that a greater proportion of SCIs result in incomplete or less severe injuries (Berkowitz, Harvey, Greene, & Wilson, 1992; DeVivo, Whiteneck, & Charles, 1995; Ditunno, Cohn, Formal, & Whiteneck, 1995; Go, DeVivo, & Richards, 1995; Stover & Fine, 1986), little research is currently available on the impact of aging with disability for this group of individuals, specifically those who are classified as grade D SCI (ASIA, 1996). Grade D SCI implies that the majority of muscles below the level of injury have some functional use and some degree of walking is typically possible. Although individuals with these types of injury may have much more function initially, preliminary evidence suggests that they may face an ever-changing health profile similar to those with more complete SCIs as they age.

In a study that looked at the short-term consequences of SCI for people with minimal injuries (Frankel D), Gerhart, Johnson, and Whiteneck (1992) found several issues of clinical concern. Analyzing data from a population-based sample of 330 individuals who were registered with the Colorado SCI surveillance program (from 1986 to 1989), 37 percent were classified as Frankel D or E at the time of discharge from acute care hospitalization. Over 75 percent of these individuals were ambulatory without orthoses or devices, and virtually all were physically independent at the time of discharge. However, on follow-up the authors found that over 80 percent of the sample population reported some problem or unmet need. Of the total, 25 percent reported pain issues; 21 percent had orthopedic issues, and 17 percent needed additional surgery; 16 percent had urinary tract problems; and 9 percent reported deterioration in strength or sensation or both. Other issues included bowel problems, gastric problems, complaints of high blood pressure, skin breakdowns, sexual difficulties, depression, and unemployability.

In a subsequent longitudinal investigation on the effects of aging with SCI, Menter and Hudson (1995) looked at 429 individuals enrolled in one of six Model Systems programs. Although age, duration of disability, and extent of neurologic impairment were found to relate to many post-injury complications, people with functionally incomplete SCIs at any level (all Frankel grade D) showed some of the most substantial changes with aging and disability. Pain was found to be a major problem with years post-injury. Menter and Hudson (1995) observed that upper extremity pain increased from a rate of 11.1 percent for those under 30 years of age to 61.1 percent for those over 45. Lower extremity pain (hips, knees, and ankles) went from 33.3 to 77.8 percent for those under 30 and over 45, respectively. This same group of people (Frankel D) also evidenced an increasing need for assistance. Below age 30, virtually none of the Frankel D study sample needed help. However, for those over 45, the authors found 27.8 percent required assistance from others.

Other findings (Hartkopp, Bronnum-Hansen, Seidenschnur, & Biering-Sorensen, 1998) have suggested that individuals who were initially less severely disabled by SCI may also be at more risk for depression, problems with psychosocial adjustment, and suicide than those with more severe levels of injury. As individuals with Frankel D SCI tend to have much shorter acute care hospital stays (DeVivo et al., 1995; Gerhart et al., 1992) and less formal rehabilitation, many may not receive the appropriate supports and health care interventions necessary to allow them to successfully reintegrate their family, social, and vocational roles and anticipate and plan for the long-term needs that many are likely to experience as a consequence of aging.

IMPLICATIONS FOR LIFE CARE PLANNING AND CASE MANAGEMENT

Although most SCIs occur among people who are relatively young, this population is rapidly aging as a result of increasing life expectancy. This trend requires that special attention be given to the aging-related needs of people with SCI. Whereas SCI was once thought to result in a relatively unchanging and static level of physical disability, there is now a growing body of literature which suggests that the process of aging interacts with SCI to compound disability (Currie, Gershkoff, & Cifu, 1993; DeVivo, Shewchuk, Stover, Black, & Go, 1992; Gerhart, Bergstrom, Charlifue, Menter, & Whiteneck, 1993; Menter & Hudson, 1995; Menter et al., 1991). This may require adaptive compensation with changing equipment, attendant care, and environmental needs (Menter & Hudson, 1995; RTC/IL, 1994).

APPENDIX F

Sexuality and Spinal Cord Injury

Sexuality has been defined as the expression of a person's femaleness or maleness through body, personality, dress, and behavior. The context of sexual rehabilitation after SCI includes body image, impairments, socialization, fertility, and role performance (Stiens, Westheimer, & Young, 1997). Sexual adjustment and functioning are major issues for many individuals. The person's sexual readjustment following injury can substantially affect his or her physical and psychosocial well-being (Cole & Cole, 1990; Drench, 1992; Lemon, 1993; McAlonan, 1996; Tepper, 1992). However, the area of sexuality for people who have sustained SCI remains one of confusion to both individuals with SCI and medical practitioners.

SEXUAL FUNCTIONING AND FERTILITY IN MEN WITH SPINAL CORD INJURY

Sexual functioning in men following SCI is impacted by both the level and severity of injury. In general, erection is more common among men who have incomplete injuries, upper motor neuron lesions, and higher level injuries (Griffith et al., 1973). Erections obtained by reflex or external stimulation are typical, while psychogenic erections in response to sexual situations occur only in a minority of men with incomplete or lower SCI (Comarr, 1977; Denil, Dana & Ohl, 1996; Denil, Ohl & Smythe, 1996; Griffith, Tomoko, & Timms, 1973; Martinez-Arizala, & Brackett, 1994).

Historically, treatment of sexual dysfunction in men with SCI has focused on restoration of erectile function (Cardenas et al., 1995). Basically, there are four methods currently available to enhance erection in men with SCI: 1) vacuum and constriction devices; 2) intracavernosal injections and intraurethral suppositories; 3) oral medications; and, 4) penile prothesis. The choice of option depends on the individual with SCI (knowledge of efficacy and safety, personal preference, visual ability and hand function and issues of bladder management), the partner (comfort or need for partner to administer the method), the health care professional (experience and biases), and availability of the option (price, pharmaceutical limitations, etc.) (Elliott, 1999). However, before the individual uses any of these erectile aids, a thorough physical examination is needed by a urologist familiar with the benefits and side effects of each method as related to SCI.

Vacuum Constriction Devices

Vacuum constriction devices have typically been considered the safest, least expensive, and probably the most widely used technique to improve erections for men with SCI (Denil, Ohl & Smythe, 1996; Ducharme & Gill, 1997). The vacuum device consists of a plastic cylinder that is placed over the penis. As a vacuum is generated within it, the penis becomes engorged with blood. Once the erection is achieved, a fitted constricting band is placed at the base of the penis to retain the blood in the penile shaft.

This technique provides satisfactory results in about 70 percent of the men with SCI who try it, and it is totally noninvasive (Denil et al., 1996). In addition, this method has the advantage of being able to be used more than once in a 24-hour period and can also be used to augment erections obtained with oral medications or as a backup technique when other erection enhancement methods have failed (Elliott, 1999). A vacuum pump device is relatively inexpensive and is generally obtained by prescription from a urologist.

There are few complications in using a vacuum constriction device as long as the techniques are carefully followed. The major complications are potential ischemic damage to the penis if the band is left on for over 30 minutes at a time, and blocked ejaculation (Denil et al., 1996; Martinez-Arizala & Brackett, 1994). However, these devices require some degree of manual dexterity. For many men with tetraplegia, the partner must be willing to assist with the procedure (Ducharme, 1999). Some of the concerns people express in using this device is that it requires planning to have the equipment on hand during sexual activity. Also, some couples find the devices intrusive.

Intracavernous Injections and Intraurethral Suppositories

Intracavernous injection of vasoactive drugs is another method for producing erections in men with SCI. Papaverine (smooth-muscle relaxant) is often mixed with other drugs, such as alprostadil and phentolamine (both alpha-blockers) for injection into the corpus cavernosum of the penis to increase blood flow and create an erection (Ducharme, 1999; Elliott, 1999; Sipski, 1997). With proper training and careful administration, side effects are minimal (Cardenas et al., 1995; Ducharme & Gill, 1997). Some of the side effects reported from injection therapy with various drugs have included priapism (painful, persistent erection requiring emergency treatment), dysesthesia (sensations of numbness, tingling, burning, or pain), ecchymosis (bruising), declining erectile quality, seizures, and intracorporeal fibrosis (Bodner, Lindan, Leffler, Kursh, & Resnick, 1987; Ducharme, 1999; Elliott, 1999; Linsenmeyer, 1991; Lloyd & Richards, 1989; Sipski, 1997).

Many men with SCI prefer this method because it is quick and does not involve bulky equipment. The drug works for about 60 to 70 percent of those who use it. Penile injections can only be used once per day, and are typically limited to no more than two or three times a week (Elliott, 1999; Northwest Regional Spinal Cord Injury System, 1996a; Zasler, 1991). Initiating this therapy requires referral to a urologist. Initially, the individual with SCI is given small doses of the pharmacologic agent, and the dose is increased until a satisfactory erection is obtained for intercourse (Earle et al., 1992; Kapoor et al., 1993). Sometimes a mixture of agents is prescribed. Erections should not persist beyond four hours.

The medicated urethral system for erection (MUSE®), an intraurethral suppository approved by the U.S. Food and Drug Administration (FDA) in 1997, is another method of delivering medication to the penis for erections. After urination the man or his partner administers a medicated pellet into the urethra, and the medication is absorbed through the lining of the urethra to the parts of the penis that are responsible for erection. The drug comes in four dosages, is much less invasive than injections, and is relatively safe and simple (Ducharme, 1997). However, preliminary studies suggest that the use of intraurethral suppositories (MUSE) is not as effective as intercavernous therapy for erection quality in men with SCI (Monga, Bernie, & Rajasekaran, 1999; Seftel, Bodner, & Krueger, 1998). Further, because of the route of administration (administered as a small intraurethral pellet into the straightened urethra lubricated with urine), there is a higher risk of the medication becoming systemic, due to venous outflow, and causing hypotension (Bodner, Haas, Krueger, & Seftel, 1999; Elliott, 1999). In general, this method may be easier than the injection method for men with tetraplegia who are able to self-catheterize. MUSE can be used up to two times in a 24-hour period (Elliott, 1999).

Oral Medications

Sildenafil (Viagra®) is an oral medication that was approved by the FDA in 1998, and appears to have a promising role in the treatment of erectile dysfunction for men with SCI who are capable of obtaining reflex erections (Derry et al., 1998; Ducharme, 1999; Glass et al., 1997; Monga et al., 1999). Urologists who are familiar with the drug and have performed early FDA testing believe that this medication will be effective for men with SCI, especially those whose lesions are not in spinal cord areas affecting sexual functioning, that is, lower thoracic or upper sacral levels (Ducharme, 1999). Initial studies using sildenafil in men with SCI demonstrated an ability to produce erections in 64 to 78 percent of individuals (Derry, Glass, & Dinsmore, 1997; Derry et al., 1998; Holmgren, Giuliana, & Hulting, 1998). Although research is limited to date, the most common side effects for men with SCI taking sildenafil were headaches, flushing of the face, indigestion, and visual disturbances (e.g., blurred vision or a blue halo effect).

Sildenafil is contraindicated in men taking nitrates, such as nitroglycerin or related cardiovascular drugs, because the risk for profound hypotension. Further, it should be prescribed with caution for men with SCI who have low baseline blood pressures. The drug is not recommended for individuals with cardiac disease (Ducharme, 1999; Monga et al., 1999). More studies on the use of sildenafil for men with SCI should be forthcoming because of its present popularity. In addition, second-generation forms of Viagra should appear in the near future.

Penile Prosthesis

Penile prostheses have also been used in treatment for erectile dysfunction in men with SCI, although this is no longer considered a treatment of choice (Cardenas et al., 1995; Ducharme, 1999; Elliott, 1999; Sipski, 1997). The rate of serious complications of penile prostheses, such as implant loss due to erosion and infection, appears to be higher in men with SCI (Denil, Ohl, & Smythe, 1996; Dietzen & Lloyd, 1992; Martinez-Arizala & Brackett, 1994; Sipski, 1997). Implants are generally classified as semirigid and inflatable. The inflatable systems seem to work best for men without sensation. Although the semirigid devices are reliable and work well for intercourse, they are also associated with higher rates of erosion problems, in which the implants work their way out through the skin (Collins & Hackler, 1988; Rossier & Fam, 1984). Further, if done in a young man, the penile implant will likely need to be replaced when the life of the prosthesis expires (Elliott, 1999).

The cost for penile prothesis typically ranges from $10,000 or more for the implant and surgery (Northwest Regional Spinal Cord Injury System, 1996a). A certain amount of time is necessary for adjustment after implant because the erections are generally different then before the injury and require practice and time to achieve a level of comfort (Durcharme & Gill, 1997). Penile implants should generally be considered permanent, since later removal can cause serious damage to the erectile tissue in the penis. In addition, because of the destruction of the corpora cavernosa, penile implant procedures preempts the future use of other erection enhancement methods with the exception of the vacuum device.

MALE FERTILITY

Male infertility is common after SCI (Brackett, Nash & Lynne, 1996; Linsenmeyer & Perkash, 1991; Sipski, 1997; Sonksen et al., 1997). As a result, men with SCI rarely father children without medical intervention (Sonksen et al., 1997). However, follow-up studies have shown that many men maintain viable sperm years after injury. Infertility in men with SCI often involves ejaculation dysfunction that creates difficulties in the sperm reaching the uterus or involves poor-quality sperm with low motility (Bors & Comarr, 1960; Sipski, 1997; Sipski & Alexander, 1992). Consequently, the odds of infertility can be substantially reduced through the use of artificial insemination using semen obtained from the individual with injury and fertility drugs for women. Vibratory stimulation and electroejaculation are two techniques found to be successful in addressing ejaculation dysfunction in men with SCI (Linsenmeyer, 1997; Monga et al., 1999; Nehra, Werner, Bastuba, Title, & Oates, 1996; Pryor, LeRoy, Nagel, & Hensleigh, 1995).

Vibratory stimulation causes a reflex action that in many cases allows the man to ejaculate. With this method, a vibrator is placed at the base or *glans* of the penis and stimulation is delivered until an ejaculation is produced. This technique is typically successful in men with SCI above T10 or with incomplete injuries and presence of a neurologically intact lower and lumbosacral cord (Brindley, 1981; Brackett, Nash, & Lynne, 1996; Nehra et al., 1998). The individual with SCI can use this technique at home, under medical supervision and the sperm can then be artificially inseminated by the physician into the woman's uterus. Between 50 to 70 percent of men with SCI above T10 were successful in achieving ejaculation using this technique (Ducharme & Gill, 1997). Although autonomic dysreflexia may be a complication of this procedure, it can be controlled with pretreatment medication.

Electroejaculation involves placing an electrode in the rectum and electrically stimulating the prostate and seminal vesicles. This technique, however, must be performed in a hospital or clinic setting because anoscopy must be performed before and after the electroejaculation (Bennett, Seager, Vasher, & McGuire, 1988). Overall, electroejaculation produces a more consist ejaculation than electrovibration (Cardenas et al., 1995). Studies tend to suggest that when assisted ejaculation procedures are combined with assisted reproductive techniques, that is, intrauterine insemination or fertilization techniques, the pregnancy rate per treatment cycle for SCI couples may approach that of natural procreation in healthy fertile couples (Nehra et al., 1996; Pryor et al., 1995; Sonksen et al., 1997; Spira, 1986). Because semen quality is critical to fertility, it is recommended that couples interested in reproduction after SCI have a semen evaluation conducted by a professional trained to obtain and analyze sperm from men with SCI and educate themselves about the rapidly growing body of work on the topic of reproduction for individuals with SCI (Rutkowski, Middleton, Truman, Hagen, & Ryan, 1995).

SEXUAL FUNCTIONING AND FERTILITY IN WOMEN WITH SPINAL CORD INJURY

Historically, the literature concerning female sexual function after SCI has been quite limited (Harrison, Glass, Owens, & Soni, 1995; Jackson & Wadley, 1999; Kettl et al., 1991; Whipple, Richards, Tepper, & Komisaruk, 1996). Possibly one reason that the effect of SCI on sexual functioning in women has been neglected is that the ratio of males to females with SCI is approximately 4:1; and in part, because the prevailing attitudes in the general public, as well as among clinicians and researchers, has been that women's physiological sexual response is less affected by disability than is that of men (Ray & West, 1984; Warnemuende, 1986; White, Rintala, Hart, & Fuhrer, 1993). In the past, when sexual function of women with SCI was studied, it was often restricted to menstruation, fertility, pregnancy, labor, and delivery (Axel, 1982; Berard, 1989; Carty & Conine, 1988; Charlifue, Gerhart, Menter, Whiteneck, & Manley, 1992; Comarr, 1976; Craig, 1990; Greenspoon & Paul, 1986; Griffith & Trieschmann, 1975; Johnston, 1982; Nosek et al., 1996; Ohry, Peleg, Goldman, David, & Rozin, 1978; Verduyn, 1986).

Orgasm can be defined as the positive experience associated with sexual contact. It is primarily an intracranial experience and is separate from ejaculation and pelvic floor reflex contraction. Recent studies indicate that many women with SCI maintain the capacity for orgasm. Charlifue et al. (1992) in their survey of 231 women with SCI reported that 50 percent were able to experience orgasm since their injuries using genital or combined genital and breast stimulation. Of the study respondents, 72 percent of the women with tetraplegia and 77 percent of those with paraplegia self-reported complete neurologic injuries. Although 69 percent of the women surveyed reported satisfaction with their post-injury sexual experiences, many noted dissatisfaction with the sexual information provided during rehabilitation and wanted more literature, counseling, and peer support.

In a study of 25 women with complete or incomplete SCI, Sipski, Alexander, and Rosen (1995) found that 52 percent were able to achieve orgasm during self- or partner-stimulation, whereas in 1978 the general belief within the medical field was that orgasm was nonexistent after SCI (Fitting, Salisbury, Davies, & Maychin, 1978). Sipski et al. (1995) concluded from their study that a large percentage of women with SCI were able to achieve orgasm regardless of the level or severity of injury. Although no consistent characteristics were identified that would allow prediction of which women with SCI would be able to achieve orgasm, the authors found that those who had achieved orgasm had a higher sex drive and a greater sexual knowledge.

Upon review of literature regarding SCI women and sexuality, it appears that the psychosocial and psychological aspects of sexuality after SCI may present as much of a barrier to a return to pre-injury sexual functioning as do the potential medical problems that complicate sexual function. Nosek et al. (1996) found that social status, higher rates of sexual activity, and psychological variables within women with SCI were associated with greater sexual satisfaction. In research that looked at the importance of sexual activity after injury, Westgren, Hultling, Levi, Seiger, and Westgren (1997) drew from a population-based study of 65 women with SCI in Stockholm, Sweden, and found that a reduction in sexual activity post-injury may be attributed to the following factors: 1) level and completeness of injury; 2) Psychological adjustment needed after SCI relegated sex to a lower priority; 3) age of injury (post-30 showed significant decline); 4) medical problems, e.g., urinary leakage, positioning problems, and spasticity. Although the authors identified a number of factors associated with decreased sexual activity after injury, the study revealed a lack of reported information and counseling on sexual matters for either the women with SCI or their partners.

As part of an overall assessment of post-injury adjustment issues, the LCP must adequately address prevention of medical problems that may interfere with sexual function and education and counseling for sexuality issues in persons with SCI and their partners. Interventions must focus on issues related to coping emotionally with changes in sexual function after SCI, strategies to assist the partner in coping emotionally with limitations on sexual activity, and providing alternatives for achieving sexual satisfaction post-injury (Westgren et al., 1997). Furthermore, all care givers should understand that sexual adjustment time varies by individual and should be trained to deal with signs of sexual distress in the individual with SCI.

Birth Control

Although women with SCI are capable of pregnancy (Baker & Cardenas, 1996), little research has examined safe and effective birth control methods (Sipski, 1997). However, the issue of birth control can be somewhat problematic for women with SCI. Barrier methods, such as diaphragms, cervical caps, etc., may be difficult to manipulate, because of decreased hand strength and loss of sensation, and require the contribution of the partner's assistance (Becker, Stuifbergen, & Tinkle, 1997; Ducharme, 1999; Welner, 1996). Intrauterine devices (IUDs) present risks for women with SCI (above the level of T6) who lack sensation and consequently are unable to notice a migration of the device out of the cervix, as well as the possibility for development of autonomic dysreflexia. Further, Jackson (1995) has pointed out that use of IUDs in women with SCI may be associated with an increased incidence of pelvic inflammatory disease.

Oral contraception is often considered contraindicated after SCI because of a high risk for thrombophlebitis (Sipski, 1997). However, the safety issues of oral contraceptives for women with SCI has not been comprehensively evaluated to date. Although a more convenient method of birth control for women with SCI may be found in the form of nonestrogenic formulations, such as Norplant® or injectable contraception, such as Depo-Provera®, Norplant may be a less desirable alternative because of the high incidence of erratic bleeding (Welner, 1996). Further, there is some concern about the long-term use of Depo-Povera as it can be associated with decreased estradiol levels in some women. A concern for women with SCI is the impact of decreased estradiol levels on bone mass.

The male condom provides another method of contraception, and does not require manual dexterity on the woman's part. In addition, the male condom can diminish the risk of sexually transmitted diseases (STDs).

Because many women with SCI have difficulty finding birth control that works for them, many simply do not use contraceptives, which unfortunately exposes them to unwanted pregnancies and STDs (Becker et al., 1997). The concern for STDs in women with SCI is an issue that must be appropriately addressed given the paucity of traditional symptoms and findings. Women with SCI who are sexually active should have routine testing for STDs. Tests for syphilis, gonorrhea, chlamydia, hepatitis, and human immunodeficiency (HIV) should be included in the workup. If an ulcer is present, herpes should also be tested for. Two issues that are of particular concern for women with SCI include sensory impairment in the pelvic area that limits self-diagnosis and physical access issues that prevent prompt intervention. Health care providers who treat women with SCI must understand and recognize the symptoms of STDs in individuals where neurologic sensations are affected (Welner, 1993, 1996).

Pregnancy and Childbirth

Women often experience amenorrhea (absence of menstrual periods) for several (3–6) months after SCI; however, menses usually eventually returns and fertility is typically restored, which allows women to conceive and bear children with nearly the same success rate as the general population (Axel, 1982; Brackett, Nash, & Lynne, 1996; Charlifue et al., 1992; Comarr, 1966; Ditunno & Formal, 1994; Jackson & Wadley, 1999; Reame, 1992; Sipski, 1991). Because pregnancy after SCI may be complicated by autonomic dysreflexia or other SCI-related factors, labor onset may be difficult to detect, and women with SCI may be at increased risk for early labor and low birth weight babies (Jackson & Wadley, 1999), it is recommended that they be monitored by a physician (Sipski, 1991). Certain medical complications are predictable and can be managed successfully. Collaboration between the obstetrician and physiatrist (specialist in physical medicine and rehabilitation) can be particularly useful during pregnancy.

Findings from various research studies addressing the management of pregnancy in women with SCI generally report good outcomes for mother and baby, with the most common complications cited being urinary tract infections, anemia, spasticity, pressure ulcers, deep venous thrombosis, autonomic dysreflexia, increased neurogenic bowel and bladder management difficulties, and problems with transfers and wheelchair propulsion (Baker & Cardenas, 1996; Baker, Cardenas & Benedetti, 1992; Cardenas et al., 1995; Charlifue et al., 1992; Cross, Meythaler, Tuel, & Cross, 1992; Feyi-Waboso, 1992; Hughes, Short, Usherwood, & Tebbutt, 1991; Jackson, 1996; Jackson & Wadley, 1999; Wanner, Rageth & Zach, 1987). Prenatal management must pay special attention to ongoing skin care, periodic checks for urinary tract infections, maintenance of regular bowel function, treatment of anemia, and prevention of unsupervised deliveries (Szasz, 1992).

Physicians also must be aware of the impact on pregnancy of the medications used by women with SCI. Medication use must be carefully monitored and some drugs may need to be given by alternative routes. As respiratory function may be impaired with the increased burden of late pregnancy or labor in women with tetraplegia or high level paraplegia, ventilatory support may also be required (Northwest Regional Spinal Cord Injury System, 1996b).

The method of delivery for women with SCI is typically determined by standard obstetrical indications, but considerations should be given to avoiding or limiting the presence of SCI complications. Women with SCI above T10 must be closely monitored because the injury may impair the ability to sense contractions; early labor may be missed by the expectant mother (Martinez-Arisala & Brackett, 1994). In addition, women with SCI at T6 or above, and who are therefore at risk for autonomic dysreflexia, should be cared for in a setting where invasive monitoring and physicians experienced with this potential complication are available (Madorsky, 1995).

Baker and Cardenas (1996) in their review of the literature found no data available for patient counseling regarding the fetal effects of SCI during pregnancy. They recommend that women be provided with preconception counseling, with specific attention given to predictable medical complications during pregnancy and the impact of pre-existing medical problems. Consultation with a maternal fetal medicine specialist should be considered for women with significant pre-existing medical problems. Obstetrical staff should be educated about the risk of pressure sores and traumatic injuries to individuals with SCI (Cross et al., 1992).

Life care planners should assess the woman's desire to have children when gathering information. If this is a possibility for the individual, some sort of allowance should be provided in the development of the LCP. Throughout the duration of the pregnancy, the woman may require more medications than a non-SCI woman, lengthier hospital stays, or increased attendant care, especially as activities of daily living (ADLs) become more difficult to perform in the third trimester. When confronted with an individual who was actively involved in parenting prior to the SCI, provisions may be required for feedings, diapering, day care, routine child care, and mobility and equipment modifications.

EDUCATIONAL INTERVENTIONS

The discussion of sex and sexuality is often neglected in the health care of people following SCI (Tepper, 1992; Zasler, 1991). However, studies have shown that sexuality plays an important role in the person's ability to cope with his or her disability (Cole & Cole, 1990; Lemon, 1993). Kreuter, Sullivan, and Sivsteen (1996) found a strong relationship between sexuality and social mobility in individuals with SCI. They recommend that rehabilitation programs emphasize support to the newly injured person to develop leisure time activities to engage in both alone and with their partner. Involvement of both partners in a counseling process post-injury is recommended.

Spica (1989) revealed the need for sexual counseling standards for individuals with SCI. The author proposed a standard of care that includes both content to be addressed with the individual with SCI and information provided to the care giver to assess the individual's needs. It is recommended that the techniques stress the importance of determining individual and family knowledge in the areas of sexual communications, methods of stimulation, and management of physical problems. The content standards suggested for sexual counseling of individuals with SCI are as follows:

- Consider the anatomy and physiology of sexual functioning
- Address sexual communication with the partner (if present)
- Adapt individual with SCI/partner to alterations in sexual performance
- Educate on alternative forms of sexual expression
- Address physical care concerns related to sexual functioning
- Assess specific gynecological/genitourinary needs
- Educate the individual with SCI/partner on sexual information and counseling for the individual and/or the partner

Depending on the individual's geographic area of residence, it may be difficult to locate a professional trained and experienced in sexual counseling who is also knowledgeable about changes after SCI. The American Association of Sex Educators,

Counselors, and Therapist (ASSECT, P.O. Box 238, Mount Vernon, IA 52314-0238) has set standards for certification of professionals working in the field of human sexuality and maintains a list of qualified professionals for specific geographic areas.

IMPLICATIONS FOR LIFE CARE PLANNING AND CASE MANAGEMENT

Although sexual desire and the ability to become sexually aroused persist after a SCI, sexual dysfunction may be present in a large number of people (Ditunno & Formal, 1994). Interdisciplinary rehabilitation that addresses body image, relationships, sexual function, fertility, and parenting can be very effective in enabling persons with SCI to achieve intimate roles with sexual partners (Stiens et al., 1997).

APPENDIX G

Mortality and Spinal Cord Injury

One of the most challenging and critical aspects of the LCP for individuals with SCI is estimation of life expectancy. Life expectancy has at least two separate influences on estimation of lifetime costs. First and most simply, the longer an individual lives, the greater the number of years of base cost, that need to be added to the lifetime cost equation. For example, if the average annual cost for an individual with a C4 complete SCI is determined to be $100,000 per year, an individual who lives 20 years will have twice the costs of an individual who lives 10 years ($2,000,000 as opposed to $1,000,000). The second factor is that as an individual ages, his or her function decreases and the per year costs likely increase. Aging with SCI brings about a new set of health problems generally raise annual costs during later years of life. This is obviously difficult to estimate and must take into account factors related to aging with disability.

The following sections outline existing mortality research and discusses their implications for life care planning. Because of the complexities involved, this information is presented to serve as a guide for understanding issues related to life expectancy and interpreting the reports of experts, rather than as a "cookbook" to be used by the life care planner in predicting life expectancy. Although this information is not sufficient to educate the life care planner to the point of making these predictions, it will provide him or her with a resource guide for understanding the parameters that must be taken into account by experts who make these evaluations. If all relevant factors have not been adequately accounted for, then it is the role of the life care planner to point out these omissions as well as their potential impact on the LCP.

MORTALITY RESEARCH

Historically, individuals did not live long after the onset of SCI, particularly with more severe injuries; urinary tract infections and other urologic complications generally led to early mortality (Breithaupt, Jousse, & Wynne-Jones, 1961; Burke, Hicks, Robbins, & Kessler, 1960; Freed, Bakst, & Barrie, 1966; Hackler, 1977; Hardy, 1976; Ravichandron & Silver, 1982). Over the past few decades, a significant body of research has indicated that the life expectancy of individuals who survive the first year after SCI has improved dramatically (DeVivo, Kartus, Stover, Rutt, & Fine, 1987; DeVivo, Stover, & Black, 1992; Krause et al., 1997b; Kiwerski, Weiss, & Chrostowska, 1981; Mesard, Carmody, Mannarino, & Ruge, 1978; Whiteneck et al., 1992). However, more recent research suggests that life expectancy over the past few decades has actually reversed, and is again on the decline (DeVivo, Krause, & Lammertse, 1999). There has also been a shift in the primary cause of death from urologic complications to pneumonia and influenza (DeVivo & Stover, 1995). There are also a substantial number of deaths caused by highly preventable causes, such as septicemia and suicide (DeVivo & Stover, 1995).

Because many people die from preventable causes, an individual's health-related behaviors impact life expectancy. For instance, Nehemkis and Groot (1980) found that when pre-death behaviors are taken into account, many deaths classified as natural on death records could be reclassified as second- or third-degree suicides. Individual behaviors include alcohol or drug abuse, sitting for ill-advised periods on pressure ulcers, or performing excessively high risk activities. Even when causes of death are not taken into account, individuals who engage in an active and satisfying lifestyle have a greater life expectancy than those who are less successful at adapting after their injuries (Krause, 1991; Krause & Crewe, 1987; Krause & Kjorsvig, 1992; Krause, Saari, & Dykstra, 1990; Krause, Sternberg, Maides, & Lottes, 1997b). This suggests that many deaths that may not appear highly preventable by looking at causes of death alone (e.g., cardiovascular, urinary tract-related) may indeed be related to an individual's behavior or level of adaptation.

Life Expectancy Tables

The most common way of estimating life expectancy in the general population is through the use of life expectancy tables. Within the general population, these tables project life expectancy based on demographic status (e.g., current age, gender, and race/ethnicity). Although multiple factors moderate how long any given individual will live (e.g., tobacco use, patterns of exercise, and the healthiness of diet), life expectancy tables do not account for these behaviors or other types of risk factors. Therefore, even in the general population, life expectancy tables provide only the most basic average predictions for a population. Accounting for risk behaviors and other factors helps to explain individual variation in longevity for a given population (in addition to that associated with demographic factors).

Much of the research on life expectancy after SCI has paralleled the life expectancy table approach, adjusting life expectancy estimates based on important parameters related to the SCI. It is necessary to account for these SCI variables because research continues to suggest that there is a diminished degree of life expectancy for people with SCI. Because there are dramatic differences in life expectancy related to severity of injury and the age at injury onset, formulas have been developed to predict average life expectancy of cohorts of people with SCI based on age at injury onset, level of injury, and Frankel grade (related to neurologic completeness of injury).

Life Expectancy after Spinal Cord Injury

In analyzing information from Model Systems, DeVivo and Stover (1995) summarized mortality data on 17,349 people with SCI. These data included standardized mortality ratios (SMR), projected life expectancy (based on the SMRs), and causes of death. The data were broken down into categories by age at injury and severity of injury. Severity of injury was broken down into four classes: 1) C1 to C4: Frankel A, B, or C; 2) C5 to C8: Frankel A, B, or C; 3) thoracic and lumbar injuries: Frankel A, B, or C; and 4) Frankel D injuries (all levels). Several sets of analyses were presented, the most relevant of which are reviewed here.

The statistical approach used is the SMR, which defines the ratio of actual deaths to expected deaths. To compute SMRs, the characteristics of a cohort of people with SCI are determined at one point in time (i.e., age at injury onset, gender, race/ethnicity, and injury characteristics). This cohort is then followed over time to determine the number of actual deaths that occur. The non-SCI related characteristics of the cohort (age, gender, race/ethnicity) are then used to identify the number of deaths that would be expected over the same time based on life expectancy tables (i.e., expected deaths). The SMR is then calculated by determining the ratio of actual deaths among the SCI cohort to expected deaths. The larger the SMR, the greater the relative mortality among the SCI cohort (a ratio of 1.0 indicates no differences).

To identify differential mortality rates between the general population and people with SCI, DeVivo and Stover (1995) used data collected through the Model Systems to develop SMRs for people with SCI. As applied to SCI, the authors calculated SMRs for individuals of different ages at injury and different severities of injury (based on both level of injury and Frankel grade). The number of actual deaths for all groups of participants studied exceeded the number of expected deaths.

However, dramatic differences existed in the size of the SMRs, depending on the age and injury characteristics of the participants. Differences also existed based on whether SMRs were calculated for all individuals who survived the first 24 hours post-injury or for all individuals who survived the first year post-injury. The SMRs were substantially higher for individuals who had survived only the first 24 hours as opposed to the first year.

Table G-1 shows that the SMRs of all individuals who survived the first year ranged from a low of 1.66 (for individuals aged 46–60 at injury onset with Frankel D injuries) to a high of 10.94 (individuals aged 0–30 at injury onset, with C1–C4 level injuries; Frankel A, B, or C). Therefore, there are substantial differences in the degree to which individuals, on average, reach full life expectancies after SCI.

DeVivo and Stover (1995) then used the SMRs to calculate average life expectancy for people of different ages at injury, again for some groups based on level of injury and Frankel grade. They again noticed dramatic differences when restricting analyses to all individuals who survived the first year as opposed to those who simply survived the first 24 hours post-injury. For example, individuals injured at the age of 30 with C1–C4 injuries (Frankel A, B or C) were expected to live an average of 16.5 years after injury, whereas those who survived the first year were expected to live 23.7 years post-injury. Because of these differences, it is generally most appropriate to use one year post-injury averages, as death during the first year post-injury substantially reduces the overall life expectancy estimate for individuals who are in good health and who are likely to survive through the first year. However, the prediction is much more complex if the individual is in poor health during the first year or has other complications.

Table G-2 presents a breakdown of life expectancy in years for individuals of varying ages at injury and varying types of injury. It is immediately clear from this table that the life expectancy estimates must be based first on an understanding of the individual's nature of injury and age. The older the individual at age of onset, the more closely he or she is to approximate a full life expectancy (again based on average), even though the individual will live a shorter duration.

It must be kept in mind that these data are based on averages for each of the groups defined by age and injury status. There will be tremendous variation between an individual's longevity and estimated longevities, with some individuals living for only a short period after injury and others living nearly full life expectancies. When using SMRs to calculate life expectancy, a substantial number of deaths early after injury produces a distribution causing these tables to underestimate the life expectancy of individuals who survive the first few years post-injury (this research has substantiated that SMRs decrease with years post-injury).

Table G-1. SMRs for Persons with SCI with First Post-Injury Year Included and Excluded by Age at Injury and Neurologic Category

First Post-Injury Year	Age at Injury	Standardized Mortality Ratio			
		C1–C4 (Frankel Grade A, B, C)	C5–C8 (Frankel Grade A, B, C)	T1–S5 (Frankel Grade A, B, C)	Frankel Grade D
Included	0–30	14.47	5.83	4.22	2.93
	31–45	16.98	7.85	4.27	2.04
	45–60	9.53	5.52	2.44	1.99
	61+	9.22	5.37	3.01	1.95
Excluded	0–30	10.94	5.07	3.86	2.58
	31–45	9.78	6.30	3.74	2.03
	45–60	5.24	3.83	1.96	1.66
	61+	3.07	3.07	2.21	1.68

(From Long-term Survival and Causes of Death by M.J. DeVivo and S.L. Stover in *Spinal Cord Injury: Clinical Outcomes from the Model Systems* by S.L. Stover et al., p. 296. Aspen Publishers, Inc., 1995. Reprinted with permission.)

Table G-2. Life Expectancy for Persons with SCI Who Survive at Least One Year Post-Injury by Current Age and Neurologic Category

Current Age	Normal*	Life Expectancy (Years)			
		C1–C4 (Frankel Grade A, B, C)	C5–C8 (Frankel Grade A, B, C)	T1–S5 (Frankel Grade A, B, C)	Frankel Grade D
5	70.8	45.0	52.0	59.5	63.0
10	65.9	40.5	47.3	53.7	58.2
15	61.0	36.1	42.6	49.0	53.4
20	56.3	32.8	38.6	44.8	49.0
25	51.6	29.9	34.7	40.8	44.7
30	46.9	26.8	30.7	36.7	40.5
35	42.2	23.7	27.0	32.7	36.1
40	37.6	20.9	23.6	28.8	31.7
45	33.0	18.4	20.4	25.1	27.5
50	28.6	15.5	17.0	21.2	23.4
55	24.4	12.8	13.8	17.3	19.5
60	20.5	11.0	11.2	13.8	15.9
65	16.9	8.8	8.8	10.9	13.2
70	13.6	6.6	6.6	8.3	10.4
75	10.7	4.7	4.7	6.1	8.0
80	8.1	3.1	3.1	4.2	6.1

*Normal values are from 1988 U.S. Life Tables for the general population.
(From Long-term Survival and Causes of Death by M.J. DeVivo and S.L. Stover in *Spinal Cord Injury: Clinical Outcomes from the Model Systems* by S.L. Stover et al., p. 298. Aspen Publishers, Inc., 1995. Reprinted with permission.)

In a more recent follow-up to this study, DeVivo et al. (1999) performed similar analyses on an expanded study sample of 28,239 individuals with SCI. There were several important findings from this study. Although the mortality rates of first-day survivors continued to be less than that observed over previous decades, the mortality rates of first-year survivors actually increased over that of recent years. Specifically, the mortality rates that had been declining from 1973 to 1992 increased 33 percent for persons injured between 1993 and 1998 relative to those injured between 1988 and 1992. Deaths due to respiratory disease were the only cause for which the relative odds increased meaningfully during the latest time period (a 76 percent increase over 1988–1992, when compared to all other causes).

Three other findings were particularly noteworthy. First, etiology of injury was included as a predictor of mortality. Analysis of first-year deaths indicated that those injured by violence had a 1.53 times greater odds of mortality during the first year as compared with those not injured by violence. However, among year-one survivors, those with a violent etiology had only 1.15 greater odds of mortality than those with nonviolent etiologies.

Second, year-one mortality was also associated with sponsor of care. Individuals covered by health maintenance organizations (HMOs) were less likely to die compared with the baseline group (other support category), whereas those on Medicare had a 2.31 times greater odds of mortality and those on Medicaid had a 1.47 greater odds of mortality during year-one. However, among year one survivors, the odds of mortality were no better for those sponsored by HMOs.

Third, for the first time in analysis of Model Systems data, life expectancy was calculated for five-year survivors in addition to one-year and one-day survivors. Although utilizing only one example (those injured at age 20), the results suggested that life expectancy of C1–C4 tetraplegics (Frankel A, B, or C) injured at age 20 is 32.9 years compared with 56.8 for the general population. For those who survive the first year to age 21, their life expectancy actually increases to 35.3 years compared to 55.9 for the general population, even though a year has passed. At five years post-injury (age 25), the life expectancy is 33 years compared with 52.1 years for the general population (i.e., it decreases only 2.3 years even though four years have passed). This trend is most notable for individuals with the most severe injuries, and is most profound for those with ventilator dependency, where the life expectancy increases dramatically with each milestone passed (15.3 years for day-one survivors; 25.9 years for year-one survivors; 28.5 years for year-five survivors). Taken together, these findings suggest a critical period after the onset of SCI during which mortality is more likely, at least for individuals with non-Frankel D cervical injuries. If individuals survive that first year, their life expectancy becomes less adversely impacted by their SCI.

Another mortality study was carried out as a collaborative study between two British hospitals and the Craig Hospital (Whiteneck et al., 1993). This study is of great relevance to predicting life expectancy after SCI, because only cases whose injuries occurred 20 or more years earlier were selected. Many individuals' injuries occurred more than 40 years prior to determination of mortality status. This is important because a large portion of individuals had the opportunity to live their full life expectancy. This is in contrast to the Model Systems study that has focused on individuals primarily within the first decade or two after the onset of SCI. As a result, the estimates based on the British study, although tempered by the fact that the sample is not from the United States, is invaluable in determining life expectancy among individuals with SCI.

A total of 412 individuals had survived from the study sample until follow-up, while 362 (43 percent) were deceased by the time of the study. The researchers broke participant samples down according to key characteristics (similar to those used in the Model Systems study). They noted across their full sample that the median survival time was 32 years. Further, 85 percent of their participants survived the first 10 years, 71 percent survived the first 20 years, 53 percent were still alive at 30 years, and 35 percent were still alive at 40 years post-injury. Obviously, the lengths of survival were determined largely by the age at injury onset, as well as by other characteristics related to injury severity.

Table G-3 summarizes the percentage of individuals surviving to four milestones in terms of years based on decades post-injury (e.g., 10 years, 20 years, 30 years, and 40 years). Participant groups were broken down based on complete or incomplete injury, injury severity, age at injury onset. Mortality rates varied as a function of these factors. For example, among individuals with complete tetraplegia, a factor known to be related to high mortality, 64 percent of those who were less than 30 at the time of injury had survived to at least their thirtieth year post-injury. In contrast, those with incomplete paraplegia had a 76 percent survival rate at 30 years post-injury. Among those injured at ages 30 to 49, the percentage of individuals with complete tetraplegia surviving 30 years was 34 percent, whereas those with incomplete tetraplegia was 47 percent. Further, among persons 50 years of age or older at injury, 53 percent of those with complete tetraplegia (N = 7) survived the first 10 years, whereas other participants had not survived by 20 years post-injury.

The authors also calculated mortality odds ratios for each of the various groups, while controlling statistically for other factors. In the 20–30-year age range, they noted an additional 7 deaths per 1,000 compared to that which would be expected in the general population, whereas in the 60–70-year age range, they noted 25 more deaths per 1,000 among individuals with SCI. When mortality ratios were calculated to take into account actual versus expected deaths, the odds of an individual injured at age 20 for mortality are 8 times that of the general population. However, by age 70 the odds of mortality dropped to 1.5 times that of the general population. This seems counterintuitive at first, except when considering that many more deaths would be expected in the 60–70 age range, as opposed to the 20-year-old range. Again, individuals who are older at injury come closer to meeting their full life expectancy, despite living fewer years post-SCI.

Table G-3. British Study of SCI Survival Rates[a]

Group	Number	Percent Surviving[b] 10 years	20 years	30 years	40 years	Median Years
<30 at Injury						
Complete Tetraplegia	66	86%	77%	64%	NA[c]	
Incomplete Tetraplegia	87	96	85	67	31	36
Complete Paraplegia	233	91	79	63	47	36
Incomplete Paraplegia	96	96	89	76	65	44[d]
30–49 at injury						
Complete Tetraplegia	33	71	42	34	NA[c]	17
Incomplete Tetraplegia	50	70	63	33	0	26
Complete Paraplegia	159	81	60	36	12	23
Incomplete Paraplegia	64	84	69	47	16	29
50+ at injury						
Complete Tetraplegia	7	53	0	0	0	10
Incomplete Tetraplegia	15	56	24	0	0	11
Complete Paraplegia	14	50	17	0	0	12
Incomplete Paraplegia	10	67	44	NA[c]	NA[c]	14

[a]First year deaths excluded from the study
[b]Using Standard Life Tables
[c]No study cases in this group have been injured for more than 40 years
[d]Estimated median survival
(From Learning from Recent Empirical Investigations by G.G. Whiteneck in *Aging with Spinal Cord Injury* by G.G. Whiteneck et al., p. 29. Demos Publishers, 1993. Reprinted with permission.)

CAUSES OF DEATH

DeVivo and Stover (1995) have also calculated causes of death for individuals who have survived the first 24 hours post-injury. They have calculated the actual percentages of death due to varying causes, as well as calculating SMRs to indicate which types of death are more common than expected among people with SCI. Therefore, the first comparisons simply indicate the most prevalent causes of death after SCI, whereas the second analysis identifies the degree to which there are a disproportionate number of certain causes of death among people with SCI, based on a comparison of causes of death in the general population.

In an analysis of the primary causes and secondary causes of death among people with SCI, DeVivo and Stover (1995) attempted to classify a total of 1,601 deaths into various diagnostic categories. After eliminating 198 who died from unknown causes (12 percent), pneumonia and influenza were found to be the primary causes of mortalities (17.7 percent) followed by nonischemic heart disease (16.5 percent) and symptoms and ill-defined conditions (15.3 percent). Septicemia also was a highly prevalent cause of death (12 percent), with several other causes ranging from 1.1 to 8.7 percent. Clearly, the decrease in causes of deaths due to urinary complications indicates a change in pattern of causes of mortality over the past few years or decades.

Although the previously described findings identify the percentages of all SCI deaths related to different causes, this does not compare the prevalence of these deaths with those which occur among the general population. To do this, DeVivo and Stover (1995) calculated SMRs with the ratio of SCI deaths to expected deaths based on the general population. This was done for all causes. The highest SMRs were for septicemia (64.2 times the general population), disease of the pulmonary circulation (47.1), pneumonia and influenza (35.6), symptoms and ill-defined conditions (13.8), and diseases of the urinary system (10.9). It is noteworthy that almost all possible causes of death were higher among the SCI sample, with the exception of homicide and legal intervention, and cancer. Other noteworthy causes of death that were

Table G-4. SMRs for Underlying Cause of Death Among Persons with SCI Who Survive at Least 24 Hours Post-Injury

Cause of Death	Actual Deaths	Expected Deaths	SMR
Septicemia	122	1.9	64.2
Cancer	71	82.0	0.9
Diseases of the Nervous System	30	5.1	5.9
Ischemic Heart Disease	91	78.4	1.2
Diseases of Pulmonary Circulation	113	2.4	47.1
Nonischemic Heart Disease	171	26.7	6.4
Cerebrovascular Disease	41	18.6	2.2
Diseases of Arteries	17	5.0	3.4
Pneumonia and Influenza	228	6.4	35.6
Other Respiratory Diseases	58	12.8	4.5
Diseases of the Digestive System	67	17.8	3.8
Diseases of the Urinary System	49	4.5	10.9
Symptoms and Ill-Defined Conditions	102	7.4	13.8
Unintentional Injuries	72	51.8	1.4
Suicide	80	16.6	4.8
Homicide and Legal Intervention	15	21.8	0.7
All Other External Causes	32	2.3	13.9
Residual	44	23.2	1.9
Unknown	198		

(From Long-term Survival and Causes of Death by M.J. DeVivo and S.L. Stover in *Spinal Cord Injury: Clinical Outcomes from the Model Systems* by S.L. Stover et al., p. 302. Aspen Publishers, Inc., 1995. Reprinted with permission.)

higher than the general population included suicide (SMR = 4.8). Unintentional injuries did not have a higher SMR than the general population (1.4).

Whiteneck et al. (1993) calculated the frequency or percentages of deaths by various causes (see Table G-5). The authors noted that genitourinary causes accounted for the greatest portion of deaths (24.3 percent). They also noted a relatively high portion of deaths caused by cardiovascular problems. The authors broke down the percentage of deaths as a function of three categories based on severity of injury: individuals with Frankel A, B, or C paraplegia; persons with Frankel A, B, or C tetraplegia; and individuals with Frankel D or E (regardless of level of lesion). A generally similar pattern was observed for the most part, although there were some differences. Genitourinary disorders were the highest cause of death for both of the groups with paraplegia and tetraplegia (Frankel A, B, or C). Between these groups, however, respiratory system disease accounted for a greater percentage of deaths among those with tetraplegia (Frankel A, B, or C). Among those with Frankel D or E level injuries, cardiovascular diseases were the most common cause of death, followed by genitourinary disorders. The authors investigated changes in patterns of death over the past few decades. Similar to the Model Systems study, they found a decrease in overall mortality over the past decade. Additionally, they identified a changing pattern in the types of deaths that occurred, with genitourinary causes decreasing during more recent decades.

Taken together, findings from the Model Systems research and the British study suggests: 1) overall life expectancy is diminished to some degree after SCI, 2) life expectancy is related to level and completeness of injury (as well as age), 3) pneumonia and influenza are the highest causes of death among people with SCI, and 4) many deaths after SCI are caused by preventable causes (septicemia and suicide). It is also not known the degree to which an individual's behavior or general activity levels were related to other causes of death, such as those related to pulmonary circulation, other respiratory diseases, diseases of the urinary system, symptoms and ill-defined conditions.

Table G-5. Distribution of Deaths by Primary Cause

Primary cause of death	Categories of Injury			
	All cases	Paraplegia ABC[a]	Tetraplegia ABC[b]	All D & E[c]
Genitourinary Disorders	88 (24.3%)	58 (28.1%)	12 (21.1%)	18 (18.2%)
Cardiovascular Diseases	84 (23.2%)	48 (23.2%)	8 (14.1%)	28 (28.3%)
Septicemia	16 (4.4%)	10 (4.9%)	4 (7.0%)	2 (2.0%)
Neoplasms	40 (11.0%)	21 (10.2%)	3 (5.3%)	16 (16.2%)
Endocrine/Blood Disorders	6 (1.7%)	3 (1.5%)	0 (0.0%)	3 (3.0%)
Respiratory System Diseases	50 (13.8%)	23 (11.2%)	11 (19.3%)	16 (16.2%)
Digestive System Disease	16 (4.4%)	8 (3.9%)	4 (7.0%)	4 (4.0%)
Nervous System Disease	2 (0.6%)	0 (0.0%)	1 (1.7%)	1 (1.0%)
Accidents and Injuries	22 (6.1%)	13 (6.3%)	6 (10.5%)	3 (3.0%)
Ill-Defined Mortality	38 (10.5%)	22 (10.7%)	8 (14.0%)	8 (8.1%)

[a]Persons with paraplegia with Frankel Grades A, B, or C (no functional motor preservation)
[b]Persons with tetraplegia with Frankel Grades A, B, or C (no functional motor preservation)
[c]Persons with paraplegia or tetraplegia with Frankel Grades D or E (functional motor preservation)
(From Learning from Recent Empirical Investigations by G.G. Whiteneck in *Aging with Spinal Cord Injury by* G.G. Whiteneck et al., p. 31. Demos Publishers., 1993. Reprinted with permission.)

LIMITATIONS OF THE LIFE EXPECTANCY TABLE APPROACH

Although the life expectancy table approach has great benefit for research purposes in following trends in life expectancy, it is very limited when applied to the individual case. The basic premise upon which all life expectancy tables approach research is that life expectancy can be predicted based on biographic characteristics alone (e.g., age, gender and race). However, even among individuals without SCI or other disabling conditions, there is wide variation in actual life expectancy or years of life lived, based on a number of factors. The majority of these factors relate to the individual's overall level of adaptation and the extent to which he or she avoids high risk behaviors (e.g., smoking, drinking) and performs necessary protective behaviors (e.g., proper exercise and nutrition). Therefore, even among individuals with no disabling condition, life expectancy tables produce only general or average estimates of how long an individual will live without regard to the many important health behaviors that may ultimately determine length of life.

As it relates to individuals with SCI, the situation is much more complex. Once an SMR is attained, this formula is used to compute the probability of living each additional year after the onset of SCI. Once an individual's probability of survival in any given year is less than 50 percent, this figure is taken as the average estimated life expectancy.

Several assumptions in this approach may lead to an incorrect estimation of life expectancy, particularly in cases of litigation, when many LCPs are developed. First, a few unusual cases where individuals die shortly after injury can skew the prediction of life expectancy dramatically. This is a problem because it has been well established that a significant portion of SCI cases are the result of violent acts or occur under conditions of alcohol or drug intoxication. The National Spinal Cord Injury Statistical Center (NSCISC) reports that 19 percent of SCI are caused by violence (NSCISC, 1997). Also, alcohol has been found to be a contributory factor to the onset of between 39 nd 50 percent of SCI (Heinemann, Donahoe, Keen, & Scholl,1988). Therefore, many SCIs occur among individuals who are prone to dangerous situations that could result in early post-injury mortality. The prediction of life expectancy for individuals without excluding people with these characteristics will be skewed downward by their presence. The extent to which these behavioral patterns led an individual to SCI also places him or her at high risk for mortality and dramatically influences life expectancy as opposed to estimates for individuals who do not share these characteristics. A recent Model Systems study found violent etiology predictive of diminished life expectancy, thus supporting this conclusion (DeVivo et al., 1999).

A second limitation is that many people who are part of these studies are indigent with no financial resources, no family to assist them, and no support systems. These circumstances are clearly different than in those cases that generally reach litigation, in which a third party is found to be responsible for the injury. In these cases, the individual will have most, if not all, of their health care needs met. These factors are not considered using the standard life expectancy estimate based on SMRs. Therefore, early mortality among individuals with no economic, familial, or health care supports also skews the life expectancy estimates for individuals who stand to have all these needs accommodated.

Finally, the data generally used to derive life expectancy estimates are from the Model Systems, in which data has been collected for less than three decades (the British data are not limited in this respect). Therefore, most cases to which an individual's life expectancy is compared will not have had the opportunity to live 25, 30, or more years post-injury. It is generally accepted that the probability of mortality for any given year is highest the closer to the time of onset of injury. In other words, the conditional probability (the probability of dying in that year) decreases over time as an individual lives with SCI. There may be a critical period during which time an individual is more prone to early mortality. However, if the individual gets through this period of time and resumes normal life activities, his or her prospects for life expectancy are very good, even with severe injuries. This is also supported by the analysis of mortality among five-year survivors in the most recent Model Systems study (DeVivo et al., 1999). Individuals who are most likely to die during this critical period are those who exhibit the maladaptive behavior patterns that led to injury in the first place. Although this has not been fully substantiated by research with SCI, it certainly has been found true in the general population.

In summary, the overriding concern of applying the life expectancy approach to individual SCI cases is that the approach will underestimate the life expectancy in many cases, particularly when the individual does not have characteristics which place him or her for risk of early mortality and does have substantial personal, familial, and economic supports. It must also be pointed out that the standard approach may overestimate life expectancy in other cases, even those reaching litigation—where there is clearly a third party responsible for the injury—if there is a pattern of high-risk behavior leading to the onset of SCI, but treatment considerations are the focus of litigation.

RESEARCH OF NON-BIOGRAPHIC OR INJURY RELATED FACTORS

Several studies have suggested that a number of nonbiographic and noninjury related factors are related to early mortality after SCI. These studies include: 1) the previously reviewed studies related to causes of death identifying many preventable deaths with appropriate self-care or general health care; 2) retrospective studies identifying a higher prevalence of self-destructive behaviors among people dying of preventable causes; and 3) prospective studies related to psychosocial, vocational, and medical adjustment to survival. These studies are important because they suggest that, for any given biographic and injury profile, there will be substantial differences in life expectancy.

Retrospective Studies

In the studies of causes of death, a relationship between poor psychological adjustment and cause of death must be inferred from data on cause of death alone. Although such a relationship might be obvious in deaths such as suicide, looking retrospectively at cause of death cannot identify the extent of the relationship between psychosocial factors and mortality. The nature or type of psychosocial factors important to survival also cannot be determined from looking at cause of death alone. Other researchers have attempted to more directly link behavior to death.

Retrospective studies have provided important insights about the factors that may underlie early mortality after SCI. These studies have identified causes of death among a sample of people with SCI (generally a quite small sample) and then reviewed pre-death records to identify if behavioral factors may have attributed to the deaths. Although plagued by difficulties in obtaining objective information in case histories, these studies have generated interesting information about correlates of early mortality, which may serve as a foundation for more sophisticated prospective studies.

Price (1973) reviewed case histories of eleven deceased persons, finding evidence of poor psychosocial adjustment among persons whose deaths appeared to be preventable (e.g., suicide, septicemia). However, the author did not have the same information on all subjects (citing Minnesota Multiphasic Personality Inventory [MMPI] results for some but not all subjects) and may have had knowledge of cause of death prior to her review of the case histories. Nehemkis and Groot (1980) studied the relationship between indirect self-destructive behavior and mortality among persons with SCI. They found that when pre-death behaviors were taken into account, many deaths categorized as natural on death certificates could be reclassified as second- or third-degree suicides. These lifestyle behaviors included alcohol or drug abuse, a lack of attention to nutrition, and sitting for ill-advised periods of time with multiple pressure sores. This study highlights the importance of considering indirect self-destructive behavior in relation to cause of death. It also highlights the limitations of death certificates, long known to be of limited reliability, in capturing the true consequences surrounding death.

Although the Price (1973) and Nehemkis and Groot (1980) studies have more directly investigated psychological and behavioral factors related to mortality, both relied on retrospective data collection. Retrospective methods are susceptible to unconscious experimenter bias, particularly when the investigator is involved in the data collection (as was the case in the Price study). This raises significant questions about their validity. Nevertheless, these studies have provided evidence for the relationship between adjustment and mortality. Still lacking is research that identifies more specific adjustment patterns related to survival.

Prospective Studies

In response to epidemiologic studies indicating the high percentage of deaths by apparently preventable causes, and retrospective studies that suggest particular behavior patterns underlie these deaths, a series of prospective studies were implemented to clarify the types of adjustment patterns that are associated with early mortality after SCI. These studies collected data on life adjustment, then investigated how these adjustment patterns were related to mortality status years later. The prospective methodology overcame issues of selective information (retrospective studies) and did not rely on looking solely at deaths that appeared preventable.

In a study by Krause and Crewe (1987), the authors obtained responses to the Life Situation Questionnaire (LSQ) from 256 participants with SCI. The LSQ was designed to measure a wide range of mostly objective information on long-term outcomes after SCI, including employment, activities, and medical treatments. It also measured satisfaction with six areas of life and asked participants to rate their overall adjustment. Eleven years later, in 1984, the authors ascertained the survival status of the participants, noting that 179 were still alive (70 percent), 46 were deceased (18 percent), and the remaining 31 could not be determined (12 percent). The deceased sample averaged 16.9 years since injury at the time of death. After statistically controlling age differences, the authors compared the survivor and deceased groups on three sets of adjustment measures: 1) psychologists' ratings of psychosocial, vocational, and medical adjustment; 2) indices of social activity, medical stability, and life satisfaction; and 3) 17 single items. Participants surviving until the 1984 follow-up had superior ratings of vocational and psychosocial adjustment, but not medical adjustment. Participants in the survivor group were more active socially, had a greater sitting tolerance, and were more likely to be working or attending school than those who had died since 1974. Somewhat surprising, none of the indicators of recent medical history (e.g., doctor visits, hospitalizations) discriminated between the survivor and deceased groups.

A replication of this study was carried out in a 1988 follow-up, 15 years after the preliminary data collection (Krause, Saari, & Dysktra, 1990). Survival status was again ascertained for all previous participants, with 161 of the original 256 participants still known to be alive, 60 deceased, and the remaining 35, who could not be located. After adding statistical controls for injury severity, survivors again showed superior adjustment on both psychosocial and vocational ratings. Somewhat less impressive, but statistically significant differences were noted on medical adjustment. Survivors also showed superior scores on each of five scales, with the most significant relationship for activities and the least significant for medical treatments. Consistent differences were found on most psychosocial variables including five of the six life satisfaction items (none of which were significant in the 11-year follow-up). In general, these results were consistent with the findings of the previous 11-year study: survivors showed superior adjustment.

Krause and Kjorsvig (1992) also analyzed the four-year prospective data collected in 1984 from 154 of the survivors from 1973, as well as an additional 193 new participants added in 1984 (a total of 347 prospective cases in 1984). By 1988, 309 of the 347 participants with 1988 data were known to be alive, 22 were deceased, and 16 could not be located. The same data analytic procedures were carried out, only using an expanded number of variables that were not available in the original study. Five more life satisfaction items and a new set of 15 problem items were also correlated with mortality status. The results over this four-year period again supported the major study findings: survivors were more active, rated their adjustment to be better, and were more satisfied with many areas of life. Recent medical history was again only marginally related to survival status. The most interesting findings were obtained with the newly added problem items as psychologically loaded problem scales (Emotional Distress and Dependency) were more highly correlated with survival status than were measures of life satisfaction. On specific items, participants who had died by 1988 had reported significantly more boredom, loneliness, and depression in 1984 than those who survived until 1988. They also reported more problems related to environmental resources including a lack of adequate transportation, conflicts with attendants, and negative attitudes towards persons with disabilities. Lastly, the deceased group reported greater problems with alcohol and drug abuse.

Another follow-up was implemented in 1996, again using prospective data collected in 1984 (Krause et al., 1997b). More sophisticated data analysis was implemented, including the use of logistic regression to identify the odds of being deceased by 1996. By 1996, 278 participants were known to be alive and 52 were deceased. After controlling for biographic and injury related characteristics, persons who were unemployed in 1985 were 2.38 times more likely than those who were employed to have died by 1996. Odds ratios were also calculated for the eight LSQ scales, with the odds ratios reflecting differences of one standard deviation on each scale. For example, an odds ratio of 2.0 for the dependency scale would indicate that individuals who scored one standard deviation higher on the scale (the difference between the 50th and 84th percentiles) were twice as likely to have died over the 11-year period. The highest odds ratios were observed for dependency (2.04) and general satisfaction (1.99); lower satisfaction scores were actually associated with a higher odds of mortality.

In summary, all three types of studies (causes of death, retrospective, prospective) have identified patterns of behavior or adjustment that are correlated with longevity, above and beyond the contributions of biographic and injury characteristics. This research has shown that individuals who are employed, more active, more satisfied with life, and who show fewer complaints of emotional distress, dependency, or health problems are likely to live significantly longer than individuals who do not share these characteristics.

Unfortunately, these studies have significant limitations. First, participants were initially studied at varying intervals after injury, rather than immediately after injury. Therefore, many deaths certainly occurred prior to selection of participants in the study. This is not a major problem, given that the intention of these studies was not to derive point estimates of life expectancy. Rather, their purpose was to identify the nature of the predictors of longevity, outside of those typically studied (i.e., biographic and injury related characteristics). Second, unlike biographic and injury characteristics which are generally stable (e.g., age at onset, race/ethnicity, or nature of injury), the characteristics used to predict mortality in prospective studies may change over time (e.g. employment status, level of dependency). Third, prospective studies cannot, at present, be used to generate point estimates of longevity. It would be preferable to be able to do so, at least for research purposes. Lastly, there is co-linearity between the predictors. In other words, the predictors used to identify individuals who are at risk for early mortality are rather highly intercorrelated (i.e., an individual who is high on life satisfaction is likely to be active and report fewer problems). As a result, the predictors are not additive in terms of their impact. For example, if an equation was generated with the goal of identifying an optimal predictive equation to derive estimates of life expectancy, the predictor that was selected first will change the significance or importance of predictors entered later; if dependency were entered first in a predictive equation, other types of predictors (e.g., employment, activities) would have a diminished relationship with mortality because of the interrelationships between dependency and these other predictors. This limitation does impact the practical utility of using these variables together in any equations, but do not change the underlying relationship between the variable and mortality (only its additive predictive value).

IMPLICATIONS FOR LIFE CARE PLANNING

Ultimately, estimating life expectancy for any given individual is no simple task. It is not enough to account for the basic biographic and injury related characteristics when doing LCPs, although this is a good starting point. It is also necessary to assess probability of satisfactory post-injury adjustment, the likelihood of return to work, and potential adverse behavior patterns. Although evaluating these factors is difficult, the best rule of thumb is that an individual's post-injury adaptations will reflect the level of adaptation shown prior to injury. Individuals who were working in professional occupations, who did not exhibit a great degree of high-risk behavior prior to injury, and those who have no responsibility in the injury are likely to have greater longevity. The availability of post-injury resources is also essential. Life expectancy tables may be used as a general guide for the average case, including those who are at high risk for early mortality, but they must be supplemented by a more complete assessment of other factors.

In cases where a third party is clearly responsible for the injury and a high settlement is possible, it is likely that the individual's life expectancy will far exceed that projected based on standard estimates (given they likely did not have risk factors leading to injury and did not otherwise have patterns of high-risk behaviors). In many cases, the actual estimate of life expectancy may not deviate greatly from that projected before the injury occurred (primarily because this estimate of life expectancy was based only on biographic characteristics).

Not all cases that reach litigation favor a greater estimated life expectancy than that produced by standard formula. Specifically, in cases where litigation is based on damages related to poor post-injury treatment after the injury, rather than on neglect surrounding the circumstances of injury, there may be great variation on how litigation is associated with life expectancy. For example, an individual who was intoxicated at the time of injury and fully contributed to the onset of injury, but whose condition was exacerbated by poor treatment in the hospital, may actually live for a shorter period of time than that projected by standard estimates. This case is clearly different than those in which the individual's injury was due to a third party.

Despite a significant body of mortality research, it is clear that predicting life expectancy is as much art as science. As with other aspects of the LCP, the life care planner's role must be to integrate multiple types of information, data sources, and expert opinions to develop the fairest and most comprehensive plan possible to best ensure post-injury longevity. Mortality is a key element to the overall plan.

APPENDIX H

Leading Complications and Concerns for Spinal Cord Injury

Collaborative planning with the spinal cord injured person, family, and various health care professionals is essential to identifying and subsequently assessing the individual's long-term needs during the LCP process. In addressing these needs and identifying specific preventive treatment interventions, the life care planner must be aware of some of the more common complications and priority health concerns faced by people with long-term SCI.

NERVOUS SYSTEM

A number of nervous system complications can occur as people with SCI age. Significant numbers of individuals report increased spasticity, weakness, fatigue, and decreases in physical function as a consequence of pain, neurologic loss, spinal cord cysts, and other recognized complications of SCI and aging (Charlifue, 1993; Lammertse, 1993). Further, people who sustained some degree of brain injury (BI) at the time of their SCI may also experience dementia, a deterioration in their mental abilities, as they age. The incidence of combined SCI/BI is estimated to be between 10 and 50 percent of the SCI population, with the variation in rates at least partially attributable to differences in how BI was defined (Davidoff, Thomas, Johnson, Berent, Dijkers, & Doljanac, 1988; Morris & Roth, 1994; Richards, Brown, Hagglund, Bua, & Reeder, 1988; Richards, Osuna, Jaworski, Novack, Leli, & Boll, 1991; Wilmot, Cope, Hall, & Acker, 1985). When BI is defined by loss of consciousness or posttraumatic amnesia alone, the observed rates are much higher than if BI is defined by the presence of residual cognitive impairment.

As these neurologic complications appear, previously mastered activities such as transferring, driving, and dressing become difficult. The secondary disabilities in which these changes result can further challenge the long-term SCI individuals' adjustment, self-esteem, and ability to participate in satisfying and rewarding activities. As a consequence of these late onset neurologic complications, persons with SCI will likely require increased personal assistance services, household help, assistive devices and equipment, environment and support services, and institutional care (Consortium for Spinal Cord Medicine, 1999a; Gerhart, 1993; Whiteneck, 1993; Winkler & Weed, 1999).

Pain

Pain is a frequently occurring complication for people with SCI. It has been estimated that between 34 and 94 percent of persons with SCI experience chronic pain post-injury (Bonica, 1991; Demirel, Yllmaz, Gencosmanoglu, & Kesiktas, 1998; Kennedy, Frankel, Gardner, & Nuseibeh, 1997; Loubser & Conovan, 1996; Rintala, Loubser, Castro, Hart, & Fuhrer, 1998; Woolsey, 1986) and that from 25 to 45 percent experience pain severe enough to significantly interfere with activities of daily living or quality of life (Britell & Mariano, 1991; Davidoff, Roth, Guarracina, Sliwa, & Yarkony, 1987; Mariano, 1992; RTC/IL, 1993a; Rose, Robinson, Ells, & Cole,

1988). People who experience chronic pain following SCI are likely to have more psychological distress and poorer employment compared to individuals without pain (Cairns, Adkins, & Scott, 1996; Kennedy et al., 1997).

Although a number of classification systems have been proposed for SCI pain (Beric, 1997; Siddall, Taylor, & Cousins, 1997), two prevalent general categories include: 1) musculoskeletal pain, which is usually associated with tendonitis, bursitis, rotator cuff impingement syndrome, epicondylitis, unstable bone fractures, joint instability, infections, osteoarthritic changes, and entrapment neuropathies such as carpal tunnel syndrome; and 2) neurogenic pain, usually described as a diffuse burning, tingling, shooting, stinging, stabbing, piercing, crushing, cutting, or dragging sensation below the level of lesion. Musculoskeletal pain is generally aggravated by activity and relieved by rest. Following SCI, it is most frequently found in the shoulders, hands, and upper and lower limbs as a result of overuse syndromes and degenerative changes. Treatment of mechanical pain generally consists of conservative care with medications, adaptive aids and equipment, surgery, management of general medical complications, and physical modalities.

Neurogenic pain is probably the most persistent type of pain and is unfortunately the most resistant to treatment (Cairns, Adkins, & Scott, 1996; Roth, 1994). Neurogenic pain is most frequently found in the legs, back, feet, thighs, and toes but also occurs in the buttocks, hips, fingers, abdomen, and neck. This type of pain is most common in individuals with incomplete lesions, central cord syndromes, and injuries caused by gunshot wounds. Neurogenic pain is more common in persons of advancing age and in individuals experiencing anxiety and adverse psychosocial situations (Cairns et al., 1996; Stormer et al., 1997). It is often the result of noxious stimuli (such as smoking, bladder and bowel distension, infections, and pressure sores), heterotopic ossification, deep venous thrombosis, fractures of the extremities, prolonged inactivity, spasticity, fatigue, depression, and changes in weather (Demirel et al., 1998).

Accurate diagnosis of the type of pain is vital for prescribing appropriate treatment interventions (CDC, 1990). Onset of neurogenic pain generally occurs within the first year after injury. Although pain complaints usually decrease both in frequency and intensity over time, controversy exists as to whether this is because of neurophysiological reasons, psychological reasons, or both (Roth, 1994).

Posttraumatic Syringomyelia (PTS)

Posttraumatic syringomyelia (PTS) is a prominent cause of late neurologic deterioration in people with SCI (Lanig & Lammertse, 1992; Rossier, Foo, Shillito, & Dyro, 1985). PTS, a progressive cystic cavitation of the spinal cord, is a neurologic complication currently estimated to occur in 1 to 8 percent of people with SCI (Bursell, Little, & Stiens, 1999; Little, 1998; Rossier et al., 1985; Roth, 1994; Vernon, Silver, & Ohry, 1982; Umbach & Heilporn, 1991). PTS occurs when fluid-filled cysts called *syrinxes* form in spinal cord grey matter. Syrinxes can develop months to years after the injury, typically starting at the level of injury and extending up, down, or in both directions within the spinal cord, causing additional damage to the nerve cells. Syrinxes are most common with upper thoracic or cervical cord injuries, but can also occur at lower levels.

A loss of awareness of pain in temperature sensation and/or change in deep tendon reflexes is the earliest sign of PTS. This can usually be detected before the onset of symptoms and is present in up to 50 percent of individuals with PTS (Biyani & El Masry, 1994). Symptoms may include a progressive loss of motor and/or sensory function, increasing spasticity, hyperhydrosis, bowel and bladder function changes, and burning, tingling pain (Lazar, 1994; Roth, 1994). These problems can lead to decreases in function in areas such as mobility and self-care. The development of PTS is typically slow and insidious in nature, and the individual with SCI may not realize a loss of function is occurring. For this reason it is imperative that routine neurologic examinations and monitoring be provided as part of a long-term follow-up care strategy (Winkler & Weed, 1999).

There appears to be no clear relationship between the development of syrinxes and the mechanisms of injury, types of early treatment, or completeness or incompleteness of the lesion, although syrinxes are more common with upper thoracic or cervical cord injuries. Magnetic resonance imaging (MRI) is the study of choice for detecting a syrinx as well as its progression and is invaluable in selecting the site of myelotomy and shunt placement (Biyani & El Masry, 1994). Treatment of the progressive form of PTS typically involves neurosurgical decompression of the syrinx cavity and shunting, in which a tube is inserted into the cyst to drain the fluid into the chest or abdomen (Biyani & El Masry, 1994; Lammertse, 1993; Little, 1998; Michals & Ramsey, 1996). Although shunts are often effective for stopping further progression of motor/sensory loss, they also require regular (annual) monitoring with routine MRI follow-up examinations to check for blockage (Biyani & El Masry, 1994). Functionally, however, many individuals show little, if any, neurologic improvement after surgery. Poor results may relate to a late clinical presentation and irreversible cord damage before surgery (Michals & Ramsey, 1996).

Spasticity

Spasticity is a neurophysiologic condition characterized by increased muscle tone and increased tendon reflexes (Lance, 1980; Leslie & Ahrendt, 1999; Maynard, Karunas, Adkins, Richards, & Waring, 1995). Spasticity is a common complication of SCI that can result in increased functional deficit by interfering with mobility, sleep, and proper positioning (CDC, 1990; Hinderer & Gupta, 1996). Spasticity may also cause pain; interfere with personal hygiene, wheelchair positioning, and sexual activities; affect the bladder, leading to trouble with kidneys; worsen pressure sores; and result in abnormal postures of the limbs, which can become permanent (contractures), making dressing and other activities difficult (Young, 1996). However, spasticity in people with SCI can also be beneficial. A degree of spasticity may improve circulation and improve muscle tone, slow the development of osteoporosis, assist with transfers and dressing, and — for some individuals with incomplete injuries, spasticity can be used to stand or walk.

Spasticity may become less prominent in many people with SCI over time (Maynard et al., 1995). Increasing spasticity is a common symptom that can result from any stimuli that would be painful if appreciated, such as urinary tract complications; pressure sores; contractures; fecal impaction; bladder distention; deep venous thrombosis; menstrual cramps; labor, delivery and pregnancy; and posttraumatic syringomyelia (Dalyan, Sherman, & Cardenas, 1998; Katz, 1994). Primary exacerbating factors of spasticity may include a persistently unstable spine and the development of posttraumatic cystic degeneration (Ditunno & Formal, 1994).

Before any treatment considerations are made, the degree of functional impairment caused by spasticity must be carefully assessed. However, Priebe, Sherwood, Thornby, Kharas, and Markowski (1996) noted that there is no widely accepted objective in comprehensive measure of spasticity available to the clinician. Current self report and clinical examination scales must be relied upon to represent various dimensions of the clinical problem of spasticity. Further, it will be necessary to determine whether the spasticity is being worsened or maintained by noxious stimuli or some other treatable complication (Katz, 1994; Young, 1996). Lesser degrees of spasticity can be managed with range of motion exercises, standing frames for prolonged stretch, hydrotherapy, and medications. More severe spasticity may require surgery, such as Intrathecal Baclofen (ITB™) pump, dorsal rhizotomy, or tendon release (CDC, 1990). Treatment for spasticity must focus on a stepped-care approach, beginning with conservative methods that have the least negative side effects and progressing to aggressive treatments with the most side effects. Common side effects of ITB therapy include sedation, with more dramatic side effects being delirium and seizures (Ditunno & Formal, 1994). The goal of treatment should be to minimize the adverse effects of spasticity without compromising function (Little & Massagli, 1993).

Fatigue

Fatigue and weakness are problems frequently experienced as late onset complications of SCI (Pentland, McColl, & Rosenthal, 1995). Fatigue not only impacts the individual's physical abilities but also affects his or her mental health. Fatigue is a significant predictor of several future problems, including depression, lower quality of life, and, in some individuals with SCI, the need for more durable medical equipment and help from others (Weitzenkamp, Gerhart, & Charlifue, 1997). Controversy continues to exist over the possible late-life risks and benefits of early-life physical activity, specifically, the various deleterious effects of inactivity versus overuse complications (Currie, Gershkoff, & Cifu, 1993). The impact of fatigue can be delayed or reduced through awareness, vigilance, active health maintenance, and wellness strategies (Whiteneck & Menter, 1993). Long-term planning for persons with SCI requires regular medical follow-up and health care support with an ongoing focus on psychosocial adjustment, equipment and lifestyle changes necessary for preserving health, energy, strength, independence, and quality of life through the aging process.

Appropriate assessment of activity and function throughout the day is necessary to treat fatigue. A complete evaluation for the complaint of fatigue requires a history and examination that includes a large variety of systems. The history should include an assessment of activity during the course of a typical day. Evaluation should also include architectural barriers and demands (Shamberg, Stiens, & Shamberg, 1997). Medical evaluation requires screening for depression, substance abuse, anemia, thyroid disease, infection, and other systemic conditions.

RESPIRATORY SYSTEM

Respiratory complications are a frequent source of morbidity and the primary cause of mortality for persons with SCI, especially those with tetraplegia and high paraplegia (Carter, 1987; DeVivo, Black, & Stover, 1993; Lanig & Lammertse, 1992; Ragnarsson, Hall, Wilmot, & Carter, 1995). Some of the more common respiratory complications such as atelectasis, ventilatory failure, bronchitis, and pneumonia are significantly related (have a higher incidence rate) to advancing age, higher neurologic levels, completeness of injury, and ventilator dependency (DeVivo & Stover, 1995; Jackson & Groomes, 1994; Ragnarsson et al., 1995). Scoliosis, a deformity that can compromise respiratory function, is a particular risk factor in children. Further, progressive kyphosis, a factor of aging with SCI that may be aggravated by increased osteoporosis, obesity, postural changes due to sitting in a wheelchair, and/or spasticity of the abdominal and chest wall, will also cause respiratory compromise. Kyphosis is most common in people with high thoracic injuries (T1–T7) (Wilmot & Hall, 1993).

For persons with high-level injuries, paralysis of the intercostal and abdominal muscles can severely limit pulmonary ventilation and the ability to cough, which increases the probability of developing life-threatening respiratory problems (Almenoff, Spungen, Lesser, & Bauman, 1995; CDC, 1990; Lanig & Lammertse, 1992). In addition, respiratory support is required for individuals whose neurologic level is C1–C3 and necessitates significant levels of skilled nursing or attendant care and frequent medical follow-up evaluations (Winkler, 1999).

Chronic alveolar hypoventilation has also been noted as a late complication of SCI, especially in individuals who may have had damage to the laryngeal structures or impaired autonomic inspiratory or bulbar muscle function. Nocturnal oxyhemoglobin desaturation, sleep disordered breathing, and late onset chronic ventilator insufficiency can occur. These complications appear to be especially prevalent in older individuals (Bach, 1993; Bach & Wang, 1994; Bonekat, Anderson, & Squires, 1990).

Strategies to prevent respiratory complications, especially in persons with high-level SCI, require regular medical evaluations to identify risk factors and detect early stages of medical problems. Annual follow-up evaluations are recommended after age 40 and should include vital capacity assessment and chest x-rays to rule out insidious respiratory problems, such as neoplasms. For individuals with high-level tetraplegia or other factors that at high risk for respiratory complications, follow-up evaluations should take place annually. In addition to vital capacity assessment and chest radiographs the evaluation should include arterial blood gases and annual sleep studies (Lanig & Lammertse, 1992). Further, prompt medical management is needed for individuals showing symptomology suggestive of more serious respiratory problems.

Treatment recommendations to prevent pulmonary infection include aggressive secretion removal, utilizing an incentive spirometer, percussion and drainage, assisted coughing, mucolytic medications, and if necessary, a bronchoscopy. If abdominal muscle tone is lost, an elastic abdominal binder may help replace the active contractible force that aids expiration (Estenne et al., 1998; Nolan, 1994; Ragnarsson et al., 1995).

Infections and tracheal stenosis must be avoided in persons who have a tracheostomy. Manually assisted coughing may be required. Further, as persons with SCI are at a higher risk for pneumonia, they must avoid crowded areas to reduce the chances of catching colds and should receive annual vaccinations for influenza. In addition, their seat backs should be adjusted to a 20-degree recline from vertical to avoid kyphosis (CDC, 1990).

MUSCULOSKELETAL SYSTEM

Musculoskeletal complications are frequently observed during long-term follow-up of people with SCI (Maynard & Weingarden, 1990). People who use wheelchairs or crutches rely heavily on their shoulder, elbow, and wrist joints and often start to develop joint problems approximately 15 years after their injuries. Overuse of these joints may cause tears in the ligaments, muscles, and tendons, and lead to dislocation. Upper extremity pain resulting from degenerative musculoskeletal conditions is a significant complication of SCI, which increases with age and duration of SCI and limits function in people with paraplegia and tetraplegia (CDC, 1990; Staas et al., 1993).

There is also evidence of higher incidence of hip and sacroiliac joint degenerative changes in individuals with SCI of greater than 20 years duration (Charlifue, 1993; Wylie & Chakera, 1988). These problems may be further compounded by the presence of heterotopic ossification or contractures. Fractures of the lower extremities caused by osteoporosis are also common long-term following injury.

As people with SCI age, they must recognize that these changes in the musculoskeletal system may change functional status. Consequently, they must be open to modifications in techniques or use of assistive devices necessary for preserving function and retaining an independent, satisfying quality of life (Waters, Adkins, Yakura, & Sie, 1993).

Upper Extremity Impairments

Upper extremity impairments resulting from injury or degenerative musculoskeletal changes are significant complications that limit function in people with paraplegia and tetraplegia who use their upper extremities for mobility as well as prehension. Even a "minor" shoulder problem can cause a marked decrease in mobility and functional independence. Further, permanent damage from such an injury may be functionally and economically equivalent to a SCI at a much higher level (Sie, Waters, Adkins, & Gellman, 1992; Waters, Sie, & Adkins, 1993).

Because individuals with SCI rely on their upper extremities for mobility in addition to prehension, an increase in degenerative conditions associated with overuse and aging can be expected (Lal, 1998; Sie et al., 1992). Further, many of the musculoskeletal injuries (i.e., rotator cuff tears, biceps tendinitis, carpal tunnel syndrome) that persons with SCI experience result from overuse and are related to the constant repetitive wrist, elbow, and shoulder movements used for transfers and mobility (Bursell et al., 1999; Stotts, 1985). The probability that a wheelchair user will experience upper extremity dysfunction increases with years of wheelchair use. Although some activities of daily living may contribute to upper extremity complications among manual wheelchair users, several studies have implicated the use of manual wheelchairs as a primary contributor (Cooper, 1998; Sie et al., 1992; Wylie & Chakera, 1988). Periodic evaluations of neurologic status may facilitate early detection and intervention for changing needs (Consortium for Spinal Cord Medicine, 1999). Treatment often includes conservative interventions and strategies that focus on changes in functional activities (transfers, wheelchair propulsion), posture, equipment, and home and work environments to minimize exacerbating factors (Goldstein, 1998; Stiens, Haselkorn, Peters, & Goldstein, 1996).

Repetitive activity and strain of the wrist extensor or flexion and extension can produce a variety of wrist injuries. Symptom complexes that are consistent with carpal tunnel syndrome can be detected with focused history and examination. Without proper wrist protection, compression neuropathy of the median nerve can occur. Carpal tunnel syndrome is a clinical diagnosis that may or may not include electrically demonstrable median neuropathy of the wrist (Limke & Stiens, 1997). A high incidence of carpal tunnel syndrome (CTS) has been reported in persons with SCI, particularly those with paraplegia. Studies have found CTS to be present in 26 to 67 percent of persons with SCI (Aljure, Eltorai, Bradley, Lin, & Johnson, 1985; Davidoff, Werner, & Waring, 1991; Gellman et al., 1988; Lammertse, 1993). Further, there is evidence to suggest that the prevalence of CTS may rise as time since injury increases. In a group of individuals with SCI who were five years post-injury, Sie et al. (1992) found 42 percent reported CTS symptoms. This increased to 63 percent in the five to nine years post-injury group, 74 percent in the 10 to 14 years post-injury group, and 92 percent in the 15 to 19 years post-injury group. Surveillance and monitoring for CTS is recommended for individuals with paraplegia who are active in transfers and manual wheelchair propulsion.

Osteoporosis

Osteoporosis is characterized by a progressive loss of bone tissue, with a resulting increase in the risk of bone fractures. Some degree of osteoporosis occurs in almost everyone who ages. It is also a common complication secondary to SCI, although the exact sequence of metabolic events resulting in bone loss following injury is still not fully understood (Szollar et al., 1997). People who have had SCI may develop osteoporosis within six months of their injury. The hips and femurs (long leg bones) are the bones most often affected (Nance et al., 1999; Szollar, 1997; Szollar et al., 1998). In addition to the SCI itself, risk factors for osteoporosis in the general population that are also risks for people with SCI include:

- Genetics—female gender, Caucasian or Asian race, light skinned or fair haired, thin and small body frames, family history of osteoporosis
- Lifestyle—cigarette smoking, excessive alcohol and caffeine consumption, lack of exercise, diet low in calcium and/or extremely high in fiber or protein
- Hormones—menopause, early surgical removal of both ovaries, hyperthyroidism, hyperparathyroidism, Vitamin D deficiency
- Medications—heparin, phenytoin (Dilantin®), phenobarbital, and corticosteriods

The average bone density loss during the first year post-SCI is about 40 to 70 percent, depending on the site and age of the individual (Nance et al., 1999). Szollar et al. (1997) observed that significant bone density loss occurs in the hip by the first year post-injury for all persons younger than 60 years and that the decline continues until 19 years after SCI. The bone that is lost as a consequence of SCI most often cannot be regained (RTC/IL, 1996). Individuals with osteoporosis generally have no symptoms until bone fractures occur. Although studies indicate a prevalence of approximately 1 to 6 percent of brittle bone-related fractures in persons with SCI, the incidence of these fractures is ten times more common in people with complete SCI compared to those with an incomplete injury (Ragnarsson & Sell, 1981; Waters, Sie, & Adkins, 1993). Anyone with osteoporosis is at risk for broken bones.

Strategies to reduce complications can include increasing physical activity and exercise (especially weight bearing activities or resistance exercises), increasing calcium intake, cessation of smoking, curtailing alcohol intake, and modifying transfer techniques. Treatment of osteoporosis may include vitamin and mineral supplements (vitamin D and calcium), estrogen replacement in post-menopausal women, and medication therapy for well-established osteoporosis (Nance et al., 1999; Pearson et al., 1997). The use of standing aids may have more positive psychological effect than physiological benefit (Kunkel et al., 1993).

Posture Problems and Contractures

Posture problems and contractures are common complications that develop in most people with SCI if not treated properly. Problems associated with posture changes and SCI range from chronic pain and fatigue to scoliosis and kyphosis as well as skin and respiratory problems. Maintenance of erect trunk posture is a frequent problem for individuals with complete tetraplegia who use wheelchairs. Without extensor support, the trunk collapses forward in a sitting position. In children with an immature skeleton, this forward collapse leads to progressive scoliosis and structural vertebral deformity (Waters, Sie, & Adkins, 1993).

Contractures occur when connective tissue, joint capsules, muscle, and tendons shorten around joints. This often results from failure to start range of motion exercises early, improper positioning of the person with SCI in bed and in the wheelchair, and failure to splint paralyzed extremities. In addition, spasticity can lead to an accelerated development of contractures. As a consequence, contractures may significantly interfere with limb positioning and the use of residual function in both the upper and lower extremities (CDC, 1990; Dalyan et al., 1998; Kunkel et al., 1993; Waters et al., 1993). Musculoskeletal problems, including contractures, curvature of the spine, and fractures, are the most commonly occurring secondary conditions associated with having lived 20 or more years with SCI (Krause, 1999).

Preventive strategies may include proper positioning of trunk and extremities (e.g., with modified cushions, solid chair backs, lateral supports, chest belts, etc.), range of motion exercises (active and passive), and rotating beds with positioning troughs for arms and legs for individuals with tetraplegia. Treatment typically involves physical therapy, progressive (dynamic) splinting, and motor point or nerve blocks for spasticity. Surgical release through tendon lengthening, osteotomies, joint replacement, and the like may be indicated in more severe cases.

Heterotopic Ossification (HO)

Heterotopic ossification (HO) is the development of ectopic bone within the soft tissues surrounding peripheral joints. HO is a fairly common complication of SCI (Arkansas Spinal Cord Commission, 1990). It can range from a small amount of bone noted as an incidental finding on an x-ray to massive bone formation around a joint, resulting in total ankylosis. A person with HO has increasingly limited or reduced range of motion in the joint. HO is a complication usually developing below the level of injury and most often affecting the hips and knees. It can also occur in the shoulders and elbows but rarely in the hands and feet. The most common time for onset of HO is between one and four months after SCI. Once individuals with SCI have experienced HO, they have a much greater likelihood of reactivating the process at some point in the future. Factors associated with reactivation of HO include fractures, kidney stones, pressure sores, and surgeries (DiLima, Hildebrandt, & Schust, 1996; Winkler & Weed, 1999).

Because the etiology is unknown, it is difficult to predict which individuals are more likely to develop HO or which are likely to have only a mild form (Arkansas Spinal Cord Commission, 1990). The incidence of HO in persons with SCI is typically cited between 20 to 30 percent (Stover, Nieman, & Tulloss, 1991). However, HO progresses to ankylosis in less than 10 percent of people with SCI. The numbers may be somewhat higher in people with tetraplegia (CDC, 1990; Waters, Sie, & Adkins, 1993).

Functional implications depend on the amount and location of the ectopic bone. At the hip, HO may affect posture, seating, lower extremity dressing, and hygiene. Skin breakdown is often a problem from either direct compression over a large mass of heterotopic bone or secondary to poor posture and seating. At the shoulder, HO may further impair upper extremity movement in the individual with tetraplegia (Goldstein 1998).

Routine medical care follow-up, serial bone scans and/or x-rays, and serum phosphorus levels (when active HO is present) are used to detect HO. Treatment, directed toward prevention of loss of motion, includes physical therapy, range of motion exercises, and medications, such as etidronate (Didronel®) and/or nonsteroidal anti-inflammatories, such as ibuprofen, indomethacin (Indocin®), and naproxen (Banovac & Gonzales, 1997; Banovac et al., 1997; Goldstein, 1998; Gonzales et al.,1993; Schurch et al., 1997). Surgical resection of bone deposits may be indicated in cases of major functional limitations from HO (Stover et al., 1991).

CARDIOVASCULAR SYSTEM

Cardiovascular complications, which can occur during both the acute and chronic phases of SCI, are major causes of morbidity and mortality. The cardiovascular complications frequently associated with SCI are autonomic dysreflexia, deep venous thrombosis (DVT) and pulmonary embolism, and coronary artery disease (Stiens, Johnson, & Lyman, 1995). Although the incidence of DVT and pulmonary emboli tend to be lower during the chronic phase of SCI (Consortium for Spinal Cord Medicine, 1999b; McKinley, Jackson, Cardenas, & DeVivo, 1999), these complications may still occur.

Orthostatic hypotension and dependent edema are also symptoms of cardiovascular dysfunction in people with SCI, although these are usually of less clinical significance (Ragnarsson et al., 1995). Orthostatic hypotension is typically associated with high level lesions and is most often noted following prolonged periods of recumbency. It is evidenced by a sudden drop in blood pressure that produces dizziness or weakness, or in severe cases, fainting. This condition may be chronic in some individuals with SCI and require intervention. Preventive measures may include abdominal binders; elastic stockings; increased sodium intake; equipment modifications, such as recline and tilt wheelchairs or elevating leg rests; and medications, such as ephedrine sulfate or fluorinated corticosteroids (Ragnarsson et al., 1995).

Dependency edema of the lower extremities is also common in people with SCI. It is generally bilateral and symmetrical, and is best managed with elevation and compression with elastic stockings. Diuretics are generally not indicated for dependency edema (Ragnarsson et al., 1995).

Autonomic Dysreflexia (AD)

Autonomic dysreflexia (AD), also known as autonomic hyperreflexia, is a potentially fatal complication of SCI characterized by exaggerated sympathetic responses to noxious (irritating) stimuli below the level of lesion, marked by symptoms such as hypertension, profuse sweating above the level of lesion, goose bumps, blurred vision, nasal congestion, pounding headache, and/or cardiac arrhythmias (Consortium for

Spinal Cord Medicine, 1997a). When a noxious stimulus occurs, a reflex is initiated that triggers blood vessel constriction and raise blood pressure (Colachis, 1992; Goetz, 1998). When the spinal cord is intact, descending inhibitory fibers can curtail or moderate sympathetic overflow in response to excessive blood pressures detected at the carotid body and other barorecptors. However, in persons with SCI, particularly at the T6 level or above, the signals which mediate vasospasm are interrupted by the injury. AD is more likely to occur in persons with complete injuries but has been seen in persons with incomplete injuries as well (Goetz, 1998; McKinley et al., 1999). AD is an emergency condition that requires immediate attention, because blood pressure can rise to dangerous levels if not controlled by outside means. Left uncontrolled, high blood pressure may cause stroke, seizures, or possibly death (DiLima et al., 1996). Because AD is a condition known to occur only with SCI, many health care professionals may not know much about it or realize how serious it can be.

Bladder distension (full bladder) and bladder/kidney complications are the most common cause of autonomic dysreflexia in people with SCI (Colachis, 1992; Selzman & Humpel, 1993). Other possible stimuli include rectal distension (fecal impaction); menses; pregnancy (especially labor and delivery); vaginitis; invasive testing; surgical or diagnostic procedures; deep vein thrombosis; fractures; drug reactions; orthostatic hypotension; ingrown toenails; burns or temperature fluctuations; sunburn; pressure sores; sexual activity; constrictive clothing, shoes, or appliances; or any painful or irritating stimuli below the level of injury (Consortium for Spinal Cord Medicine, 1997a; Goetz, 1998; Yarkony, 1994b). Typically, the management of AD focuses on quick identification and elimination of noxious stimuli that may produce symptoms, prompt suppression of elevated blood pressure, and prevention of recurrent episodes (Ragnarsson et al., 1995). It is important that care givers be educated about AD and capable of responding rapidly when an episode occurs.

Blood pressure must be carefully monitored with injuries at or above T6 and routine medical reevaluations are very important, even if the individual does not have AD symptoms. Medications, such as phenoxybenzamine (Dibenzyline®), may be prescribed if the person has frequent, recurring AD. If AD occurs at predictable times, such as with bowel care, the person may use a topical anesthetic such as lidocaine jelly during the procedure or nitropaste prior to an anticipated AD episode. If necessary, surgical treatment, including rhizotomy or sacral neurectomy, may be indicated in life-threatening, recurring AD. Epidural anesthesia is the treatment of choice for AD during labor and delivery. Also, because fetal heart rate may rise during the mother's AD, heart-rate monitoring of mother and fetus is important (Chanaud, 1997).

Deep Venous Thrombosis (DVT)

Deep venous thrombosis (DVT) and subsequent pulmonary embolism (PE) most commonly occur during the first year following SCI as a consequence of paralysis and immobilization associated with decreased vascular tone and hypercoagulability (Kim et al., 1994; McKinley et al., 1999; Ragnarsson et al., 1995). The period of highest risk for development of DVT appears to be during the first three to six months after onset of SCI (Schmitt, Midka, & McKenzie, 1995). Findings from Model Systems studies indicate that DVT occurs slightly more often in persons with paraplegia than in those with tetraplegia and more commonly in those with complete injuries than with incomplete injuries (McKinley et al., 1999; Ragnarsson et al., 1995).

Prevention and early detection of DVT is preferable to treatment and is critical in the management process. Physical methods of prophylaxis typically include gradient elastic stockings and intermittent pneumatic compression devices. Pharmacologic prophylactic treatment during the acute phase of SCI, usually involving lower limb compression and anticoagulation therapy, generally begins within the first 14 days after injury when the risk of DVT is thought to be greatest (Merli et al.,

1988). Prophylactic treatment is typically continued for at least three months (Consortium for Spinal Cord Medicine, 1999b), although this is no guarantee that DVT will not occur. Once DVT has been diagnosed, full anticoagulation is generally recommended as the treatment of choice. This is usually continued for three months for DVT without PE and for six months if PE is present. This same length of anticoagulation treatment is indicated for any subsequent episodes of DVT or PE as well (Merli, 1992; Ragnarsson et al., 1995).

Coronary Artery Disease (CAD)

Evidence suggests that many coronary artery disease (CAD) risk factors may be magnified by SCI (Bauman, 1997; Bauman, Raza, Spungen, & Machac, 1994; Dallmeijer, Hopman, & Van der Woude, 1997; Yarkony, Formal, & Cawley, 1997; Yekutiel, Brooks, Ohry, Yarom, & Carel, 1989). Drawing from the National SCI Database, DeVivo and Stover (1995) identified CAD as the second leading underlying cause of death for persons with tetraplegia and the leading underlying cause of death for persons with paraplegia and persons with Frankel grade D injuries. A collaborative study by Craig Hospital and two British SCI centers (Whiteneck, 1993) revealed that CAD was the leading cause of mortality among persons with SCI who were more than 30 years post-injury (46 percent of all deaths) and among those over 60 years of age (35 percent of all deaths). The study sample was drawn from people in the United Kingdom and represents the largest investigation conducted to date of persons who were more than 20 years post-SCI.

Bauman (1997) found that persons with SCI are generally more insulin-resistant than the non-SCI population. This results in multiple metabolic abnormalities that can increase the risk of developing atherosclerotic-ischemic heart disease. Specifically, these abnormalities include the development of noninsulin dependent diabetes mellitus, impaired glucose tolerance, high blood pressure (hypertension), high blood fat levels (triglycerides), with a lower level of high-density lipoprotein cholesterol (HDL-C), and relatively high levels of low-density lipoprotein cholesterol (LDL-C). Certain physical changes associated with SCI contribute to the metabolic abnormalities that increase the risk of CAD; these include the loss of muscle mass because of atrophy below the level of injury, an increase in body fat, and a general decrease in the ability to maintain cardiovascular or aerobic fitness (Bauman & Spungen, 1994; Dallmeijer et al., 1997; Kocina, 1997; Krum, Howes, & Brown, 1992).

The CAD risk factors appear to differ as a function of injury level (Kemp, Bauman, Adkins, Spungen, & Krause, 1999). People with paraplegia have been found to have higher total cholesterol, low density lipids (LDL), and triglycerides when compared to those with tetraplegia. However, specific mechanisms for the interaction of risk factors after SCI are not fully understood and may include psychologic factors. For example, nondepressed individuals with tetraplegia showed higher cholesterol levels (total, LDL, triglycerides) than people with tetraplegia who were depressed, whereas nondepressed individuals with paraplegia had lower cholesterol levels than individuals with paraplegia who were depressed. This is a new area of research that will no doubt unfold over the next few years as a major area of concern for people with SCI.

Any long-term, health care planning for individuals with SCI must incorporate appropriate preventive strategies to detect and reduce the risk of developing CAD. Specific strategies include proper annual medical follow-up care, maintaining a healthy diet, not smoking, avoiding excessive use of alcohol, participating in regular physical exercise, and appropriate equipment modification (Bauman, 1997; Janssen et al., 1997). Medical follow-up care should include regular screening tests for diabetes and insulin resistance and treatment of anomalies (Bauman, 1997). Laboratory tests to determine blood lipid levels are useful on an annual basis. Electrocardiography is recommended to evaluate for suspected CAD, particularly for individuals with tetraplegia (Stiens, Johnson, & Lyman, 1995). Because of sensory perception deficits in individuals with complete SCI above T5 levels, the clinician must be especially vigilant in checking for coronary ischemia. Reliance on symptoms alone in patients with interruption of sensory pathways is insufficient to detect CAD at a stage that is most effectively treated (Stiens et al., 1995). Silent ischemia can present without symptoms or with very nonspecific symptoms such as autonomic dysreflexia, nausea, or arm pain. Persantive stress testing should be utilized to rule out ischemic compromise to sections of the myocardium. The recent development of high-speed CT scans to detect CAD may also be useful for people with SCI because they cannot participate in traditional cardiac stress testing. Chest radiography should be considered to detect changes that may suggest congestive heart failure (Stiens et al., 1995).

Individuals with high-level SCI may also be susceptible to bradycardia, tachycardia, or even asystole (cardiac standstill) during tracheal suction. These arrhythmias are more common during the first two months after SCI. A careful history should be taken to determine if any past episodes of arrhythmias have occurred. A negative history of arrhythmias does not assure the problem will not occur in the future. Individuals at risk include persons with higher-level SCI, tracheostomy or ventilator dependent individuals, and older persons. Individuals at risk require personnel who have received proper training in how to avoid body stimulation and the proper suction techniques to use, as well as training in how to respond to an arrhythmia. Treatments may include the administration of Atropine IV, chronic use of theophylline, CPR, or the placement of a pacemaker in individuals who have repeated episodes.

GASTROINTESTINAL SYSTEM

Studies of the gastrointestinal (GI) system and changes in the GI tract after SCI document a high prevalence of post-injury complications (Glickman & Kamm, 1996; Stone, Nino-Murica, Wolfe, & Perkash, 1990). Although the incidence has been found to vary greatly among people with SCI, GI tract complications include, but are not limited to, gastrointestinal hemorrhage, gastric ulcerations, ileus, cholelithiasis, esophageal problems, autonomic dysreflexia, pain, abdominal distention, diverticulosis, hemorrhoids, fecal impaction, constipation, diarrhea, delayed bowel evacuation, and fecal incontinence (Albert, Levine, Balderston, & Cotler, 1991; Apstein & Dalecki-Chipperfield, 1987; Gore, Mintzer, & Calenoff, 1981; Neumayer, Bull, Mohr, & Putnam, 1990; Soderstrom & Ducker, 1990; Stiens, 1998; Stinneford, Keshavarzian, Nemchasky, Doria, & Durkin, 1993; Stone et al., 1990; Watson, 1981). However, as Cosman, Stone, and Perkash (1993) suggest, age, level and completeness of injury, time since injury, pre-injury GI function, diet, and quality of long-term care are all likely to affect GI function and occurrence of complications following SCI.

Asymptomatic cholelithiasis is more prevalent for individuals with SCI that for the general population (Moonka, Stiens, Eubank, & Stelzner, 1999). The prevalence of gallstones after injury, as determined in cross-sectional studies, has been estimated to be as high as 30 percent, making it up to three times more likely than in the general population. Risk factors for cholelithiasis in people with SCI include decreased intestinal transit rate, which delays the enterohepatic circulation of bile salts; catabolic changes after SCI that could mobilize protein, calcium, and cholesterol into bile; and gallbladder stasis from impaired neural and hormonal control (Ketover, Ansel, Goldish, Roche, & Gebhard, 1996; Stiens, 1998; Stiens et al., 1997). Follow-up medical care suggests annual ultrasound surveillance for stone formation and evidence of inflammation, along with annual renal scanning. Prophylactic cholecystectomy is not necessary because persons with SCI typically present with symptoms in sufficient time for cholecystectomy (Moonka et al., 1999; Stiens, 1998).

Although many of the GI tract complications, such as gastroduodenal hemorrhage, paralytic ileus, and pancreatitis, appear to be more prevalent in the early phases post-SCI, lower tract dysfunction tends to be the most common long-term GI complications for people with SCI (Cardenas, Farrell-Roberts, Sipski, & Rubner, 1995; CDC, 1990; Linsenmeyer & Stone, 1993). Lower tract dysfunction can be a source of inconvenience, frustration, and expense, especially for individuals with high-level injuries who require attendant support (Stiens, Bierner-Bergman, & Goetz, 1997). Between 27 to 61 percent of people with SCI report bowel dysfunction (constipation, incontinence, and difficulties with evacuation) as a major life-limiting problem (Glickman & Kamm, 1996; Han, Kim, & Kwon, 1998; Stone et al., 1990). Further, these problems become more evident as individuals age after injury and can impact their independence, self-esteem, work, and personal relationships (Consortium for Spinal Cord Medicine, 1998; Frost, 1994; Glickman & Kamm, 1996; Krotoski & Bennett, 1996; White, Rintala, Hart, & Fuhrer, 1993).

Menter et al. (1997) analyzed data on outcomes of bowel management from 221 British long-term survivors as part of a longitudinal collaborative study on aging with SCI between two British SCI treatment centers and Craig Hospital. All of the participants in this population-based sample were at least 20 years post-SCI. From comprehensive assessments and extensive interviews, 42 percent of the sample population reported constipation, 35 percent reported gastrointestinal pain, and 27 percent complained of bowel accidents. The physicians in this study diagnosed significantly more hemorrhoids among individuals using primarily suppositories and enemas to manage their bowels and more constipation among persons with paraplegia and those using digital stimulation, manual evacuation, or increased abdominal pressure in their bowel care routines. Fecal incontinence and diarrhea were diagnosed three times more often in participants with tetraplegia as in other neurologic groupings.

There is presently little information available on functional assessment related to bowel care for people with SCI. Model Systems data revealed that of the 1,758 individuals who were discharged from 1988 through 1992, 30.4 percent of those with both complete or incomplete injuries required assistance with bowel management. The level of assistance varied by severity of injury, ranging from 78 percent for individuals with complete tetraplegia who required complete assistance to 11.8 percent for those with complete paraplegia. Of individuals with complete paraplegia, 53.3 percent managed their bowel care with modified assistance (Cardenas et al., 1995).

After interviewing 758 people with SCI, Berkowitz, Harvey, Greene, and Wilson (1992) found that 35.7 percent of all respondents required assistance with bowel care. People with tetraplegia were three times more likely to report the need for assistance than individuals with paraplegia (59.2 percent compared to 16.3 percent).

In general, individuals with SCI at or above the C5 level will be dependent for all physical aspects of bowel care. Although people with C6 and C7 level injuries may perform bowel care without assistance for related areas such as clothing management and transfer skills, many opt for assistance to save time and energy and to prevent frustration (Consortium for Spinal Cord Medicine, 1998).

Studies of the effects of medications on bowel function specific to SCI have been limited to date. In general, however, the use of antibiotics can change the balance of the colon microflora and result in soft stool or diarrhea. Medications that have anticholinergic properties have the potential to slow bowel motility, resulting in constipation or even adynamic ileus. Drugs commonly used to manage a neurogenic bladder, such as oxybutynin (Ditropan®) and propantheline (Pro-Banthine®), may decrease bowel motility. A number of antidepressant drugs, such as amitriptyline, also have anticholinergic effects. Narcotic pain medications can result in constipation, due to the slowing of bowel motility. Certain medications used for treatment of spasticity may also have an effect on bowel function (Consortium for Spinal Cord Medicine, 1998).

The goals of an effective bowel management program are to minimize or prevent incontinence, to evacuate stool at a regular and predictable time, and to minimize the secondary complications of colonic overdistension, fecal impaction, and diverticuli (Consortium for Spinal Cord Medicine, 1998; Stiens, 1998; Zejdlik, 1992). A bowel program can take months to establish and requires careful management to maintain. It is important that a bowel management routine is designed and revised with participation of the individual with SCI. Stiens (1998) outlines a number of factors that should be considered in individualizing a bowel program. These include:

- Dietary modulation of stool consistency with fiber and liquid intake
- Increased physical activity
- Regular scheduling of bowel care time and frequency
- Adaptive equipment (e.g., commode chair, digital stimulation devices, etc., based on individual's functional status and home/community environmental needs)
- Oral medications (that either promote or inhibit bowel function)
- Rectal medications (suppositories)

With the exception of a small number of studies on rectal stimulants (Stiens, 1995; House & Stiens, 1997) and prokinetic medications, and some studies on dietary fiber, systematic testing of these components for individuals with SCI is lacking (Consortium for Spinal Cord Medicine, 1998). In addition to safety and effectiveness, the design of a bowel program also must consider personal goals, life schedules, role obligations of the individual and family caregiver, self-rated quality of life, and the need for and availability of attendant care (Consortium for Spinal Cord Medicine, 1998).

GENITOURINARY SYSTEM

Impairments in bladder and pelvic floor function after SCI interact to produce problems with storage and voluntary voiding of urine. As a result, there may be difficulties with bladder emptying, excessively high pressures, infection, stone formation, and renal damage. Secondary complications of SCI related to the bladder are common. While urinary tract infections and kidney failure were once a leading cause of death in people with SCI, better medical treatment and surveillance strategies, antibiotics, and improved bladder management programs have reduced death from urinary problems to an infrequent cause of mortality (Apple & Hudson, 1990; DeVivo, Black, & Stover, 1993; Lanig, 1993). However, urological problems, particularly urinary tract infections (UTIs), continue to be one of the most frequently occurring complications for people with SCI (Cardenas & Hooton, 1995; Waites, Canupp, & DeVivo, 1993). Further, with the emergence of extremely resistant strains of bacteria it might be anticipated that both morbidity and cost of treatment will increase.

Other genitourinary system complications include calculi, uretheral tears, hydronephrosis, bladder dilation, bladder trabeculations, chronic cystitis, prostatitis, and epidimyorchidis. Bladder cancer is more common among people with SCI than in the general population (Bickel, Culkin, & Wheeler, 1991; Broeker, Klein, & Hackler, 1981; El Masri & Fellows, 1981; Hackler, 1977). The most commonly quoted overall incidence of bladder cancer in people with SCI seems to be around 150 in every 5,000, or 3 percent (Hammond et al., 1998) compared to about one person in every 5,000 for the general population. Even though bladder cancer may be 100 times more frequent for people with SCI than the general population, it still is not that common. Further, the pathophysiology and natural history of bladder malignancy in the neurogenic bladder secondary to SCI is not well understood (Lanig, 1993).

Historically, most factors that increase a person's risk of bladder cancer after SCI seem to relate to chronic or repeated bladder irritation, such as frequent UTIs, bladder stones, smoking, and long-term use of indwelling catheters (Dolin, Darby, & Beral, 1994; El Masri & Fellows, 1981; Kantor et al., 1984; Kaufman et al., 1977; Locke, Hill, & Walzer, 1985). However, some researchers believe that the incidence of bladder cancer in the aging population with SCI may be more a function of the "era of care," and that given the current antibiotic and anticholinergic drugs and catheters made from safer, nonrubber materials, the incidence rates may be lower among more recently injured individuals (El Masri & Fellows, 1981). Although the degree of risk for bladder cancer among people with SCI may still be controversial, long-term surveillance strategies recommend that individuals should have a regular scheduled (every 1-2 years) cystoscopy (and bladder biopsy, as indicated) after ten years of continued indwelling catheter use or, if the individual is at high risk, a smoker, over age 40, or has a history of recurrent UTIs (Cardenas, Mayo, & King, 1996; Goetz & Little, 1998).

Although findings indicate that UTIs remain one of the most common secondary medical complications following SCI, most literature suggests that many UTIs that lead to further complications may be prevented with proper evaluations and bladder management (Cardenas, Farrell-Roberts, Sipski, & Rubner, 1995; Goetz & Little, 1998; Lanig, 1993). Whereas many genitourinary complications are considered to be related to methods for bladder management, there is no consistent consensus about an optimal method (Maynard & Weingarden, 1990). Further, as people with SCI age, long-term planning efforts must address their changing urinary management needs within the context of age-related physical, physiological, and psychosocial considerations (Lanig, 1993). In determining the method of urinary management for people with SCI, consideration must be given to the person's functional abilities and/or attendant support as well as his or her preference and motivation. Other factors that must be considered include living environment, lifestyle, and time since injury (Jackson & DeVivo, 1992).

The rationale for choice of bladder drainage method is based on the premises of maximizing independence of the user, success in prevention of incontinence or leaking, and prevention of complications. Minimizing the presence of a foreign body in the bladder and the amount of equipment required is desirable. Pharmacologic adjuncts to drainage methods are often required to prevent bladder spasm, increase sphincter tone, and prevent bacterial overgrowth. The least invasive situation is that of voluntary voids or sensory signaled, reflex-triggered, and/or Valsalva voiding. This is possible in some individuals who are sensory and motor incomplete. If individuals have unplanned reflex voids, anticholinergic medications such as oxybutynin are helpful. The next less invasive situation is intermittent catheterization, which requires education of the user, dexterity to perform the catheterization, and adherence with the protocol. This allows regular bladder emptying with an interim catheter-free state. If the bladder is contractible and the sphincter offers little resistance, condom catheter drainage into a leg bag is effective. Sphincterotomy is a surgical option to reduce outflow resistance. Constant indwelling catheterization can be maintained with a Foley catheter through the urethra or a suprapubic catheter surgically placed through the abdominal wall. Fluid intake should be high to constantly flush urine through the system to prevent bacterial overgrowths.

Although intermittent catheterization (IC) has contributed to a reduction in morbidity after SCI, this method requires that an individual have adequate hand function or assistance to be able to empty the bladder every four to six hours. Anatomic considerations make IC more difficult for women with SCI. Persons with upper motor neuron bladders who use IC commonly require an anticholinergic drug to inhibit contractions and to increase bladder storage (Goetz & Little, 1998).

External or condom catheters are often found to be the most practical method for men with high-level tetraplegia and limited hand function. In general, condom catheters should be changed on a daily basis. Individuals who are obese or those with a small, retractile penis may have difficulty retaining a condom. Penile prosthesis are occasionally implanted to facilitate use of a condom catheter (Goetz & Little, 1998).

Indwelling catheters may be either urethral or suprapubic. The catheter must be changed at least monthly and the bedside or leg bag cleaned daily. Indwelling catheters are used if other options are not feasible. Urethral catheters should generally not be used in the presence of a penile prosthesis because of the risk of erosion. Potential complications of indwelling urethral catheters include prostatitis, epididymitis, dislodgement, erosion of the urethra, and accidental inflation of th catheter balloon in the urethra. Although the degree of increased risk of bladde cancer is controversial for individuals using indwelling catheterization, people with SCI should undergo a cystoscopy after ten years of continued indwelling catheter use or five years if at high risk (i.e., smoker, over age 40, recurrent UTIs) (Cardenas, Mayo, & King, 1996). For women, suprapubic catheters are generally used only if other methods of management are unsuccessful as a result of complications.

Based on data from the National Spinal Cord Injury Statistical Center (NSCISC), Cardenas et el. (1995) analyzed the amount of assistance required for different methods of bladder management. The authors found that, based on FIM ratings, 58.7 percent of all one-year post-injury individuals on intermittent catheterization (N = 1059) were independent (modified or complete independence) while 41.3 percent required some level of assistance. For individuals using an indwelling catheter (N = 180), only 19.4 percent were independent compared with 80.6 percent requiring assistance. The use of an external collector was about evenly divided between individuals who were independent (47.0 percent) and those who required some level of assistance (53.0 percent).

Using 15 years of follow-up data from the Model Systems programs, Cardenas et al. (1995) examined the method of bladder management over time. From this study, the authors identified the most predominate trend for men to be a decline in the use of intermittent catheterization from 36.4 percent at discharge from initial rehabilitation to 6.8 percent at 15 years post-injury. For women, the use of intermittent catheterization declined from 38.6 percent at discharge to 18.5 percent at 15 years, and there was a concurrent increase in the use of indwelling catheterization from 33.2 percent at discharge to 52.3 percent at 15 years. For men, this trend was seen in the use of condom drainage, which increased from 22.2 percent at discharge to 35.6 percent at 15 years post-SCI. These findings may have implications when looking at long-term planning for attendant care needs.

Periodic evaluation of the genitourinary system is important to preserve renal function and reduce morbidity and mortality (Cardenas et al., 1995). Medical follow-up requires regular (every 12–24 months) comprehensive genitourinary evaluations, unless clinical signs and symptoms necessitate earlier evaluation (Lanig, 1993). Periodic evaluations typically include urodynamic testing (used in cases of voluntary or spontaneous voiding), ultrasound (renal, ureters, bladder), abdominal radiography, 24-hour urine for creatinine clearance, urinalysis, post void residuals if the individual self-voids, and other tests of renal function, as needed, such as renal radionucleotide scan. Intravenous pyelograms are no longer performed on a routine basis and should be used as indicated by other test results. Cystoscopy is generally performed in individuals after use of an indwelling catheter for more than ten years or if the individual is at high risk for bladder cancer, such as smokers, over age 40, or history of frequent UTIs (Goetz & Little, 1998). In addition, comprehensive gynecological evaluation for women with SCI must include annual pelvic examination, Pap smear, and breast examination (Lanig, 1993).

SKIN

The skin is the largest organ system of the body. It is responsible for regulation of body temperature, sensation (touch, pain, and temperature), fluid regulation, and protection from bodily harm. Skin problems can limit a person's ability to care for himself or herself or to function on the job (Berkowitz, Harvey, Greene, & Wilson, 1992).

SCI produces a variety of deficits that affects skin function and puts the skin at risk for breakdown. Paralysis below the level of injury limits mobility and can result in excessive prolonged pressure on skin over bony prominences. Interruption of sensory pathways prevents perception of injury to the skin. Damage to the sympathetic nervous system affects piloerection, sweating, and autoregulation of blood flow to the skin.

Skin complications, particularly pressure sores, are a common problem for people with SCI and one of the largest medical care expenses, leading to hospitalization and extended bed rest (Burns & Betz, 1999). Pressure sores are areas of skin or soft tissue damage caused by excessive or prolonged pressure. Pressure sores are one of the leading causes of frequent disruptions in routine life activities that can interfere with personal independence and mobility (CDC, 1990; Stover, Hale, & Buell, 1994). After a SCI, there is poor regulation of blood flow through capillaries, with resulting decreased cutaneous response to focal pressure. The end result can be skin breakdown and pressure sores. This pressure cuts off the blood supply to the skin, causing ischemic infarction (RTC/IL, 1993b). Pressure sores commonly develop in areas over the buttocks, sides of hips, knees, ankles, heels, toes, and other bony areas of the body. Pressure sores are usually grouped into four categories or grades, ranging from grade 1 (minor) to grade 4 (severe) (Enis & Sarmiento, 1973; Stover & Fine, 1986).

Rehabilitative management to prevent pressure sores requires reestablishment of skin–brain sensory connection and development of habits of skin protection. The sensory connection can be done by visually inspecting the area at least twice daily with a mirror. Skin protection programs include regular use of emollients, avoidance of moisture exposure, use of pressure distributing cushions, and regular pressure releases — are movements to redistribute pressure over the skin done with lifting the body part briefly or through wheelchair seating adjustments.

Gerhart, Charlifue, Menter, Weitzenkamp, and Whiteneck (1997) outlined characteristics that placed people with SCI at risk for pressure sores: individuals with paraplegia were more than three times more likely than other SCI individuals; those with abnormal pulses in the feet and lower extremities were at greater risk; and those who did not work had three times more pressure sores than those who were working. Garber, Rintala, Rossi, Hark, and Fuhrer (1996) also noted that previous ulcers, taking less responsibility for skin care, and being less satisfied with activities of life were associated with incidence of pressure sores. More severe ulcers occured among people who are non-white, older, less mobile, less educated, and older at time of injury (Garber et al., 1996). Other population-based research has found pressure sores to be associated with lower levels of education, utilization of prescription medication for pain and spasticity, a history of incarceration or suicidal ideation, smoking, being underweight, unemployment, and being single (Krause, Vines, Farley, Sniezek, & Coker, 1999). Clearly these wounds have etiologies that are multifactorial, and rehabilitative efforts to reduce handicap can be helpful in prevention.

Byrne and Salzberg (1996) critically evaluated the medical, nursing, and nutritional research literature to identify the principle risk factors for development of pressure sores in people with SCI. The authors found that pressure sores are an underestimated health care problem, in terms of costs and productivity, for individuals with SCI. These data suggested an annual incidence of pressure sores among people with SCI of between 23 and 30 percent, and that up to 85 percent will develop a pressure sore at some point during their lifetimes. As Byrne and Salzberg (1996) discovered an overwhelming number (more than 200) of risk factors reported in the literature, the authors were subsequently able to pare this down to 15 major risk factors consistently identified across studies for development of pressure sores in people with SCI (see Table H-1). In spite of a concerted effort to prevent them in environments such as inpatient SCI units, one study recorded a prevalence of up to 25 percent for any grade 2 or greater pressure sore (Hammond, Bozzocco, Stiens, Buhrer, & Lyman, 1994).

The psychosocial adjustment of persons with SCI can also have a major impact on pressure sore development (Krause, 1998; Yarkony & Heinemann, 1995). Anderson and Andberg (1979) found that people who do not follow through on self-care requirements because of depression, lack of motivation, or alcohol and substance abuse are at greatest risk of developing pressure sores. Pressure sores, in turn,

Table H-1. Major Risk Factors for Pressure Sores in People with SCI

Severity of SCI	Preexisting Conditions	Malnutrition and Anemia
• Decreased level of activity • Immobility • Completeness of SCI • Urine incontinence/moisture • Autonomic dysreflexia/severe spasticity	• Advanced age • Tobacco use/smoking • Pulmonary disease • Cardiac disease/abnormal electrocardiogram • Diabetes/poor glycemic control • Renal disease • Impaired cognitive function • Residing in a nursing home/hospital	• Hypoalbuminemia/hypoproteinemia • Anemia

may also have a negative impact on psychosocial adjustment (Gordon, Harasymiw, Bellile, Lehman, & Sherman, 1982).

Complications from pressure sores can include local and systemic infection, dehydration, anemia, pelvic abscess, malignancy, and lengthy periods of medical treatment and hospitalizations. Model Systems studies estimate that individuals with SCI who have pressure sores incur hospital charges of three to four times those of other individuals with SCI and average at least an additional $15,000 per year in health care costs. These costs can increase to more than $30,000 for grade 4 sores (DeVivo, 1998; Dixit, Martin, Hendricks, & Cardenas, 1998; Feldman, 1994) and require months of skilled care. These figures do not reflect the indirect costs incurred by the individual as a result of having less contact with family and friends as well as disrupted employment or job loss secondary to pressure sore complications. In extreme cases, pressure sores can be a potentially fatal complication of SCI (Yarkony, 1994c).

Although prevention is the best management for pressure sores, this is not always possible. Whereas prolonged pressure is an important factor in the development of pressure sores for people with SCI, other factors that must be considered include shear force, skin temperature, moisture, nutritional status, local tissue integrity and viability, altered sensation, and psychological status (CDC, 1990; Mawson, Biando, Neville, Linares, Winchester, & Lopez, 1988). In addition, with the neurotrophic skin changes that occur with age, people with SCI become more susceptible to pressure sores and often require lifestyle changes that necessitate increased vigilance and willingness to use preventive methods (Yarkony, 1993).

Preventive strategies include educating the individual with SCI and caregiver, decreasing the amount and time that pressure is applied, being mobile, keeping dry, frequently shifting positions, and performing self inspections (Ditunno & Formal, 1994). Supplies needed by individuals with SCI to treat pressure sores include mirrors, antibiotics, antiseptics, saline solution, gauze, and topical enzyme preparations. Equipment that is recommended to aid in pressure sore prevention includes special mattresses, cushions for wheelchairs, wheelchair pushup monitors, and reclining or tilt wheelchairs.

Because a pressure sore develops deep inside the tissues (close to the bone), by the time that there is break in the skin, tissue damage may be far more extensive than it may appear. Pressure sore education should, therefore, focus on early detection, and the individual should be encouraged to have a second person check his or her skin. Most importantly, medical attention should be sought immediately for even a small break in the skin.

PSYCHOSOCIAL FUNCTION

Learning to live with disability is a lifelong process of adaptation and can present different problems at different stages throughout the individual's life (Stiens et al., 1997; Trieschmann,1988). Studies suggest that there are significant risks of substance abuse and self-neglect in persons with SCI. Further, people with SCI are more likely to be distressed, depressed, and anxious, and may perceive their future as out of their control, especially during the first few years post-injury (Craig, Hancock, & Dickson, 1994; Craig, Hancock, Dickson, & Chany, 1997; DeVivo, Black, Richards, & Stover, 1991; Elliott & Macleod, 1988; Elliott & Frank, 1996; Fuhrer, Rintala, Hart, Clearman, & Young, 1993; Hancock et al.,1993; Macleod, 1988). Recent research (Kemp, Krause, & Adkins, 1999) suggests that depression is highly prevalent after injury, even among individuals who have lived for long periods with SCI, particularly those of Hispanic origin. A more recent study with 1,391 individuals with SCI found even higher rates of depression, with the highest rates among minorities (particularly minority women), individuals who were older at injury, those with less than 12 years of education, and those who had lived either the shortest or longest duration with SCI (Krause, Kemp, & Coker, 1999). In addition, individuals who have difficulty coping with their disability may have much higher risks for experiencing medical complications caused by behavioral (e.g., noncompliance) and psychosocial (e.g., adaptation) issues (Heinemann & Hawkins, 1995). Individuals who have the most difficulty adapting to life with SCI are those who are middle-aged or older at the time of injury (CDC, 1990; Krause, 1998).

Kennedy, Lowe, Grey, and Short (1995) found a positive correlation between age and depression, suggesting that those with earlier onset of SCI adjust better to the lifestyle long-term. However, the authors also noted that within this same group there was a negative correlation at six weeks post-injury between depression and age suggesting that older individuals handle initial impact of the injury better. Other research (Kemp, Krause, & Adkins, 1999), however, has found aging factors unrelated to the likelihood of depression, although the sample size was substantially smaller than a second study (Krause et al., 1999), which found multiple aging factors related to depression, including a curvilinear relationship between depression and years lived post-injury.

In addressing the adjustment aspects of SCI, particular attention must be given to the issues of choice and self-control when planning the individual's long-term goals and needs. Further, in evaluating adjustment issues, consideration must be given to the family and the person's support system. Friends and other peer systems must be included as an integral part of the individual's support network, particularly for adolescents (Staas et al., 1993). Kennedy et al. (1995) found a high quality of social support to be associated with greater psychological well-being. They concluded that coping strategies and group membership are more important than functional independence and marital satisfaction, suggesting that cognitive and behavioral styles are very important in post-injury adjustment.

Treatment decisions for persons with SCI must be based upon an accurate diagnosis that differentiates between organic and functional etiologies (Elliott & Frank, 1996). Counseling and psychotherapy preferably should be done by someone with experience with the disabled population, preferably SCI (Mourer, 1999). The use of medications such as antidepressants will depend on the degree of depression, its effect on function, the time since injury, and history of depression and medication usage.

Substance use and abuse is an adjustment issue that is often overlooked among people with SCI and can contribute to increased morbidity. It is therefore important to ensure that close monitoring of substance use patterns in persons who are prescribed sedating, tranquilizing, or narcotic medications be incorporated into the long-term planning needs (Heinemann, Doll, Armstrong, Schnoll, & Yarkony, 1991; Young, Rintala, Rossi, Hart, & Fuhrer, 1995).

IMPLICATIONS FOR LIFE CARE PLANNING AND CASE MANAGEMENT

A comprehensive LCP, by providing for effective and efficient medical and health-related professional support systems as well as attendant or nursing services, should positively influence the issue of complications by reducing their frequency, severity, and cost (Deutsch, 1992). Consequently, a schedule of periodic follow-up assessment is essential to monitor, maintain, and improve the health of persons with SCI and to maximize their opportunities for community integration, avocational or vocational achievement, and psychosocial adjustment.

As part of the RRTC on Aging with SCI project, Craig Hospital has developed a health assessment instrument (*Wellness and Risk Assessment Profile*, or *WRAP*) that is available to individuals with SCI as well as practitioners. Information is obtained through completion of a 42-item questionnaire by the person with SCI. The responses are then analyzed by computer to estimate the individual's probability of risks for various medical, functional, or psychosocial complications during the next three years. The risk model calculations are based on extensive longitudinal research by Craig Hospital of a population-based sample of British people (> 225) with SCI of 20 or more years duration. Responses to the self-administered questionnaire are used to provide a user-generated 10 to 15-page report that communicates the level of risk in key areas specific to his or her situation and recommends changes that must be targeted to lessen these risk factors.

The WRAP instrument lends itself for incorporation into the LCP and case management process with its emphasis on promotion of health and minimization of secondary conditions to SCI. It can be accessed through Craig Hospital (Research Department, 3425 South Clarkson Street, Englewood, CO 80110; 303/789-8202; www.craig-hospital.org) and is also available in a self-contained computer program that can be loaded onto a personal or laptop computer.

APPENDIX I

Costs Associated with Complications Secondary to Spinal Cord Injury

Costs are highly correlated with severity of injury. Data collected from a prospective population-based study of 115 people with SCI by the Colorado Spinal Cord Injury Early Notification System (Johnson, Brooks, & Whiteneck, 1996) showed that individuals with high tetraplegia experienced the highest costs for respiratory and neurologic complications; those with low tetraplegia had the highest costs associated with skin and neurologic complications; persons with paraplegia had the highest expenses in the categories of neurologic, skin, and musculoskeletal complications; and individuals with incomplete injury experienced their highest costs in the areas of musculoskeletal, skin, and neurologic complications (Johnson et al., 1996).

Overall, findings from this study (Johnson et al., 1996) demonstrate that the costs associated with treating complications secondary to SCI are over six times greater than those incurred from routine medical evaluations. However, these figures may be somewhat conservative, because the study indicates that many of the potentially high-cost complication categories were identified when they were in less severe and less costly stages, thus supporting the need for preventive strategies and closer routine follow-up care. Table I-1 summarizes the average charge incurred by body system complication during the first two years post-SCI.

Berkowitz, O'Leary, Kruse, and Harvey (1998) demonstrate some of the costs incurred from complications secondary to SCI in their study of economic consequences of injury. The authors present their findings as annual medical care costs

Table I-1. Charges Associated with General Follow-up Evaluation and Specific Body System Complications (1992 Dollars)

Source of Complication	Frequency (Number of Occurrences)	Frequency for Which Costs Could Be Associated	Average Charge Per Occurrence
Urological/Bladder/Renal	60	23	$1,167
Skin	43	14	17,301
Pain	38	8	233
Gastrointestinal	37	6	841
Muscular/Spasticity	34	9	1,268
Neurologic	33	8	22,321
Orthopedic	28	14	12,601
Circulatory	19	7	7,484
Concomitant Injury	19	19	2,957
Injury	16	9	9,001
Respiratory	14	8	13,274
Psychological	12	8	2,628
Endocrine	11	0	—
Gynecological	9	0	—
Fatigue	1	0	—

(Adapted by permission of the publisher from Cost of Traumatic Spinal Cord Injury in a Population-based Registry by R.L. Johnson, G.A. Brooks, and G.G. Whiteneck, *Spinal Cord*, p. 477. International Medical Society of Paraplegia, 1996.)

based on utilization rather than actual costs. Respondents were asked to recall medical experiences over the last year, when they were treated, at what type of facility, where they admitted (to critical care unit), surgery, and number of follow-up appointments necessary. The authors then calculated the annual costs of medical care from *Healthcare Cost and Utilization Project* data from the *Nationwide Inpatient Sample (NIS) Release 1*, Mutual of Omaha Insurance Company, and data published by the Department of Veterans Affairs in the *Federal Register*. Hospital charges were estimated based upon surgical and nonsurgical diagnosis-related groups (DRGs). Physician charges for inpatient services were based on 50 percentile fees for such services from the Practice Management Information Corporation (PMIC) physician fees guide. Table I-2 is a breakdown of daily hospital charges incurred for selected DRGs associated with complications secondary to SCI.

The University of Alabama (UAB) Model System, Spain Rehabilitation Center (DeVivo,1998) conducted a study of 206 people injured between 1973 and 1996 and initially treated at the UAB Model System, to determine the most frequent causes of rehospitalizations for complications and the average charge per episode. Urinary tract complications (primarily urinary tract infections) were the total leading cause for rehospitalization. Skin conditions (almost always pressure sores) ranked second, and respiratory complications (predominately pneumonia) ranked third (see Table I-3).

When these data were analyzed by level of injury, urinary tract complications accounted for one-third of the hospitalizations for people with tetraplegia. Respiratory complications and skin conditions ranked second and third for those with tetraplegia. For persons with paraplegia, urinary tract complications accounted for a smaller percentage of hospitalizations, but still ranked first; skin conditions ranked second and respiratory complications ranked third. In terms of time since injury, respiratory complications were found to cause proportionately more hospitalizations during the first five years post-injury than in later years. Urinary tract complications and psychosocial problems caused proportionately more hospitalizations in later years.

Table I-2. Hospital Charges Based on Diagnosis-Related Groups (DRGs)

DRG Group	Mean Charges per Day for DRG Group (adjusted $)*
Skin and wound problems — nonsurgical	$1,105
Skin and wound problems — surgical	1,822
Urinary tract problems — nonsurgical	1,489
Urinary tract problems — surgical	2,056
Circulatory problems — nonsurgical	1,436
Circulatory problems — surgical	2,411
Respiratory problems — nonsurgical	1,459
Respiratory problems — surgical	1,893
Muscular/joint stress problems — nonsurgical	1,152
Muscular/joint stress problems — surgical	2,136
Wheelchair injuries — nonsurgical	1,530
Wheelchair injuries — surgical	2,059
GI problems — nonsurgical	1,332
GI problems — surgical	1,292
Spinal cord/disc problems — nonsurgical	1,107
Spinal cord/disc problems — surgical	2,529
Other SCI-related problems — nonsurgical	1,353
Other SCI-related problems — surgical	2,074
Peripheral nerve problems — nonsurgical	1,642
Psychiatric problems — nonsurgical	732

*Adjusted using the 1997 CPI-U BLS. Hospital and Related Services
(From Direct Costs of Spinal Cord Injury in *Spinal Cord Injury: An Analysis of Medical and Social Costs* by Berkowitz, O'Leary, Kruse & Harvey, p. 47. Demos Medical Publishing, 1998. Reprinted with permission.)

Table I-3. Primary and Secondary Causes of Rehospitalization (%)

Complications	Primary	Secondary	Total
Urinary tract	29.6%	12.8%	42.4%
Skin	16.6	12.1	28.7
Respiratory system	12.6	4.2	16.8
Nervous system	8.4	8.2	16.6
Digestive system	8.2	6.8	15.0
Injury	6.3	0	6.3
Psychosocial	4.7	2.8	7.5
Musculosketal	4.4	4.0	8.4
Cardiovascular	3.5	1.6	5.1
Endocrine/blood	2.1	8.6	10.7
Other	3.6	0.2	3.8

(From DeVivo, M.J. *Rehospitalization Costs of Individuals with Spinal Cord Injury*. Research Update. Birmingham, AL: University of Alabama at Birmingham, RRTC in Secondary Conditions of SCI, September 1998.)

Table I-4. Charges per Hospitalization (1997 Dollars)

Cause	Days	Charge
Skin	19.8	$37,272
Musculoskeletal	14.0	34,126
Cardiovascular	7.4	22,600
Nervous system	6.9	22,296
Digestive system	10.9	22,137
Respiratory system	7.5	14,726
Injury	8.2	13,651
Urinary tract	7.3	11,794
Psychosocial	9.0	8,135
Endocrine/blood	5.4	6,647

(From DeVivo, M.J. *Rehospitalization Costs of Individuals with Spinal Cord Injury*. Research Update. Birmingham, AL: University of Alabama at Birmingham, RRTC in Secondary Conditions of SCI, September 1998.)

In looking at the costs for hospitalization, the study found skin complications to be the most expensive to treat. Musculoskeletal conditions ranked second, followed by cardiovascular, nervous (mostly cases of autonomic dysreflexia), and digestive system conditions. Respiratory conditions ranked as sixth most expensive, followed by injuries, urinary tract, psychosocial (predominantly related to substance abuse or severe depression), and endocrine or blood conditions. It should be noted that the charges calculated in this study did not include physician fees. Table I-4 provides a breakdown of the average length of stay and charge per episode.

IMPLICATIONS FOR LIFE CARE PLANNING AND CASE MANAGEMENT

Aside from the direct economic impact, complications secondary to SCI can also exact a high personal toll in terms of disrupting the individual's ability to live independently and productively. In addition to resulting absences from school, work, and family life, complications and resultant hospitalizations can compromise many of the functional gains made during rehabilitation (American Congress of Rehabilitation Medicine, 1993). Because many of the conditions that necessitate hospitalization and loss of productivity may be preventable, particularly those related to pressure sores, urinary tract infections, and psychosocial problems, it is critical that the LCP focus on strategies to prevent complications, to the extent possible.

APPENDIX J

Health Issues for Women with Spinal Cord Injury

Although population-based studies indicate that approximately 20 to 30 percent of SCIs occur in women, research-based literature on issues of gender and SCI has not been well studied (Go, DeVivo, & Richards, 1995; Krotoski, Nosek, & Turk, 1996; Trieschmann, 1988). Historically, the little research related to women with SCI has focused mainly on the physiologic aspects of pregnancy and childbirth and not on the impact of disability on overall health and ability to function in society (Nosek, 1997; Quigley, 1995). As Nosek (1997) points out, little is known about the effect of hormone cycles on recovery from SCI or the exacerbation of autoimmune disorders; the course of osteoporosis over the lifespan of women with mobility impairments; the diagnosis and treatment of breast cancer in women who cannot access mammography equipment; adaptive techniques for caring for small children; or behaviors that enhance the health of women with severe physical impairments (p. S1). In addition to the anatomic differences that women with SCI may face, both social and familial roles may be dramatically altered for women who have sustained injury.

SECONDARY CONDITIONS IN WOMEN WITH SPINAL CORD INJURY

A population-based study by the Arkansas Spinal Cord Commission (1996), designed to investigate long-term outcomes in people with SCI (128 women and 522 men), found that women with SCI reported different rates of certain secondary conditions than men and that many times these conditions affect women differently than men. For example, women in this study were found to report a greater interference of their regular activities (such as mobility and personal relationships) by secondary conditions than men. Women were also found to spend more out-of-pocket on health care, were more likely to be supporting children, and were more likely to receive paid assistance than men. Women with SCI also showed much less independence than men with regard to availability, accessibility, and use of transportation. The respondents in this study were drawn from the state-mandated registry of all persons with SCI and interviewed in their place of residence by case managers. All of the participants were over 18 years of age and at least one year post-injury.

Nervous System

Approximately 60 percent of both female and male respondents in this study reported chronic pain related to SCI. In general, the study found that chronic pain always or often interferes with the daily activities (relationships, mobility, and sleep) in about one-third of both women and men. Although chronic pain was a problem across gender, female respondents reported a greater proportion of fatigue (55.9 percent) or tiring easily during normal activities, than males (43.2 percent). The study found no appreciable difference between female and male respondents regarding the incidence of posttraumatic syringomyelia. While approximately 84 percent of both female and male respondents reported spasticity, approximately 20 percent stated that the muscle spasms were of enough severity to often interfere with ADLs, leisure, relationships, mobility, and sleep.

Respiratory System

In terms of post-injury respiratory problems, the respondents reported nearly the same proportion of physician-diagnosed pneumonia. However, the female respondents were more likely to be hospitalized for pneumonia (24.2 percent) and reported more respiratory problems (26.2 percent) than males. Non-white females were further found to report a greater proportion of both physician-diagnosed pneumonia and hospitalization, as well as respiratory difficulties. Not surprisingly, those women who used tobacco reported a higher proportion of both diagnosed pneumonia and hospitalization.

Musculoskeletal System

With the exception of osteoporosis, physician-diagnosed muscle and bone conditions (contractures, osteoporosis, rotator cuff tear, heterotopic ossification, and carpal tunnel syndrome) were found to affect women and men in approximately the same proportions. As is common in the general population, female respondents in this study reported a much higher incidence of osteoporosis. Although the percentage was approximately the same for females and males (approximately 40 percent) reporting limitations in range of motion, women reported substantially more interference with daily activities than men. Overall, the female respondents were also found to experience a higher rate of leg fractures since injury than their male counterparts. However, a breakdown by neurologic level of injury revealed that women with tetraplegia sustained a greater proportion of arm and other fractures than women with paraplegia, who reported a greater proportion of leg fractures.

Cardiovascular System

Females reported a higher proportion of several conditions relating to the cardiovascular system than did their male counterparts. While the male respondents evidenced a larger percentage of those with high blood pressure, female respondents showed a greater percentage of those with low blood pressure (31.0 percent), heart disease (5.6 percent), heart attack (4.0 percent), and high cholesterol (14.4 percent). In addition, non-white females had a higher percentage of low blood pressure, stroke, heart attack, and high cholesterol than white females. Female respondents in this study also reported a greater percentage of anemia (21.4 percent) than males (10.3 percent), which is common in the general population. Females reported a lower percentage of autonomic dysreflexia (23.0 percent) than males (30.3 percent).

Gastrointestinal System

The only digestive system problem that showed a noticeable gender difference in this study was gallbladder disease. The female respondents reported an incidence rate over twice that of males for gallbladder disease (11.4 percent for women and 5.1 percent for men). Overall, women with paraplegia experienced a greater proportion of digestive system problems (stomach ulcers, bowel ostomy, gallbladder disease, hemorrhoids, rectal bleeding, and gas) than women with tetraplegia.

Genitourinary System

The frequency of urinary tract infections (UTIs) was a considerable problem for women in this study. Women reported a substantially higher rate (29.4 percent) of multiple episodes (more than three within the last year) of UTIs than men (17.1 percent). In terms of bladder management, women who were able to void on their own or who used intermittent catheterization appeared to have the least trouble with UTI.

Skin

Although the women in this study reported rates of pressure sores at a similar proportion to men, the pressure sores affected women to a greater extent than men with regard to interfering with activities of daily living (ADLs), leisure, relationships, mobility, and sleep. Women who were single (43.4 percent) or separated (33.3 percent) were found to have a much higher proportion of hospitalizations for pressure sores than those who were widowed (20.0 percent), married (23.9 percent), or divorced (27.3 percent).

Psychosocial Functioning

A higher percentage of women (72.2 percent) than men (60.7 percent) in this study reported that they had experienced depression in the last year. While there is a proportional difference at the mild level of depression (48.4 percent for females and 38.0 percent for males), similar rates of depression between genders was found at the moderate and severe levels. An examination of race and neurologic level of injury revealed a smaller percentage of non-white females (60.0 percent) than white females (75.2 percent) had experienced depression during the previous year. However, non-white females experienced a higher percentage of depression at the moderate level (16.0 percent), although white females experienced higher rates of depression at the mild (51.5 percent) and severe level (10.9 percent). Although women with tetraplegia reported an overall lower percentage of depression in the year previous to the study (65.8 percent), they reported a greater percentage of moderate depression (14.6 percent) than women with paraplegia. Women with paraplegia showed a higher percentage of mild (50.6 percent) and severe depression (11.8 percent). Overall, females who were divorced reported the highest rates of depression (81.8 percent), while females who were single reported the lowest rates (62.1 percent).

In terms of suicide, the study demonstrated a lower percentage of women (34.9 percent) than men (39.7 percent) with SCI had thought about committing suicide since their injury, but a greater percentage of women (9.5 percent) than men (5.9 percent) had attempted suicide since injury. A breakdown by race revealed that a higher percentage of white females had thought about committing suicide since injury (37.6 percent), but a greater percentage of non-white females had attempted suicide since injury (12.0 percent). Further, the study found that women with tetraplegia were more likely to have thought of committing suicide (43.9 percent) and more likely to have attempted suicide (12.2 percent) since injury.

Although a lower percentage of females (18.3 percent) than males (24.3 percent) in this study reported that they had been a victim of crime post-injury, the male respondents were more likely to be a victim of robbery or theft, or assault and battery, while female respondents were more likely to report sexual abuse and crimes such as neglect. Overall, non-white women and women with paraplegia were more likely to have been victimized by crime since injury.

HEALTHCARE ACCESS AND DISABILITY IN WOMEN

The need for health promotion has been acknowledged as an important strategy for enhancing and maintaining health and independence and promoting quality of life for persons with disability (U.S. Preventive Health Services Task Force, 1989). Although women with SCI face similar barriers to accessing medical treatment (transportation, attendant care, etc.) as men, there are additional barriers that women may face because of a lack of understanding of treatment for women in this population. Nosek and Howland (1997) analyzed findings by the National Study of Women with Physical Disabilities about the rates of screening for breast and cervical cancers among able-bodied women and those with disabilities, most commonly SCI. In their survey of 843 women, 31 percent had been refused care by a physician due to their disability. Those who obtained appointments reported that complete examinations were often not performed (perhaps attributable to the doctor's belief that the women's disability precludes sexual activity) or were discontinued if spasticity or autonomic hyperreflexia became a problem. For pelvic examinations, severity of disability and race were found to impact the examinations performed. Of women with disabilities who had not had mammograms, 34.1 percent reported that they were unable to get in the position required; 25 percent had not been told by a doctor that they should get one; and 23.5 percent had a belief that their risk of getting breast cancer was very low. Mammograms performed were often complicated by the lack of radiologists and mammography technicians training on techniques for manipulating equipment and positioning the patient for a complete mammogram.

QUALITY OF LIFE ISSUES

Tate, Rile, Perna, and Roller (1997) assessed quality of life (QOL) and life satisfaction among women with physical disabilities to identify factors predictive of QOL and life satisfaction in both men and women. The authors found that women and men with physical disabilities emphasize different aspects of their lives when evaluating QOL and life satisfaction. Women named health and functional well-being as the best predictors of QOL, while men named emotional well-being. Therefore, health care providers may be required to target different aspects of the individual's life when teaching SCI adjustment based upon the gender of the person. When comparing men and women on seven subjective well-being scales, Krause (1998c) found only one significant difference; women reported greater subjective well-being and quality of life when related to interpersonal relations.

Quigley (1995) reviewed the impact of SCI in the lives of women and identified a need to encourage the practitioner to recognize the role of negotiation, which may be critical to the rehabilitation of women with SCI. In addition, Quigley points out that educating the female patient on returning to the pre-injury environment is a continual and active process of redefinition and negotiation. The author concluded that the personality of the individual with SCI and the availability of social support are important components of reconciliation of problems of re-entry into the community following SCI.

IMPLICATIONS FOR LIFE CARE PLANNING AND CASE MANAGEMENT

Because women make up a minority of the total SCI population, many medical practitioners are less familiar with the complications of physical examinations of women. Female consumers with SCI and medical practitioners should be educated on the specific factors that may complicate the process of seeking medical treatment and the risks associated with undetected medical conditions. The life care planner and case manager must not only understand the gender-specific medical examinations necessary and the schedule of these examinations, but should seek practitioners who are familiar with the treatment of women's health issues and are comfortable treating this group within the SCI population.

APPENDIX K

Employment After Spinal Cord Injury

From the perspective of a LCP, the economic benefits of employment may often be secondary to either health or intrinsic benefits; however, individuals with SCI who are employed enjoy a higher quality of life, including greater satisfaction with nearly all aspects of life (Krause, 1990, 1992a). This higher level of quality of life is also reflected in self-ratings of life adjustment, the number of problems experienced, and overall health of the individual. Of greater importance, return to gainful employment has been associated with a significantly greater likelihood of surviving SCI over an extended period of time (Krause, 1991; Krause, Sternberg, Maides, & Lottes, 1997a).

In cases where employment is either not possible or not a desired goal, performing nonpaid productive activities such as homemaking, school attendance, or volunteering may be a viable option. However, these types of activities are generally not associated with the same levels of intrinsic and extrinsic benefits as those that have been identified in relation to competitive types of employment (Krause, 1990). Therefore, it is the responsibility of the life care planner to evaluate the viability of competitive employment, not just for economic benefit, but also in making projections about what may be expected in terms of health and quality of life for the individual over the years and decades following injury.

Several studies have attempted to identify an overall employment rate for individuals with SCI. Employment rates have been found to depend largely on the composition of the participant sample and the nature of their biographical characteristics, such as their age at injury and race/ethnicity. Injury characteristics, including severity of injury and the number of years since injury, are also important predictors of employment. Finally, years of education are very important to return to work.

It is important to differentiate between return to work and the ability to sustain work. Current employment rates reflect the percentage of people who have sustained work (i.e., those who were working at the time of the particular study). Return to work is truly measured by whether an individual has worked at any time since injury. These rates are always higher than current rates. Further, the discrepancy between current and post-injury employment rates can be compared among subgroups (or cohorts) with different characteristics to determine what characteristics are associated with difficulty in maintaining employment.

Data from the National Spinal Cord Injury Statistical Center (NSCISC) (DeVivo, Richards, Stover, & Go, 1991) show employment rates ranging from 12.6 percent for individuals two years post-injury to 38.3 percent for those who were twelve years post-injury. Similarly, Stover and Fine (1986) noted employment rates between 14 to 28 percent 5 years post-injury. In a study that used a highly educated nonmodel systems sample, Krause (1992b) found that over 80 percent of all participants who had lived 25 or more years with SCI had worked at some time since the injury (see Figure K-1). Other research, although not consistently finding such high employment rates, has clearly shown that the probability of having returned to gainful employment at some time since injury increases with years since injury (Krause & Anson, 1996a; Krause et al., 1997a). Consequently, studies that look at individuals shortly after injury seem to produce artificially low employment rates, whereas those that investigate individuals who have been injured for two or three decades find much higher employment rates. Similarly, post-injury employment

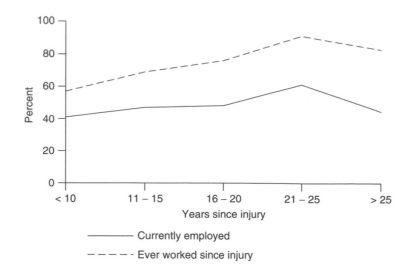

Figure K-1. Percent currently working and ever worked as a function of years since injury.

rates (i.e., ever worked since injury) are higher than current employment rates, which require individuals to both return to employment and to sustain employment.

Rather than attempt to predict future employment based on research of large samples of people with SCI, it is a more prudent strategy for the life care planner to identify those specific characteristics of the individual which increase or decrease the likelihood of return to work. Although this may appear to be a daunting task, a body of research exists that may direct the life care planner to the more relevant assessment factors.

Of the many factors found to predict return to gainful employment after SCI, none is more important than educational level (Alfred, Fuhrer, & Rossi, 1987; DeJong, Branch, & Corcoran, 1984; DeVivo, Rutt, Stover, & Fine, 1987; Dvonch, Kaplan, Grynbaum, & Rusk, 1965; El Ghatit & Hanson, 1978; El Ghatit & Hanson 1979; Geisler, Jousse, & Wynne-Jones, 1966; Goldberg & Freed, 1982; Krause, 1992, 1996, 1998). Overall level of education, including both pre- and post-injury education, is associated with a greater likelihood of return to work (El Ghatit & Hanson, 1978, 1979; Felton & Litman, 1965). These differences are neither small nor insignificant. For example, one study (Krause et al., 1997a) found the current employment rate of individuals with fewer than 12 years of education to be 11 percent, whereas 75 percent of all individuals with 16 or more years of education were employed (the rates for a second sample were 8 percent and 52 percent respectively; see Figure K-2). When looking at employment rates over the entire time post-injury, the picture is equally dramatic. Individuals with 16 or more years of education have an excellent chance of returning to gainful employment post-injury, although it may take some time and the person may be unable to sustain continuous employment. In contrast, individuals with fewer than 12 years of education are not likely to return to gainful employment or maintain employment after the injury. In terms of the LCP, increasing an individual's education level, if possible, is the single most important factor in facilitating return to work.

Severity of injury is another predictor of post-injury employment status. Individuals with less severe injuries tend to be more likely to return to employment (Castle, 1994; DeVivo & Fine, 1982; El Ghatit & Hanson, 1978; Geisler et al., 1966; Krause, 1992b; Stover & Fine, 1986), but are not necessarily more likely to sustain employment or work more hours at their job (El Ghatit & Hanson, 1979; Krause & Anson, 1996a). Some evidence suggests that individuals with less severe injuries may be more likely to attempt a return to work, but do not maintain employment (Krause et al., 1997a). Individuals with paraplegia have the added advantage of having an increased probability of returning to the same job that they had at the time of injury. In general, retraining seems to be essential in returning to work

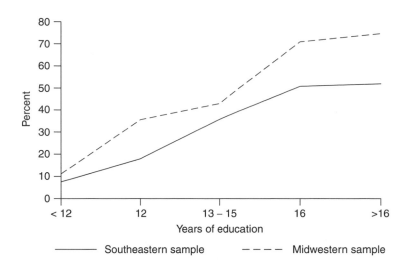

Figure K-2. Percent currently working as a function of years of education.

for individuals with more severe injuries, such as complete tetraplegia, except in cases where an individual already has extensive education. Retraining may also account for an increased amount of time between the onset of injury and start of employment.

A younger age at injury has also been associated with a greater likelihood of return to work. Figure K-3 summarizes the percentage of participants from two different samples who returned to work at some time since injury as a function of age at injury onset (Krause et al., 1997a). In this study, participants were grouped into cohorts, starting with 18 years and younger at injury onset. Although the percentages differ between the two samples for any given cohort (i.e., the overall employment rates differed), the pattern was the same—the older the individual was at injury onset the less likely he or she was to return to work. In the Midwestern sample (identified through two Minnesota hospitals), 92 percent of individuals who were injured prior to age 18 had worked at some point since injury, whereas only 25 percent of those who were over 45 had done so. In the Southeastern sample, whereas 64 percent of those injured prior to 18 had worked at some point since injury, only 11 percent of those injured over the age of 55 had done so (only the Southeastern sample had sufficient cases to form an older-than-55-at-injury cohort).

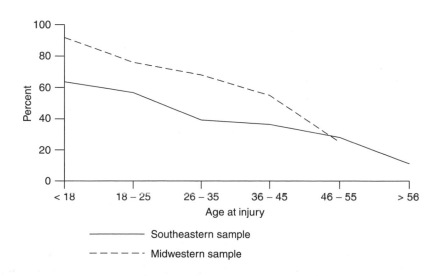

Figure K-3. Percent ever worked since injury as a function of age at injury.

The advantages for those who are younger at injury is probably at least partially the result of the greater time period for re-training and increasing their education. Additionally, because individuals who are injured at a younger age are not as deeply into their careers, it may be easier for them to change occupations. However, their needs for services throughout their lifetime may be more pronounced. For those injured prior to starting work or a career path, there is greater room for formulating, rather than changing, career choices. Vocational interests tend to be highly stable after about the age of 25 (Campbell, 1971), and longitudinal research on people with SCI suggests that their interests are equally or more stable than those of their nondisabled peers (Rohe & Krause, 1997), even when the interests are incongruent with the limitations imposed by injury (i.e., if the individual is unable to use his or her hands, yet has interests in activities that require physical strength or manual dexterity). People who are over 50 at injury often may need to look at avocational alternatives rather than gainful employment.

Chronologic age is also associated with the differential probability of working (DeJong, Branch, & Corcoran, 1984; DeVivo & Fine, 1982; Dvonch et al., 1965; El Ghatit & Hanson, 1979; Geisler et al., 1966). Figure K-4 summarizes the relationships identified between age with both current employment and employment since injury among a sample of participants from the Midwest (Krause, 1992b). The most significant finding is an apparent divergence between current employment and ever employed since injury in the age cohort 51–60. Whereas 74 percent of individuals in this age group had worked at some time since injury, only 38 percent were currently working (a significant decrease compared with other age cohorts). This suggests that people with SCI may tend to leave the work force earlier than the traditional retirement age. It is important for the life care planner to account for the likelihood of an early departure from the work force and to identify resources, as necessary, to smooth the transition to retirement.

Data regarding the role of gender in employment is somewhat contradictory. Studies consistently find women to have lower employment rates at the time of injury (Krause & Anson, 1996b; Krause et al., 1997a). However, there has been mixed evidence for employability after injury, with some studies finding men more likely to be employed (James, DeVivo & Richards, 1993) and some finding women more likely to be employed (Krause & Anson, 1996b). Early studies were confounded by including homemaking in the definition of employment. In terms of hours spent per week working, employed women with SCI tend to work fewer hours on average than men who are employed (Krause & Anson, 1996a). This may suggest that work has a different meaning for women as opposed to men, at least among a certain portion of people with SCI.

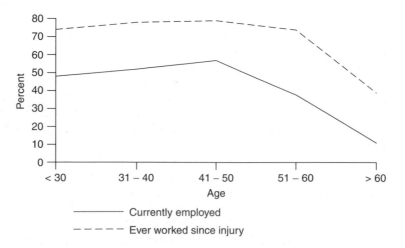

Figure K-4. Percent currently working and ever worked since injury as a function of chronologic age.

Race/ethnicity also plays a role in return to gainful employment after SCI. Minorities, generally African-Americans, have consistently been found to have lower employment rates after SCI (James et al., 1993). There has also been some evidence for an interaction between race/ethnicity and gender, because white males have often been found more likely to return to work than white females (the evidence has been mixed), whereas African-American females have generally been found to have a greater probability of returning to gainful employment than African-American males (Krause & Anson, 1996a). A more recent report from the Model Systems data identifies substantial differences in employment rates between Caucasians and minority participants, with particularly poor outcomes observed among African-Americans (Krause et al., 1999). Males had higher employment rates for all racial/ethnic groups studied, except African-Americans, where females had higher rates. Differences in education alone do not account for the racial/ethnic differences in return to employment. Whites were found to be twice as likely to be employed after SCI, even after controlling for differences in education (Krause et al., 1997a).

Not all individuals who work post-injury do so on a full-time basis. A recent Model Systems employment study (Krause et al., 1999) found that approximately half of all employed participants were working 30 or more hours per week. This study focused on all individuals from the Model Systems who completed the Craig Handicap Assessment Reporting Technique (CHART) as part of their routine follow-up. There were initially 3,756 participants, although this decreased to 2,980 after eliminating all individuals who were not in the active work age group (defined by being a non-student between the ages of 18 and 61). Although 56.3 percent of employed participants at the first year post-SCI were working a minimum of 30 hours per week, this figure increased to 81.7 percent for employed participants at year two. Based on five-year intervals (i.e., 5, 10, 15, or 20 years post-injury), the remaining cohorts reported rates of full-time employment (based on 30 or more hours per week) that ranged from 75.3 to 84.4 percent. Other non-Model Systems research also found high full-time employed rates. For example, Krause et al. (1998) found that employed participants averaged 37 hours per week at work and had worked at their current job an average of 7.6 years. In a second study (Krause & Anson, 1996), employed participants averaged 37.6 hours per week at work. In short, it appears that many individuals who return to work post-injury do so on a full-time basis, with some working more or less hours.

Work life expectancy is also an important issue for the LCP. Unfortunately, surprisingly little research has directly focused on the issue of work life expectancy, and the research that does exist is generally cross-sectional and indirect (i.e., work life expectancy was not the intention of the study). Studies that have investigated both current and post-SCI work status (ever worked since injury) have found that starting work after SCI does not ensure continued employment post-injury (Krause et al., 1997a). The only evidence of work life expectancy comes from studies (Krause and Anson, 1996a; Krause et al., 1997a) that compare current and post-injury employment rates as a function of age (years since injury). However, the findings from these studies are mixed.

There are three aspects to work life expectancy: 1) time between injury onset and return to work, 2) continuity of work once started, and 3) time to retirement. Berkowitz et al. (1998) found that the average time between injury and initiating work was 3.8 years. No research was identified that addressed the issue of continuity of work.

There are many barriers to work for people with SCI and other disabilities, which may be environmental, attitudinal, or financial. Krause and Anson (1996b) investigated perceived reasons for not working among a sample of unemployed participants with SCI. Physical limitations and other health issues were the most commonly cited reasons for not working (60 percent), and emotional issues or lack of interest were the least frequently cited reasons (10 percent and less). However, loss of benefits and inaccessibility of the work environment were frequently cited reasons for not working (28 and 23 percent respectively). The types of barriers cited also varied as a function of individual characteristics. For example, African-Americans were more likely to cite employer prejudice and inadequate transportation or other resources as reasons for not returning to work. In summary, a number of barriers make returning to work difficult for people with SCI and other disabling conditions.

IMPLICATIONS FOR LIFE CARE PLANNING

Being employed and/or productive are fundamental to adult life. Therefore employment or other productive activities (e.g., volunteering, education, hobby, church-going) should be a core element in the overall LCP, not simply for economic reasons, but also for intrinsic ones. After SCI, increasing the likelihood of an individual returning to gainful employment also increases the likelihood of more favorable outcomes in terms of overall health, satisfaction with life, overall quality of life, and even life expectancy.

APPENDIX L

Common Mobility Equipment Needs for Spinal Cord Injury

Table L-1 summarizes some of the most commonly used equipment for mobility by level of injury. Because changes and advances in equipment and technology are made, the equipment identified has been kept fairly generic. This information was adapted from the Consortium for Spinal Cord Medicine (1999a) study on outcomes following SCI.

Table L-1. Common Mobility Equipment Needs by Level of Injury

Level of Injury	Wheelchair	Bed Mobility	Toilet / Tub / Shower	Other
C1–C3	Power recline/tilt wc with head, chin, or breath control; manual recliner; vent tray; pressure relief cushion; postural support and head control devices as indicated	Full electric hospital bed with Trendelenburg feature and side rails; speciality or pressure relief mattress may be indicated; power or mechanical lift with sling; transfer board	Padded/reclining shower/commode chair (if roll-in shower available); handheld shower	Two ventilators (bedside, portable); suction equipment; generator/battery backup; mouth stick, hightech computer access, environmental control unit (ECU); hand splints may be indicated
C4	Power recline/tilt wc with head, chin, or breath control; manual recliner; vent tray; pressure relief cushion; postural support and head control devices as indicated	Full electric hospital bed with Trendelenburg feature and side rails; speciality or pressure relief mattress may be indicated; power or mechanical lift with sling; transfer board	Padded/reclining shower/commode chair (if roll-in shower available); handheld shower	See C1–C3 if not ventilator free; tilt table; hydraulic standing table; mouth stick, hightech computer access, ECU, hand splints may be indicated
C5	Power recline/tilt wc with arm drive control; lightweight manual wc (rigid or folding) with handrim modifications; pressure relief cushion; posture support devices	Full electric hospital bed with Trendelenburg feature with patient control; side rails; speciality or pressure relief mattress may be indicated; power or mechanical lift with sling; transfer board	Padded/reclining shower/commode chair or padded transfer tub bench with commode cutout; handheld shower	Adaptive devices as indicated; hydraulic standing frame

(continued overleaf)

227

Table L-1. (*continued*)

Level of Injury	Wheelchair	Bed Mobility	Toilet / Tub / Shower	Other
C6	Lightweight manual wc (rigid or folding) with modified rims; power recline or standard upright power wc; pressure relief cushion; postural support devices	Full electric hospital bed; side rails; full to king standard bed may be indicated; pressure relief mattress or overlay may be indicated; mechanical lift; transfer board	Padded tub bench with commode cutout or padded shower/commode chair; handheld shower; other adaptive devices as indicated	Adaptive devices as indicated; hydraulic standing frame
C7–C8	Lightweight manual wc (rigid or folding) with modified rims; pressure relief cushion; postural support devices	Full electric hospital bed or full to king standard bed; pressure relief mattress or overlay may be indicated; transfer board	Padded tub bench with commode cutout or padded shower/commode chair; handheld shower; other adaptive devices as indicated	Adaptive devices as indicated; hydraulic or standard standing frame
T1–T9	Lightweight manual wc (rigid or folding); pressure relief cushion; postural support devices as indicated	Full to king standard bed; pressure relief mattress or overlay may be indicated; may or may not require transfer board	Elevated padded toilet seat or padded tub bench with commode cutout; handheld shower	Standing frame
T10–L1	Lightweight manual wc (rigid or folding); pressure relief cushion; postural support devices as indicated	Full to king standard bed; pressure relief mattress or overlay may be indicated	Padded standard or raised padded toilet seat; padded transfer tub bench; handheld shower	Standing frame; forearm crutches or walker; knee-ankle-foot orthosis (KAFO)
L2–S5	Lightweight manual wc (rigid or folding); pressure relief cushion; postural support devices as indicated	Full to king standard bed	Padded toilet seat; padded tub bench; handheld shower	Standing frame; KAFO or ankle-foot orthosis (AFO); forearm crutches or cane as indicated

Assumptions:

(1) The SCI is motor complete and circumstances are optimal

(2) There are no significant constraining factors such as obesity, advancing age, preexisting disabilities, or other medical conditions or complications

(3) Appropriate attendant care is available

(Adapted from *Outcomes Following Traumatic Spinal Cord Injury: Clinical Practice Guidelines for Health-Care Professionals* by the Consortium for Spinal Cord Medicine, pp. 13–20. Paralyzed Veterans of America, 1999. Adapted with permission.)

IMPLICATIONS FOR LIFE CARE PLANNING AND CASE MANAGEMENT

In addition to independence, safety, easier care, and improved or maintained health are realistic outcomes when appropriate equipment is available and used (ASIA, 1993). However, a decline in strength along with joint degeneration caused by overuse combine to diminish the mobility capabilities of people with SCI as they age (Waters, Sie, & Adkins, 1993). These declines necessitate changes in equipment and assistance (Gerhart et al., 1993).

APPENDIX M

Personal Assistance Guidelines for Spinal Cord Injury

Projecting an accurate estimate of assistance levels requires close coordination and clarification with the individual, family, and treatment team members on the actual life-demand needs. Findings from the PVA sponsored Consortium for Spinal Cord Medicine study (1999a) offer some guidelines for hours of personal care and homemaking assistance that may be appropriate to each level of injury (see Table M-1). These guidelines were based on consensus of clinical experts, available literature on functional outcomes, and data compiled from Uniform Data Systems (UDS) and the National Spinal Cord Injury Statistical Center (NSCISC). The hours were determined representative of the skilled and unskilled and paid and unpaid hours of assistance required for individuals who were one year post-SCI.

Table M-1. Hours Per Day of Assistance by Level of Injury and FIM™ Instrument

Level of Injury	Assistance Required	FIM™a	NSCISC Median[b]	NSCISC Interquartile Range[c]
C1–C3	24-hour attendant care to include homemaking	24 hrs/day	24 hrs/day	12–24 hrs/day
C4	24-hour care to include homemaking	24 hrs/day	24 hrs/day	16–24 hrs/day
C5	Personal care[d]: 10 hrs/day Homemaking[e]: 6 hrs/day	16 hrs/day	23 hrs/day	10–24 hrs/day
C6	Personal care: 6 hrs/day Homemaking: 4 hrs/day	10 hrs/day	17 hrs/day	8–24 hrs/day
C7–C8	Personal care: 6 hrs/day Homemaking: 2 hrs/day	8 hrs/day	12 hrs/day	2–24 hrs/day
T1–T9	Homemaking: 3 hrs/day	2 hrs/day	3 hrs/day	0–15 hrs/day
T10–L1	Homemaking: 2 hrs/day	2 hrs/day	2 hrs/day	0–8 hrs/day
L2–S5	Homemaking: 0–1 hr/day	0–1 hr/day	0 hrs/day	0–2 hrs/day

[a]Expected FIM™ instrument outcomes based on expert clinical consensus
[b]Median FIM estimates, as compiled by NSCISC
[c]Interquartile range for NSCISC FIM data
[d]Personal care includes hands-on delivery of all aspects of self-care and mobility, as well as safety interventions
[e]Homemaking activities include meal planning and preparation and home management
(Adapted from *Outcomes Following Traumatic Spinal Cord Injury: Clinical Practice Guidelines for Health-Care Professionals* by the Consortium for Spinal Cord Medicine, pp. 13–20. by Paralyzed Veterans of America, 1999. Adapted with permission.)

IMPLICATIONS FOR LIFE CARE PLANNING AND CASE MANAGEMENT

The hours identified in Table M-1 were based on what may be needed for a person with motor-complete SCI, given optimal circumstances one year post-injury. These estimates do not reflect changes in assistance that may be required over time nor do they take into account other medical conditions, complications, age, obesity, cognitive abilities, psychosocial, and environmental factors. In using these data, the life care planner or case manager must be aware that these estimates are not intended to be prescriptive, but rather to serve as a guideline for understanding the personal assistance needs that may be anticipated in the LCP process.

APPENDIX N

Wheelchair Sports and Recreation Associations

Table N-1 list some of the adaptive sports and recreational activities in which people with SCI might participate, along with their respective associations. These organizations are valuable sources of more information regarding programs, equipment, adaptations, etc. (PVA, 1997).

Table N-1. Wheelchair Sports and Recreation Associations

Activity	Association
Aerobics/Physical Fitness	Disabled Sports USA 451 Hungerford Drive, Suite 100 Rockville, MD 20850
Air Guns	National Wheelchair Shooting Federation c/o Wheelchair Sports, USA 3595 East Fountain Boulevard, Suite L-1 Colorado Springs, CO 80910
All-Terrain Vehicles	Wheelchair Motorcycle Association 101 Torrey Street Brockton, MA 02401
Archery	Wheelchair Archery, USA c/o Wheelchair Sports, USA 3595 East Fountain Boulevard, Suite L-1 Colorado Springs, CO 80910
Basketball	National Wheelchair Basketball Association c/o Charlotte Institute of Rehabilitation 1100 Blythe Boulevard Charlotte, NC 28203
Billiards	National Wheelchair Poolplayers Association 30872 Puritan Livonia, MI 48154
Bowling	American Wheelchair Bowling Association 6264 North Andrews Avenue Ft. Lauderdale, FL 33309
Camping	United States National Park Service 800 North Capitol, NW Washington, DC 20002
Canoeing	American Canoe Association 7432 Alban Station Boulevard, Suite B-232 Springfield, VA 22150
Fencing	United States Fencing Association 1 Olympic Plaza Colorado Springs, CO 80909

(continued overleaf)

Table N-1. Wheelchair Sports and Recreation Associations

Activity	Association
Fishing	Paralyzed Veterans of America 801 Eighteenth Street, NW Washington, DC 20006
Flying	Freedom's Wings International 1832 Lake Avenue Scotch Plains, NJ 07076
	International Wheelchair Aviators 1117 Rising Hill Escondido, CA 92029
Football	Universal Wheelchair Football Association U.C. Raymond Walters College 9555 Plainfield Road Cincinnati, OH 45236
Golf	Association of Disabled American Golfers P.O. Box 280649 Englewood, CO 80228-0649
Handcycling	Crank Chair Racing Association 3294 Lake Redding Drive Redding, CA 96003
	United States Handcycling Federation c/o Wheelchair Sports, USA 3595 East Fountain Boulevard, Suite L-1 Colorado Springs, CO 80910
Hockey	United States Sled Hockey Association 21 Summerwood Court Buffalo, NY 14223
Horseback Riding	North American Riding for the Handicapped Association P.O. Box 33150 Denver, CO 80233-3150
Hunting	National Rifle Association Disabled Shooting Services 11250 Waples Mill Road Fairfax, VA 22030
Motorcycling	National Handicap Motorcyclist Association 315 West 21st Street, Suite 6F New York, NY 10011
	Wheelchair Motorcycle Association 101 Torrey Street Brockton, MA 02401
Quad Rugby	United States Quad Rugby Association 990 Logan Street, # 205 Denver, CO 80203
Racquetball	United States Racquetball Association 1685 West Uyntah Colorado Springs, CO 80904
Road Racing	Wheelchair Track and Field — USA 2351 Parkwood Road Snellville, GA 30278
Rowing	United States Rowing Association 201 South Capitol Avenue, Suite 400 Indianapolis, IN 46225

Table N-1. (*continued*)

Activity	Association
Sailing	Access to Sailing 6475 East Pacific Coast Highway Long Beach, CA 90803
Scuba Diving	Handicapped Scuba Association 1104 El Prado San Clemente, CA 92672
Shooting	National Wheelchair Shooting Federation c/o Wheelchair Sports, USA 3595 East Fountain Boulevard, Suite L-1 Colorado Springs, CO 80910
	National Rifle Association Disabled Shooting Services 11250 Waples Mill Road Fairfax, VA 22030
Skiing	Disabled Sports USA 451 Hungerford Drive, Suite 100 Rockville, MD 20850
Softball	National Wheelchair Softball Association 1616 Todd Court Hastings, MN 55033
Swimming	United States Wheelchair Swimming, Inc. c/o Wheelchair Sports, USA 3595 East Fountain Boulevard, Suite L-1 Colorado Springs, CO 80910
Table Tennis	American Wheelchair Table Tennis Association 23 Parker Street Port Chester, NY 10573
Tennis	United States Tennis Association 70 West Red Oak Lane White Plains, NY 10604-3602
Track and Field	Wheelchair Track and Field — USA 2351 Parkwood Road Snellville, GA 30278
Waterskiing	Water Skiers With Disabilities Association 799 Overlook Drive Winter Haven, FL 33884
Weightlifting	United States Wheelchair Weightlifting Federation 39 Michael Place Levittown, PA 19057

APPENDIX O

Guidelines for Follow-up Care of Spinal Cord Injury

The following tables summarize some general guidelines for relevant follow-up assessments appropriate during the lifetime care of persons with SCI. These data are drawn from evidence-based studies, professional opinions and clinical experience of a number of recognized SCI experts. These recommendations are for healthy persons with SCI. For individuals who have already experienced or are at risk for specific complications, additional assessments may be needed.

A MODEL SYSTEM GUIDELINES

Table O-1. Basic SCI Follow-Up Every 1–3 Years

Suggested Assessments:

Full history and physical review by physician
Weight
Blood pressure and pulse
Vital capacity (VC) lungs (T6 and above)
Blood
   Complete blood count (CBC)
   Electrolytes and glucose (fasting)
   Cholesterol/HDL, triglycerides (fasting)
Cardiac risk assessment starting at age 40
Urologic evaluation
   Urine analysis
   Urine culture and sensitivity (if UA positive)
   Upper tract evaluation
     Renogram or
     Ultrasound or
     Intravenous pyelogram (IVP)
     Lower tract evaluation
   Cystogram
     Cystoscopy
     Post-void residual (if voiding)
Motor and sensory neurologic evaluation (strength and sensory)
Nursing evaluation
Physical therapy evaluation (range of motion, strength, seating, transfers, gait)
Occupational therapy evaluation (activities of daily living, adaptive equipment)
Psychological/social evaluation (depression, substance abuse screen)
   Leisure activity assessment

Table O-2. Age-Specific SCI Follow-Up: Women and Men

Suggested Assessments:

WOMEN

Breast examination and review of self-examination procedure

Gynecological exam	Annually
Papanicolaou smear	Annually
Breast mammography	Screen at age 35, then every 1–3 years (depending on screen and family history)
FSH determination (when unable to determine menopause due to surgical procedures)	Annually, starting at age 45 until menopause documented

MEN

Testicular examination	Annually
Prostate digital evaluation	Annually, starting at age 45
Prostatic specific antigen (blood)	Annually, starting at age 45

Table O-3. Recommended SCI Follow-Up after Age 45: Men and Women

In addition to the suggested assessments in Tables O-1 and O-2, the following assessments are also suggested:

Assessment	*Repeat Years*
Heart	
Electrocardiogram(EKG)	1–3 (after age 40)
Stress EKG	3–5 (depending on history, physical, and family)
Lungs, Chest[a]	
Radiogram, x-ray	1–3
Bowel	
Fecal occult blood	Annually
Flexible sigmoidoscopy	1–5
Audiometry	5
Visual evaluation	5
Diabetes evaluation	
Glucose tolerance test (3 hour oral)	Depending on family history and clinical findings
Vaccinations[b]	
Influenza (if no allergy to egg/ egg products)	Annually
Diphtheria/tetanus boosters	10
Pneumococcal (pneumovax)	5

[a]More often if smoker or in presence of other respiratory impairment
[b]For individuals at increased risk of respiratory infection from pneumococcal bacteria.
(From Where Do We Go From Here by G.G. Whiteneck and R.R. Menter in *Aging with Spinal Cord Injury* by G.G. Whiteneck, et al., pp. 367–368. Demos Publishers, 1993. Reprinted with permission.)

DEPARTMENT OF VETERANS AFFAIRS GUIDELINES

The Department of Veterans Affairs (VA) clinical practice guidelines recommend a yearly, interdisciplinary SCI examination that consists of no less than the following examinations (see Table O-4).

IMPLICATIONS FOR LIFE CARE PLANNING AND CASE MANAGEMENT

Although guidelines can be written that take into account variables in clinical settings, resources, or common patient characteristics, these guidelines cannot

Table O-4. SCI Follow-up Care Guidelines by the Department of Veterans Affairs (VA)

Medical History
Physical examination to include:
  Sensory and motor level reflex functions
  Skeletal changes
  ADL function changes (use of FIM™ instrument recommended)
  Skin integrity
  Cardiovascular assessment
  Pulmonary function
  Digital rectal examination
  Stool for occult blood
Dental evaluation
Psychosocial assessment (including vocational rehabilitation potential/readiness and
  sexuality)
Rehabilitation — physical and occupational therapist functional evaluation (changes
  due to aging included)
Chest x-ray as indicated
Tonometry (when over age 35)
Electrocardiogram (EKG), when indicated
Complete blood count (CBC) chemical profile (including lipids) — UA C/S to include
  acid phosphatase/prostatic specific antigen (for individuals over age 40)
Urinary tract evaluation (function and morphology)
  Creatine clearance
  Urinary cytology
  Renal sonogram
  Computerized renal scan, when indicated
  Intravenous pyelogram (IVP), when indicated
  Cystoscopy with biopsy, when indicated, especially in individuals with indwelling
  catheters
  Urodynamics evaluation (every 3 years, or more frequently if indicated)
Abdominal sonogram (gall bladder and aorta), when indicated
Rectosigmoidoscopy (over age 40)/colonoscopy, when indicated
Health promotion, such as:
  Immunization (pneumovax (once), influenza)
  Anti-smoking information
  Substance abuse screening and counseling
  Purified protein derivative (PPD)
Dietary and nutritional assessment
WOMEN, to include:
  Pelvic examination
  Pap smear
  Breast examination
  Mammogram (over age 40)

(From Department of Veterans Affairs. Veterans Health Administration Manual M-2 (Clinical Affairs, Part XXIV Spinal Cord Injury Services), 1994.)

address the unique needs of each individual nor the combination of resources available to a particular community or health care professional or provider. Consequently, deviations from general clinical practice guidelines may be justified by individual circumstances. Thus, guidelines must be applied based on individual needs using professional judgment (National Guideline Clearinghouse, 1998).

APPENDIX P

Ethical Issues for Life Care Planning

Ethics are an essential guide for the work of life care planning for people with catastrophic injuries such as SCI. Ethics is a process through which life care planners become aware, enhance, inform, expand, and improve their ability to respond effectively to individuals with disability (Blackwell, 1995a, 1995b, 1999; Pope & Vasquez, 1991). By practicing ethically, the life care planner furthers the welfare of the person with SCI.

The term *ethics* generally refers to a system of moral principles of conduct that guide the behavior of an individual or profession. These are principles that are considered to be fundamental, in that they are proved to have enduring, permanent value (Beauchamp & Childress, 1994; Blackwell, 1999; Corey, Corey & Callanan, 1998; Covey, 1989). Although they may be reflected in the formal standard of a professional association, in the civil or criminal law, or in the administrative guidelines of certification and licensing boards, ethics are not static codes (Granello & Witner, 1998; Pope & Vasquez, 1991). Codes may serve as a useful point of reference, but the complexity of ethical dilemmas and the obsolescence of any static document in an ever-changing work environment of legal, technical, and social developments require that decisions be placed in a broader process of ethical decision-making (Tarvydas, 1987).

Although ethical codes are necessary, they are not sufficient for exercising ethical responsibility. This responsibility falls upon the life care planner, who must continually evaluate his or her actions against the purpose of the life care planner's discipline with the actual needs of those people whom the discipline was created to serve (Blackwell, Havranek & Field, 1996; Corey et al., 1993).

Not only is the life care planner responsible for the judgments and ethics of his or her professional activities, but also for the real life effect these activities have on the individual and family involved in the long-term planning and decision making process. Underlying this responsibility is the need on the part of life care planners to maintain integrity, objectivity, independence, and competency in their work and conclusions.

INTEGRITY

Integrity requires an uncompromising adherence to moral and ethical principles. As such, practitioners who perform life care planning services must perform all aspects of their professional responsibilities with the highest degree of integrity, including the dissemination of findings and conclusions (Blackwell, Martin, & Scalia, 1994). Life care planners often work in an environment in which adversarial and advocatorial pressures exist and where there is often an absence of specific rules, standards, or guidelines. To meet these challenges, practitioners must frequently call on integrity and conscience. They must be honest, fair, and respectful of others. Integrity can tolerate an occasional error and the honest difference of opinion, but it cannot tolerate deceit or subordination of judgment or principles (Blackwell, 1999). It is imperative that the life care planner understand his or her responsibility to protect the person with disability whom he or she is serving.

OBJECTIVITY AND INDEPENDENCE

Objectivity is critical for life care planners in all professional dealings. In developing LCPs, they must be free from conflicts of interest and possess an independence that will not jeopardize their objectivity. Life care planners must keep in mind that they are not advocates for the preconceived agendas of either an individual with injury or the payor; their role is to use their knowledge to develop and then advocate for a LCP that is comprehensive in nature and meets and anticipates the person's unique long-term needs (Blackwell, 1995a, 1999). Their opinions and services should be of the same quality and character regardless of who is paying for the professional's services. Objectivity and independence are never static. These qualities evolve with constant assessment of the individual's needs and the practitioner's responsibilities.

PROFESSIONAL CARE AND COMPETENCE

Technical standards of the profession—whether written or implied—must be observed at all times by practitioners providing life care planning services. Life care planners should continually strive to improve their competence and the quality of their expertise in the field of life care planning and discharge that expertise to the best of their ability. Competence represents the attainment and maintenance of a level of knowledge and understanding that enables practitioners to render services with quality, acumen, and clarity. Competence is not only the recognition of one's knowledge, it is also the recognition and affirmation of the limitations and range of that knowledge. Consequently, life care planners should accept only cases that they can perform with technical competence (Blackwell, 1995a, 1999). LCP professionals should take reasonable steps to avoid negative consequences and should adhere to accepted standards in research and treatment protocol and informed consent, and understand the potential limitations or biases in assessment devices. As the LCP involves other interdisciplinary team practitioners, the life care planner must also respect and understand the areas of competence of these other professionals and work in full cooperation with them to best meet the needs of the individual with SCI (Blackwell et al., 1994).

CONCLUSION

In summary, maintaining an ethical awareness of obligations and responsibilities is not always as simple as it may seem. Nonetheless it is necessary if the life care planning process is to further the best interests of the individual with disability as well as those of the larger society. In essence, sound ethical behavior on the part of the life care planning practitioner is the hallmark of a sound life care plan (Blackwell, 1995a, 1995b, 1999).

REFERENCES

Abrams, K.S. (1981). Impact on marriage of adult-onset paraplegia. *Paraplegia*, **19**, 253–259.

Acton, P.A., Farley, T., Freni, L.W., Ilegbodu, V.A., Sniezek, J.E., Wohlleb, J.C. (1993). Traumatic spinal cord injury in Arkansas, 1980 to 1989. *Arch Phys Med Rehab* **74**, 1035–1040.

Agency for Health Care Policy and Research. (1996). *Hospital Inpatient Statistics, 1996*, (AHCPR Publication No. 99-0034). Rockville, MD: Author.

Alander, D.H., Parker, J., Stauffer, E.S. (1997). Intermediate-term outcome of cervical spinal cord-injured patients older than 50 years of age. *Spine*, **22**, 1189–1192.

Albert, T., Levine, M., Balderston, R., Cotler, J. (1991). Gastrointestinal complications in spinal cord injury. *Spine*, **16**, S522–525.

Alfred, W.G., Fuhrer, M.J., Rossi, C.D. (1987). Vocational development following severe spinal cord injury: a longitudinal study. *Arch Phys Med Rehab* **68**, 854–857.

Aljure, J., Eltorai, I., Bradley, W., Lin, J.E., Johnson, B. (1985). Carpal tunnel syndrome in paraplegic patients. *Paraplegia*, **23**, 182–186.

Almenoff, P.L., Spungen, A.M., Lesser, M., Bauman, W.A. (1995). Pulmonary function survey in spinal cord injury: influences of smoking and level of completeness of injury. *Lung*, **173**, 297–306.

American Congress of Rehabilitation White Paper (1993). Addressing the post-rehabilitation health care needs of persons with disabilities. *Arch Phys Med Rehab* **74**, S8–14.

American Spinal Injury Association. (1993). Durable medical equipment for the patient with spinal cord injury: a task force report of the American Spinal Injury Association. Chicago: Author.

American Spinal Injury Association. (1996). International standards for neurological and functional classification of spinal cord injury, revised 1996. Chicago: Author.

Anderson, T.P., Andberg, M.M. (1979). Psychosocial factors associated with pressure sores. *Arch Phys Med Rehab* **60**, 341–346.

Anson, C.A., Shepherd, C. (1996). Incidence of secondary complication in spinal cord injury. *Intl J Rehab Res* **19**, 55–66.

Apple, D.F., Hudson, L.M. (eds.). (1990). *Spinal Cord Injury: The Model*. Atlanta, GA: The Georgia Regional Spinal Cord Injury Care System, Shepard Center for Treatment of Spinal Injuries, Inc.

Apstein, M., Dulecki-Chipperfield, K. (1987). Spinal cord injury as a risk factor for gallstone disease. *Gastroenterology*, **92**, 966–968.

Arkansas Spinal Cord Commission. (1990). Fact sheet 1: Heterotopic ossification in spinal cord injury. Little Rock, AR: Author.

Arkansas Spinal Cord Commission. (1996). Identifying secondary conditions in women with spinal cord injury. Little Rock, AR: Author.

Atterbury, J.L., Groome, L.J. (1998). Pregnancy in women with spinal cord injuries. *Nursing Clin N Am* **33**, 603–613.

Axel, S. (1982). Spinal cord injured women's concerns: menstruation and pregnancy. *Rehabilitation Nursing*, **7**, 10–15.

Bach, J.R. (1993). Inappropriate weaning and later onset ventilatory failure of individuals with traumatic quadriplegia. Paraplegia, **31**, 430–438.

Bach, J.R., Wang, T.G. (1994). Pulmonary function and sleep disordered breathing in traumatic tetraplegics: a longitudinal study. *Arch Phys Med Rehab* **75**, 79–84.

Baker, E.R., Cardenas, D.D. (1996). Pregnancy in spinal cord injured women. *Arch Phys Med Rehab* **77**, 501–507.

Baker, E.R., Cardenas, D.D., Benedetti, T.J. (1992). Risks associated with pregnancy in spinal cord-injured women. Obstetrics and Gynecology, **3**, 425–428.

Batavia, A.I. (1990). Implications of the current knowledge database. In D.F. Apple L.M. Hudson (eds.), *Spinal Cord Injury: The Model* (pp. 127–129). Atlanta, GA: The Georgia Regional Spinal Cord Injury Care System, Shepard Center for Treatment of Spinal Injuries, Inc.

Bauman, W.A. (1997). Carbohydrate and lipid metabolism in individuals after spinal cord injury. *Topics in Spinal Cord Injury Rehabilitation*, **2**, 1–22.

Bauman, W.A., Raza, M., Spungen, A.M., Machac, J. (1994). Cardiac stress testing with thallium-201 imaging reveals silent ischemia in individuals with paraplegia. *Arch Phys Med Rehab* **75**, 946–950.

Bauman, W.A., Spungen, A.M. (1994). Disorders of carbohydrate and lipid metabolism in veterans with paraplegia or quadriplegia: a model of premature aging. *Metabolism*, **43**, 949–956.

Bauman, W.A., Spungen, A.M., Zhong, Y., Rothstein, J.L., Petry, C., Gordon, S.K. (1992). Depressed serum high density lipoprotein cholesterol levels in veterans with spinal cord injury. *Paraplegia*, **30**, 697–703.

Bayakly, A.R., Lawrence, D.W. (1992). Spinal cord injury in Louisiana: 1991 annual report. New Orleans, LA: Louisiana Office of Public Health.

Beauchamp, T.L., Childress, J.F. (1994). *Principles of Biomedical Ethics* (4th ed.). New York: Oxford University Press.

Becker, H., Stuifbergen, A., Tinkle, M. (1997). Reproductive health care experiences of women with physical disabilities: a qualitative study. *Arch Phys Med Rehab* **78**, 526–533.

Bennett, C.J., Seager, S.W., Vasher, E.A., McGuire, E.J. (1988). Sexual dysfunction and electroejaculation in men with spinal cord injury: a review. *J Urol* **139**, 453–456.

Berard, E.J.J. (1989). The sexuality of spinal cord injured women: physiology and pathophysiology: a review. *Paraplegia*, **27**, 99–112.

Beric, A. (1997). Post-spinal cord injury states. *Pain*, **72**, 295–298.

Berkowitz, M., Harvey, C., Greene, C.G., Wilson, S.E. (1992). *The Economic Consequences of Traumatic Spinal Cord Injury*. New York: Demos Publications.

Berkowitz, M., O'Leary, P., Kruse, D.L., Harvey, C. (1998). *Spinal Cord Injury: An Analysis of Medical and Social Costs*. New York: Demos Medical Publishing, Inc.

Bersoff, D.N. (1995). *Ethical Conflicts in Psychology*. Washington, DC: American Psychological Association.

Bickel, A., Culkin, D.J., Wheeler, J.S. (1991). Bladder cancer in spinal-cord-injured patients. *The J Urol* **146**, 196–197.

Biyani, A., El Masry, W.S. (1994). Post-traumatic syringomyelia: a review of the literature. *Paraplegia*, **32**, 723–731.

Blackmer, J. (1997). Orthostatic hypotension in spinal cord injured patients. *J Spinal Cord Med* **20**, 212–216.

Blackwell, T.L. (1995a). An ethical decision making model for life care planners. *The Rehabilitation Professional*, **3**, 18,28.

Blackwell, T.L. (1995b). Ethical principles for life care planners. *Inside Life Care Planning*, **1**, 1,9.

Blackwell, T.L. (1999). Ethical issues in life care planning. In R.O. Weed (ed.), *Life Care Planning and Case Management Handbook* (pp. 399–406). Boca Raton, FL: CRC Press.

Blackwell, T.L., Havranek, J.E., Field, T.F. (1996). Ethical foundations for rehabilitation professionals. *NARPPS Journal*, **11**, 7–12.

Blackwell, T.L., Martin, W.E., Scalia, V.A. (1994). *Ethics in Rehabilitation: A Guide for Rehabilitation Professionals*. Athens, GA: Elliott and Fitzpatrick, Inc.

Blackwell, T.L., Millington, M.J., Guglielmo, D.E. (1999). Vocational aspects of life care planning for people with spinal cord injury. *Work: A Journal of Prevention, Assessment, and Rehabilitation*, **13(1)**, 13–19.

Blackwell, T.L., Weed, R.O., Powers, A.S. (1994). *Life Care Planning for Spinal Cord Injury: A Resource Manual for Case Managers*. Athens, GA: Elliott and Fitzpatrick, Inc.

Blankstein, A., Shmueli, R., Weingarten, I., Engel, J., Ohry, A. (1985). Hand problems due to prolonged use of crutches and wheelchairs. *Ortho Rev* **14**, 29–34.

Bodner, D.R., Haas, C.A., Krueger, B., Seftel, A.D. (1999). Intraurethral alprostadil for treatment of erectile dysfunction in patients with spinal cord injury. *Urology*, **53**, 199–202.

Bodner, D.R., Lindan, R., Leffler, E., Kursh, E.D., Resnick, M.I. (1987). The application of intracavernous injection of vasoactive medications for erection in men with spinal cord injury. *J Urol* **138**, 310–311.

Bonekat, H.W., Andersen, G., Squires, J. (1990). Obstructive disorder breathing during sleep in patients with spinal cord injury. *Paraplegia*, **28**, 392–398.

Bonica, J.J. (1991). Introduction: Sementic, epidemiologic, and educational issues. In K.L. Casey (ed.), *Pain and Central Nervous System Disease: The Central Pain Syndromes* (pp. 13–29). New York: Raven Press.

Bors, E., Comarr, A. (1960). Neurological disturbances of sexual function with special reference to 529 patients with spinal cord injury. *Urological Survey*, **110**, 191–221.

Bracken, M.B., Freeman, D.H., Hellenbrand, K. (1981). Incidence of acute traumatic hospitalized SCI in the United States, 1970–77. *Am J Epidemiology* **15**, 477–479.

Brackett, N.L., Nash, M.S., Lynne, C.M. (1996). Male fertility following spinal cord injury: facts and fiction. *Physical Therapy*, **76**, 1221–1229.

Bregman, S., Hadley, R.G. (1976). Sexual adjustment and feminine attractiveness among spinal cord injured women. *Arch Phys Med Rehab* **57**, 448–450.

Breithaupt, D.J., Jousse, A.T., Wynne-Jones, M. (1961). Late cause of death and life expectancy in paraplegia. *Can Med Assoc J* **85**, 73–77.

Brenes, G., Dearwater, S., Shapera, R., LaPorte, R.E., Collins, E. (1986). High density lipoprotein cholesterol concentrations in physically active and sedentary spinal cord injured patients. *Arch Phys Med Rehab* **67**, 445–450.

Brindley, G.S. (1981). Reflex ejaculation under vibratory stimulation in paraplegic men. *Paraplegia*, **9**, 299–302.

Britell, C.W., Mariano, A.J. (1991). Chronic pain in spinal cord injury. *Phys Med Rehabilitation* **5**, 71–82.

Broeker, B.H., Klein, F.A., Hackler, R.H. (1981). Cancer of the bladder in spinal cord injury patients. *The J Urol* **125**, 196–197.

Brown, J.S., Giesy, B. (1986). Marital status of persons with spinal cord injury. *Social Science and Medicine*, **23**, 313–322.

Bureau of Epidemiology. (1993). Utah spinal cord injury surveillance summary, 1989–1991. Salt Lake City, UT: Utah Department of Health.

Burke, M.H., Hicks, A.F., Robbins, M., Kessler, H. (1960). Survival of patients with injuries to the spinal cord. *J A M A* **172**, 121–124.

Burns, S.P., Betz, K.L. (1999). Seating pressures with conventional and dynamic wheelchair cushions in tetraplegia. *Arch Phys Med Rehab* **80**, 566–571.

Bursell, J.P., Little, J.W., Stiens, S.A. (1999). Electrodiagnosis in spinal cord injured persons with new weakness or sensory loss: central and peripheral etiologies. *Arch Phys Med Rehab* **80**, 904–909.

Butt, L., Fitting, M. (1993). Psychological adaptation. In G.G. Whiteneck et al. (eds.), *Aging with Spinal Cord Injury* (pp. 199–210). New York: Demos Publications.

Byrne, D.W., Salzberg, C.A. (1996). Major risk factors for pressure ulcers in the spinal cord disabled: a literature review. *Spinal Cord*, **34**, 255–263.

Cairns, D.M., Adkins, R.H., Scott, M.D., (1996). Pain and depression in acute traumatic spinal cord injury: origins of chronic problematic pain? *Arch Phys Med Rehab* **77**, 329–335.

Campbell, D.P. (1971). *Handbook for the Strong Vocational Interest Blank*. Palo Alto, CA: Stanford University Press.

Canter, M.B., Bennett, B.E., Jones, S.E., Nagy, T.F. (1994). *Ethics for Psychologists: A Commentary on the APA Ethics Code*. Washington, DC: American Psychological Association.

Cardenas, D.D., Farrell-Roberts, L., Sipski, M.L., Rubner, D. (1995). Management of gastrointestinal, genitourinary, and sexual function. In S.L. Stover et al. (eds.), *Spinal Cord Injury: Clinical Outcomes from the Model Systems* (pp. 120–144). Gaithersburg, MD: Aspen Publishers, Inc.

Cardenas, D.D., Hooton, T.M. (1995). Urinary tract infections in persons with spinal cord injury. *Arch Phys Med Rehab* **76**, 272–280.

Cardenas, D.D., Mayo, M.E., King, J.C. (1996). Urinary tract and bowel management in the rehabilitation setting. In R.L. Braddom (ed.), *Phys Med Rehab*. (pp. 555–569). W.B. Saunders Company.

Carter, R.E. (1987). Respiratory aspects of spinal cord injury management. *Paraplegia*, **25**, 262–266.

Carty, E.A., Conine, T.A. (1988). Disability and pregnancy: a double dose of disequilibrium. *Rehab. Nursing*, **13**, 85–87.

Castle, R. (1994). An investigation into the employment and occupation of patients with a spinal cord injury. *Paraplegia*, **32**, 182–187.

Centers for Disease Control. (1990). First colloquium on preventing secondary disabilities among people with spinal cord injuries. Atlanta, GA: Author.

Charlifue, S.W. (1993). Research into the aging process. In G.G. Whiteneck et al. (eds.), *Aging with Spinal Cord Injury* (pp. 9–21). New York: Demos Publications.

Charlifue, S.W., Gerhart, K.A. (1991). Behavioral and demographic predictors of suicide after traumatic spinal cord injury. *Arch Phys Med Rehab* **72**, 488–492.

Charlifue, S.W., Gerhart, K.A., Menter, R.R., Whiteneck, G.G., Manley, M.S. (1992). Sexual issues of women with spinal cord injuries. *Paraplegia*, **30**, 192–199.

Charlifue, S.W., Weitzenkamp, D.A., Whiteneck, G.G. (1999). Longitudinal outcomes in spinal cord injury: aging, secondary conditions, and well-being. *Arch Phys Med Rehab* **80**, 1429–1434.

Chanaud, C.M. (1997). Autonomic dysreflexia. *Paraplegia News*, **51**, 76–80.

Colachis, S.C., III. (1992). Autonomic hyperreflexia with spinal cord injury. *J Am Paraplegia Soc* **15**, 171–186.

Cole, T.M. (1994). Prevention of secondary disabilities after brain injury and spinal cord injury: Implications for future research. *Preventive Medicine*, **23**, 670–675.

Cole, T.M., Cole, S.S. (1990). Rehabilitation of problems of sexuality in physical disability. In E.H. Wickland, Jr. (ed.), *Krusen's Handbook of Physical Medicine and Rehabilitation* (4th ed., pp. 988–1008). Philadelphia: W.B. Saunders Company.

Collins, J.G. (1986). Types of injuries and impairments due to injuries. *Vital and Health Statistics — Series 10: Data from the National Health Survey*, **159**, 1–74.

Collins, K.P., Hackler, R.H. (1988). Complications of penile prostheses in the spinal cord injured population. *J Urol* **140**, 984–985.

Colorado Department of Public Health and Environment and Rocky Mountain Regional Spinal Injury System. (1997). *1996 Annual Report of the Spinal Cord Injury Early Notification System*. Denver, CO: Colorado Department of Transportation Printing Office.

Comarr, A.E. (1966). Observations on menstruation and pregnancy among female spinal cord injured patients. *Paraplegia*, **3**, 263–272.

Comarr, A.E. (1976). Sexual response of paraplegic women. *Medical Aspects of Human Sexuality*, **10**, 124–128.

Comarr, A.E. (1977). Sexual function in patients with spinal cord injury. In P.S. Pierce, V.H. Nickel (eds.). *The Total Care of Spinal Injury* (pp. 171–185). Boston: Little Brown and Company.

Consortium for Spinal Cord Medicine. (1997a). *Clinical Practice Guidelines: acute management of autonomic dysreflexia*. Patients with spinal cord injury presenting to health-care facilities. Washington, DC: Paralyzed Veterans of America.

Consortium for Spinal Cord Medicine. (1997b). *Clinical Practice Guidelines: Prevention of thromboembolism in spinal cord injury*. Washington, DC: Paralyzed Veterans of America.

Consortium for Spinal Cord Medicine. (1998a). *Clinical Practice Guidelines: Neurogenic bowel management in adults with spinal cord injury*. Washington, DC: Paralyzed Veterans of America.

Consortium for Spinal Cord Medicine. (1998b). *Depression Following Spinal Cord Injury: A clinical practice guideline for primary care physicians*. Washington, DC: Paralyzed Veterans of America.

Consortium for Spinal Cord Medicine. (1999a). *Outcomes Following Traumatic Spinal Cord Injury: Clinical practice guidelines for health-care professionals*. Washington, DC: Paralyzed Veterans of America.

Consortium for Spinal Cord Medicine. (1999b). *Prevention of Thromboembolism In Spinal Cord Injury*. Washington, DC: Paralyzed Veterans of America.

Consortium for Spinal Cord Medicine. (1999c). *Depression: What you should know. A guide for people with spinal cord injury*. Washington, DC: Paralyzed Veterans of America.

Cooper, R.A. (1998). *Wheelchair Selection and Configuration*. New York: Demos Medical Publishing, Inc.

Cooper, R.A., Boninger, M.L., Rentschler, A. (1999). Evaluation of selected ultralight manual wheelchairs using ANSI/RESNA standards. *Arch Phys Med Rehab* **80**, 462–467.

Cooper, R.A., Robertson, R.N., Lawrence, B., Heil, T., Albright, S.J., VanSickle, D.P., Gonzalez, J. (1996). Life-cycle analysis of depot versus rehabilitation manual wheelchairs. *J Rehab Res Dev* **33**, 45–55.

Corbet, B. (1995). Consumer involvement in research: Inclusion and impact. In S.L. Stover et al. (eds.), *Spinal Cord Injury: Clinical Outcomes from the Model Systems* (pp. 213–233). Gaithersburg, MD: Aspen Publishers, Inc.

Corey, G., Corey, M.S., Callanan, P. (1998). *Issues and Ethics in the Helping Professions* (5th ed.). Pacific Grove, CA: Brooks/Cole.

Cosman, B.C., Stone, J.M., Perkash, I. (1993). The gastrointestinal system. In G.G. Whiteneck et al. (eds.), *Aging with Spinal Cord Injury* (pp. 117–127). New York: Demos Publications.

Covey, S.R. (1989). *The Seven Habits of Highly Effective People*. New York: Simon and Schuster.

Craig, A.R., Hancock, K.M., Dickson, H.G. (1994). A longitudinal investigation into anxiety and depression in the first two years following spinal cord injury. *Paraplegia*, **32**, 675–679.

Craig, A.R., Hancock, K., Dickson, H., Chang, E. (1997). Long-term psychological outcomes in spinal cord injured persons: Results of a controlled trial using cognitive behavior therapy. *Arch Phys Med Rehab* **78**, 33–38.

Craig, D.I. (1990). The adaptation to pregnancy of spinal cord injured women. *Rehabilitation Nursing*, **15**, 6–10.

Crewe, N.M., Athelstan, G.T., Krumberger, J. (1979). Spinal cord injury: a comparison of preinjury and postinjury marriages. *Arch Phys Med Rehab* **60**, 252–256.

Crewe, N., Krause, J. (1988). Marital relationships and spinal cord injury. *Arch Phys Med Rehab* **69**, 435–438.

Cross, L.L., Meythaler, J.M., Tuel, S.M., Cross, A.L. (1992). Pregnancy, labor and delivery post spinal cord injury. *Paraplegia*, **30**, 890–892.

Currie, D.M., Gershkoff, A.M., Cifu, D.X. (1993). Geriatric rehabilitation: mid- and late-life effects of early-life disabilities. *Arch Phys Med Rehab* **74**, S413–416.

Dallmeijer, A.J., Hopman, M.T.E., van der Woude, L.H.V. (1997). Lipid, lipoprotein, and apolipoprotein profiles in active and sedentary men with tetraplegia. *Arch Phys Med Rehab* **78**, 1173–1176.

Dalyan, M., Sherman, A., Cardenas, D.D. (1998). Factors associated with contractures in acute spinal cord injury. *Spinal Cord*, **36**, 405–408.

Danek, M., Conyers, L., Enright, M., Munson, M., Brodwin, M., Hanley-Maxwell, C., Gugerty, J. (1996). Legislation concerning career counseling and job placement for people with disabilities. In E.M. Szymanski, R.M. Parker (eds.), *Work and Disability: Issues and Strategies in Career Development and Job Placement* (pp. 39–78). Austin, TX: Pro-Ed, Inc.

Dattilo, J., Caldwell, L., Lee, Y., Kleiber, D. (1998). Returning to the community with a spinal cord injury: implications for therapeutic recreation specialists. *Therapeutic Recreation Journal*, **32**, 13–27.

Davidoff, G., Roth, E., Guarracina, M., Sliwa, J., Yarkony, G. (1987). Function-limiting dysesthetic pain syndrome among traumatic spinal cord injury patients: a cross-sectional study. *Pain*, **29**, 39–48.

Davidoff, G.N., Roth, E.J., Richards, J.S. (1992). Cognitive deficits in spinal cord injury: epidemiology and outcome. *Arch Phys Med Rehab* **73**, 275–284.

Davidoff, G., Thomas, P., Johnson, M., Berent, S., Dijkers, M., Doljanac, R. (1988). Closed head injury in acute traumatic spinal cord injury: incidence and risk factors. *Arch Phys Med Rehab* **69**, 869–872.

Davidoff, G., Werner, R., Waring, W. (1991). Compression mononeuropathies of the upper extremity in chronic paraplegia. *Paraplegia*, **29**, 17–24.

Davies, T.D., Beasley, K.A. (1999). *Accessible Home Design: Architectural Solutions for the Wheelchair User*. Washington, DC: Paralyzed Veterans of America.

DeJong, G., Branch, L.G., Corcoran, P.J. (1984). Independent living outcomes in spinal cord injury: multivariate analyses. *Arch Phys Med Rehab* **65**, 66–73.

DeJong, G., Brannon, R.W., Batavia, A.I. (1993). Financing health and personal care. In G.G. Whiteneck et al. (eds.), *Aging with Spinal Cord Injury* (pp. 275–294). New York: Demos Publications.

DeLisa, J.A., Martin, G.M., & Currie, D.M. (1993). Rehabilitation medicine: Past, present and future. In J.A. DeLisa (Ed.), *Rehabilitation medicine: Principles and practice* (2nd ed. pp. 28–40). Philadelphia: J.B. Lippincott Company.

DeLisa, J., Stolov, W.C. (1981). Significant body systems. In W.C. Stolov, M.R. Clowers (eds.), *Handbook of Severe Disability: A Text for Rehabilitation Counselors, Other Vocational*

Practitioners, and Allied Health Professionals (pp. 19–54). Seattle, WA: University of Washington.

DeLoach, C., Greer, B. (1981). *Adjustment to Severe Physical Disability: A Metamorphosis*. New York: McGraw Hill.

Demirel, G., Yllmaz, H., Gencosmanoglu, B., Kesiktas, N. (1998). Pain following spinal cord injury. *Spinal Cord*, **36**, 25–28.

Denil, J., Ohl, D.A., Smyth, C. (1996). Vacuum erection device in spinal cord injured men: patient and partner satisfaction. *Arch Phys Med Rehab* **77**, 750–753.

Department of Veterans Affairs. (1994). *Veterans Health Administration Manual M-2* (clinical affairs part XXIV spinal cord injury services). Washington, DC: Author.

Department of Veterans Affairs. (1998). *Medical Care of Persons with Spinal Cord Injury*. Washington, DC: Author.

Department of Veterans Affairs. (1999, February 25). News release: VA to study spinal cord injury care. Washington, DC: Author.

Derry, F., Dinsmore, W., Fraser, M., Gardner, B., Glass, C., Maytom, M., Smith, M. (1998). Efficacy and safety of oral sildenafil (Viagra) in men with erectile dysfunction caused by spinal cord injury. *Neurology*, **51**, 1629–1633.

Derry, F., Glass, C., Dinsmore, W. (1997). Sildenafil (Viagra®): an oral treatment for men with erectile dysfunction caused by traumatic spinal cord injury—a 28-day, double blind placebo controlled, parallel-group, dose-response study [Abstract]. *Neurology*, **48**, A215.

Deutsch, P.M. (1990). *A Guide to Rehabilitation Testimony: The Expert's Role as an Educator*. Orlando, FL: Paul M. Deutsch Press, Inc.

Deutsch, P.M. (1992). Life expectancy in catastrophic disability: issues and parameters for the rehabilitation professional. *NARPPS Journal & News*, **7**, 58–61.

Deutsch, P.M. (1996). *Ethics and Life Care Planning*. Unpublished manuscript.

Deutsch, P.M., Raffa, F.A. (1981). *Damages in Tort Actions* (Vols. 8–9). New York: Matthew Bender.

Deutsch, P.M., Sawyer, H.W. (eds.). (1999). *A Guide to Rehabilitation*. Purchase, NY: AHAB Press, Inc.

DeVivo, M.J. (1998). *Research Update: Rehospitalization Costs of Individuals with Spinal Cord Injury*. Birmingham, AL: UAB-Spain Rehabilitation Center.

DeVivo, M.J., Black, K.J., Richards, S., Stover, S.L. (1991). Suicide following spinal cord injury. *Paraplegia*, **29**, 620–627.

DeVivo, M.J., Black, K.J., Stover, S.L. (1993). Causes of death during the first 12 years after spinal cord injury. *Arch Phys Med Rehab* **74**, 248–254.

DeVivo, M.J., Fine, P.R. (1982). Employment status of spinal cord injured patients 3 years after injury. *Arch Phys Med Rehab* **63**, 200–203.

DeVivo, M.J., Fine, P.R. (1985). Spinal cord injury: its short-term impact on marital status. *Arch Phys Med Rehab* **66**, 501–504.

DeVivo, M.J., Fine, P.R., Maetz, H.M., Stover, S.L. (1980). Prevalence of spinal cord injury: a re-estimation employing life table techniques. *Arch Neurology* **37**, 707–708.

DeVivo, M.J., Hawkins, L.N., Richards, J.S., Go, B.K. (1995). Outcomes of post-spinal cord injury marriages. *Arch Phys Med Rehab* **76**, 130–138.

DeVivo, M.J., Jackson, A.B., Dijkers, M.P., Becker, B.E. (1999). Current research outcomes from the model spinal cord injury care systems. *Arch Phys Med Rehab* **80**, 1363–1364.

DeVivo, M.J., Kartus, P.L., Stover, S.L., Rutt, R.D., Fine, P.R. (1987). Seven year survival following spinal cord injury. *Arch Neurology* **44**, 872–875.

DeVivo, M.J., Krause, J.S., Lammertse, D.P. (1999). Recent trends in mortality and causes of death among persons with spinal cord injury. *Arch Phys Med Rehab* **80**, 1411–1419.

DeVivo, M.J., Richards, J.S. (1996). Marriage rates among persons with spinal cord injury. *Rehab Psychol* **41**, 321–338.

DeVivo, M.J., Richards, J.S., Stover, S.L., Go, B.K. (1991). Spinal cord injury: rehabilitation adds life to years. *West J Med* **154**, 602–606.

DeVivo, M.J., Rutt, R.D., Stover, S.L., Fine, P.R. (1987). Employment after spinal cord injury. *Arch Phys Med Rehab* **68**, 494–498.

DeVivo, M.J., Shewchuk, R.M., Stover, S.L., Black, K.J., Go, B.K. (1992). A cross- sectional study of the relationship between age and current health status for persons with spinal cord injury. *Paraplegia*, **30**, 820–827.

DeVivo, M.J., Stover, S.L. (1995). Long-term survival and causes of death. In S.L. Stover et al. (eds.), *Spinal Cord Injury: Clinical Outcomes from the Model Systems* (pp. 289–316). Gaithersburg, MD: Aspen Publishers, Inc.

DeVivo, M.J., Stover, S.L., Black, K.J. (1992). Prognostic factors for 12-year survival after spinal cord injury. *Arch Phys Med Rehab* **73**, 156–162.

DeVivo, M.J., Whiteneck, G.G., Charles, E.D. (1995a). The economic impact of spinal cord injury. In S.L. Stover et al. (eds.), *Spinal Cord Injury: Clinical Outcomes from the Model Systems* (pp. 234–271). Gaithersburg, MD: Aspen Publishers, Inc.

Deyoe, F. (1972). Spinal cord injury: long-term follow-up of veterans. *Arch Phys Med Rehab* **53**, 523–529.

Dietzen, C.J., Lloyd, L.K. (1992). Complications of intracavernous injections and penile prostheses in spinal cord injured men. *Arch Phys Med Rehab* **73**, 652–655.

Dijkers, M. (1997). Measuring quality of life. In M. Fuhrer (ed.), *Assessing Medical Rehabilitation Practices: The Promise of Outcomes Research* (pp. 153–179). Baltimore: Paul H. Brookes Publishing Co.

Dijkers, M. (1999). Correlates of life satisfaction among persons with spinal cord injury. *Arch Phys Med Rehab* **80**, 867–876.

Dijkers, M., Abela, M.B., Gans, B.M., Gordon, W.A. (1995). The aftermath of spinal cord injury. In S.L. Stover et al. (eds.), *Spinal Cord Injury: Clinical Outcomes from the Model Systems* (pp. 185–212). Gaithersburg, MD: Aspen Publishers, Inc.

Dijkers, M., Yavuzer, G. (1999). Short versions of the telephone motor functional independence measure for use with persons with spinal cord injury. *Arch Phys Med Rehab* **80**, 1477–1484.

DiLima, S.N., Hildebrandt, U., Schust, C.S. (1996). *Spinal Cord Injury: Patient Education Manual*. Gaithersburg, MD: Aspen Publishers, Inc.

Ditunno, J.F., Cohen, M.E., Formal, C., Whiteneck, G.G. (1995). Functional outcomes. In S.L. Stover et al. (eds.), *Spinal Cord Injury: Clinical Outcomes from the Model Systems* (pp. 170–184). Gaithersburg, MD: Aspen Publishers, Inc.

Ditunno, J.F., Formal, C.S. (1994). Chronic spinal cord injury. *N Eng J Med* **330**, 550–556.

Ditunno, J., Stover, S., Murray, F., Ahn, J. (1992). Motor recovery of the upper extremities in traumatic quadriplegia: a multicenter study. *Arch Phys Med Rehab* **73**, 431–436.

Dixit, B., Martin, G., Hendricks, H., Cardenas, D. (1998). Outcomes of an inpatient pressure ulcer protocol on a spinal cord injury service. *Journal of Spinal Cord Medicine Abstracts*, **21**, 152.

Dolin, P.J., Darby, S.C., Beral, V. (1994). Paraplegia and squamous cell carcinoma of the bladder in young women: findings from a case-control study. *British Journal of Cancer*, **90**, 167–168.

Donovan, W.H. (1981). Spinal cord injury. In S.L. Stolov, M.R. Clowers (eds.), *Handbook of Severe Disability: A Text for Rehabilitation Counselors, Other Vocational Practitioners, and Allied Health Professionals* (pp. 65–82). Seattle, WA: University of Washington.

Drench, M.E. (1992). Impact of altered sexuality and sexual function in spinal cord injury: a review. *Sexuality and Disability*, **10**, 3–14.

Ducharme, S.H. (1997). Injection alternatives. *Paraplegia News*, **51**, 27–29.

Ducharme, S. (May, 1999). *Sexuality and Spinal Cord Injury*. Session presented at the annual conference on Spinal Cord Injury: Issues and Answers by Contemporary Forums, Seattle, WA.

Ducharme, S.H., Gill, K.M. (1997). *Sexuality after Spinal Cord Injury*. Baltimore: Paul H. Brookes Publishing Co.

Dvonch, P., Kaplan, L.I., Grynbaum, B.B., Rusk, H.A. (1965). Vocational findings in postdisability employment of patients with spinal cord dysfunction. *Arch Phys Med Rehab* **46**, 761–766.

Earle, C.M., Keogh, E.J., Ker, J.K., Cherry, D.J., Tulloch, A.G., Lord, D.J. (1992). The role of intracavernosal vasoactive agents to overcome impotence due to spinal cord injury. *Paraplegia*, **30**, 273–276.

El Ghatit, A.Z., Hanson, R.W. (1975). Outcome of marriages existing at the time of a male's spinal cord injury. *J Chron Dis* **28**, 383–388.

El Ghatit, A.Z., Hanson, R.W. (1976). Marriage and divorce after spinal cord injury. *Arch Phys Med Rehab* **57**, 470–472.

El Ghatit, A.Z., Hanson, R.W. (1978). Variables associated with obtaining and sustaining employment among spinal cord injured males: a follow-up of 760 veterans. *J Chron Dis* **31**, 363–369.

El Ghatit, A.Z., Hanson, R.W. (1979). Educational and training levels and employment of the spinal cord injured patient. *Arch Phys Med and Rehab* **60**, 405–406.

Elliott, S.L, (1999, May). Assessment and treatment of male sexual dysfunction in men with spinal cord injury. Session presented at the annual conference on Spinal Cord Injury: Issues and Advances by Contemporary Forums, Seattle, WA.

Elliott, T.R., Frank, R.G. (1996). Depression following spinal cord injury. *Arch Phys Med Rehab* **77**, 816–823.

El Masri, W.S., Fellows, G. (1981). Bladder cancer after spinal cord injury. *Paraplegia*, **19**, 265–270.

Engel, G. (1982). Sounding board: The biopsychosocial model and medical education—who are to be the teachers? *New England Journal of Medicine*, **13**, 802–805.

Enis, J.E., Sarmiento, A. (1973). The pathophysiology and management of pressure sores. *Ortho Rev* **2**, 25–34.

Ergas, Z. (1985). Spinal cord injury in the United States: a statistical update. *Central Nervous System Trauma*, **2**, 19–30.

Estenne, M., VanMuylem, A., Gorini, M., Kinnear, W., Heilporn, A., Detroyer, A. (1998). Effects of abdominal strapping on forced expiration in tetraplegic patients. *Am J Res Criti Care Med* **157**, 95–98.

Federal Register. (December 9, 1999). Notice of proposed funding priority for fiscal years 2000–2001 for model spinal cord injury centers, 64(236), 69153–69158.

Feldman, D. (April, 1994). Skin complications other than pressure ulcers following spinal cord injury. *UAB-RRTC Research Update Newsletter*, 1–5.

Felton, J.S., Litman, M. (1965). Study of employment of 222 men with spinal cord injury. *Arch Phys Med Rehab* **46**, 809–814.

Feyi-Waboso, P.A. (1992). An audit of five years' experience of pregnancy in spinal cord damaged women: a regional unit's experience and a review of the literature. *Paraplegia*, **30**, 631–635.

Fine, P.R., Kuhlemeier, K.V., DeVivo, M.J., Stover, S.L. (1979). Spinal cord injury: an epidemiological perspective. *Paraplegia*, **17**, 237–250.

Fitting, M., Salisbury, S. Davies, N., Mayclin, D. (1978). Self-concept and sexuality of spinal cord injured women. *Arch Sex Behav* **7**, 143–156.

Fordyce, W.E. (1964). Personality characteristics in men with spinal cord injury as related to manner of onset of disability. *Arch Phys Med Rehab* **45**, 321–325.

Foreman, P.E., Cull, J., Kirkby, R.J. (1997). Sports participation in individuals with spinal cord injury: demographic and psychological correlates. *Intl J Rehab Res* **20**, 159–168.

Formal, C.S., Crawley, M.F., Stiens, S.A. (1997). Spinal cord injury rehabilitation: three functional outcomes. *Arch Phys Med Rehab* **78**, S59–64.

Frankel, H., Hancock, D., Hyslop, G., Melzak, J., Michaelis, L., Unger, G., Vernon, J., Walsh, J. (1969). The value of postural reduction in the initial management of closed injuries to the spine with paraplegia and tetraplegia. *Paraplegia*, **7**, 179–192.

Freed, M.M., Bakst, H.J., Barrie, D.L. (1966). Life expectancy, survival rates, and causes of death in civilian patients with spinal cord trauma. *Arch Phys Med Rehab* **47**, 457–463.

Frost, F.S. (1994). Gastrointestinal dysfunction in spinal cord injury. In G.M. Yarkony (ed.), *Spinal Cord Injury: Medical Management and Rehabilitation* (pp. 27–39). Gaithersburg, MD: Aspen Publishers, Inc.

Fuhrer, M.J., Garber, S.L., Rintala, D.H., Clearman, R., Hart, K.A. (1993). Pressure ulcers in community-resident persons with spinal cord injury: prevalence and risk factors. *Arch Phys Med Rehab* **74**, 1172–1177.

Fuhrer, M.J., Rintala, D.H., Hart, K.A., Clearman, R., Young, M.E. (1993). Depressive symptomatology in persons with spinal cord injury who reside in the community. *Arch Phys Med Rehab* **74**, 255–260.

Galvin, J.C., Scherer, M.J. (1996). *Evaluating, Selecting, and Using Appropriate Assistive Technology*. Gaithersburg, MD: Aspen Publishers, Inc.

Gans, B.M. (1993). Rehabilitation of the pediatric patient. In J.A. DeLisa (Ed.), *Rehabilitation Medicine: Principles and Practice* (2nd ed., pp. 623–641). Philadelphia: J.B. Lippincott Company.

Garber, S.L., Rintala, D.H., Rossi, D., Hark, K.A., Fuhrer, M.J. (1996). Reported pressure ulcer prevention and management techniques by persons with spinal cord injury. *Arch Phys Med Rehab* **77**, 744–749.

Garland, D.E., Stewart, C.A., Adkins, R.H. (1992). Osteoporosis following spinal cord injury. *J Orthop Res* **10**, 371–378.

Geders, J.M., Gaing, A., Bauman, W.A., Korsten, M.A. (1995). The effect of cisapride on segmental colonic transit time in patients with spinal cord injury. *Am J Gastroenterology* **90**, 285–298.

Geisler, W.O., Jousse, A.T., Wynne-Jones, M. (1966). Vocational re-establishment of patients with spinal cord injury. *Medical Services Journal of Canada*, **22**, 698–709.

Geisler, W.O., Jousse, A.T., Wynne-Jones, M., Breithaupt, D. (1983). Survival in traumatic spinal cord injury. *Paraplegia*, **21**, 364–373.

Gellman, H., Chandler, D., Petrasek, J., Sie, I., Adkins, R., Waters, R. (1988). Carpal tunnel syndrome in paraplegic patients. *J Bone and Joint Surg* **70**, 517–519.

Georgia Central Registry. (1993). *Spinal Cord Disabilities and Traumatic Brain Injury.* Warm Springs, GA: Roosevelt Warm Springs Institute for Rehabilitation.

Gerhart, K.A. (1993). Changing the adaptive environment. In G.G. Whiteneck et al. (eds.), *Aging with Spinal Cord Injury* (pp. 343–352). New York: Demos Publications.

Gerhart, K.A. (1996). Spasticity: friend or foe? *Paraplegia News*, **50**, 17–21.

Gerhart, K.A., Bergstrom, E., Charlifue, S.W., Menter, R.R., Whiteneck, G.G. (1993). Long-term spinal cord injury: functional changes over time. *Arch Phys Med Rehab* **74**, 1030–1034.

Gerhart, K.A., Charlifue, S.W., Menter, R.R., Weitzenkamp, D.A., Whiteneck, G.G. (1997). Aging with spinal cord injury. *American Rehabilitation*, **23**, 19–26.

Gerhart, K.A., Johnson, R.L., Whiteneck, G.G. (1992). Health and psychosocial issues of individuals with incomplete and resolving spinal cord injuries. *Paraplegia*, **30**, 282–287.

Gerhart, K.A., Lammertse, D.P. (1997). Bladder cancer: a complex puzzle. *Paraplegia News*, **51**, 21–25.

Glass, C., Derry, F., Dinsmore, W., Fraser, M., Gardner, B., Maytom, M., Orr, M., Osterloh, H., Smith, M. (1997). Sildenafil (Viagra™): an oral treatment for men with erectile dysfunction caused by traumatic spinal cord injury—a double-blind, placebo-controlled, single-dose, two-way crossover study using rigiscan [Abstract]. *J Spinal Cord Med* **20**, 145.

Glickman, S., Kamm, M.A. (1996). Bowel dysfunction in spinal cord injury patients. *Lancet*, **347**, 1651–1653.

Go, B.K., DeVivo, M.J., Richards, J.S. (1995). The epidemiology of spinal cord injury. In S.L, Stover et al. (eds.), *Spinal Cord Injury: Clinical Outcomes from the Model Systems* (pp. 21–55). Gaithersburg, MD: Aspen Publishers, Inc.

Goetz, L.L. (1998). Autonomic dysreflexia. In M.C. Hammond (ed.), *Medical Care of Persons with Spinal Cord Injury* (pp. 23–27). Washington, DC: Department of Veterans Affairs.

Goetz, L.L., Little, J.W. (1998). Genitourinary system. In M.C. Hammond (ed.), *Medical Care of Persons with Spinal Cord Injury* (pp. 61–68). Washington, DC: Department of Veterans Affairs.

Goldberg, R.T., Freed, M.M. (1982). Vocational development of spinal cord injury patients: an 8-year follow-up. *Arch Phys Med Rehab* **63**, 207–210.

Goldstein, B. (1998). Musculoskeletal system. In M.C. Hammond (ed.), *Medical Care of Persons with Spinal Cord Injury* (pp. 69–79). Washington, DC: Department of Veterans Affairs.

Gordon, W.A., Harasymiw, S., Bellile, S., Lehman, L., Sherman, B. (1982). The relationship between pressure sores and psychosocial adjustment in persons with spinal cord injury. *Rehab Psychol* **27**, 185–191.

Gordon, J.L., Kohl, C.A., Areti, M., Complin, R.A., Vulpe, M. (1996). Spinal cord injury increases the risk of abdominal aortic aneurysm. *American Surgeon*, **62**, 249–252.

Gore, R., Mintzer, R., Calenoff, L. (1981). Gastrointestinal complications of spinal cord injury. *Spine*, **6**, 538–544.

Graitcer, P.L., Maynard, F.M. (eds.). (1990). First colloquium on preventing secondary disabilities among people with spinal cord injuries. Atlanta, GA: Centers for Disease Control.

Granello, P.F., Witmer, J.M. (1998). Standards of care: potential implications for the counseling profession. *J Counsel Develop* **76**, 371–380.

Granger, C.V., Fiedler, R.C. (1997). The measurement of disability. In M.J. Fuhrer (ed.), *Assessing Medical Rehabilitation Practices: The Promise of Outcomes Research* (pp. 103–126). Baltimore: Paul H. Brookes Publishing Co.

Greenspoon, J.S., Paul, R.H. (1986). Paraplegia and quadriplegia: special considerations during pregnancy and labor and delivery. *Am J Obstet Gynecol* **155**, 738–741.

Griffith, E.R., Tomoko, M.A., Timms, R.J. (1973). Sexual function in spinal cord injured patients: a review. *Arch Phys Med Rehab* **54**, 539–543.

Griffith, E.R., Trieschmann, R.B. (1975). Sexual functioning in women with spinal cord injury. *Arch Phys Med Rehab* **56**, 18–21.

Haas, J.F. (1993). Ethical issues in rehabilitation medicine. In J.A. DeLisa (ed.), *Rehabilitation Medicine: Principles and Practice* (2nd ed., pp. 28–39). Philadelphia: J.B. Lippincott Company.

Habeck, R., Lynch, R.T. (1997). Vocational rehabilitation counseling. In B.A. O'Young, M.A. Young, S.A. Stiens (eds.), *Physical Medicine and Rehabilitation Secrets: a Socratic Textbook* (pp. 145–150). Philadelphia: Hanley and Belfus.

Hackler, R.H. (1977). A 25-year prospective mortality study in the spinal cord injured patient: comparison with the long term living paraplegic. *J Urol* **117**, 486–488.

Hall, K.M., Cohen, M.E., Wright, J., Call, M., Werner, P. (1999). Characteristics of the functional independence measure in traumatic spinal cord injury. *Arch Phys Med Rehab* **80**, 1471–1476.

Hall, K.M., Knudsen, S.T., Wright, J., Charlifue, S.W., Graves, D.E., Werner, P. (1999). Follow-up study of individuals with high tetraplegia (C1–C4) 14 to 24 years post-injury. *Arch Phys Med Rehab* **80**, 1507–1513.

Hamilton, B.B., Granger, C.V., Sherwin, F.S., Zielezny, M., Tashman, J.S. (1987). A uniform national data system for medical rehabilitation. In M.J. Fuhrer (ed.), *Rehabilitation Outcomes: Analysis and Measurement* (pp. 137–147). Baltimore: Paul H. Brookes Publishing Co.

Hammond, M.C. (ed.). (1998). *Medical Care of Persons with Spinal Cord Injury*, Washington, DC: Department of Veterans Affairs.

Hammond, M.C., Bozzocco, V.A., Stiens, S.A., Buhrer, R., Lyman, P. (1994). Pressure ulcer incidence on a spinal cord injury unit. *Advances in Wound Care*, **6**, 57–60.

Han, T.R., Kim, J.H., Kwon, B.S. (1998). Chronic gastrointestinal problems and bowel dysfunction in patients with spinal cord injury. *Spinal Cord*, **36**, 485–490.

Hancock, K.M., Craig, A.R., Martin, J., Dickson, H.G., Chang, E. (1993). Anxiety and depression over the first year of spinal cord injury: a longitudinal study. *Paraplegia*, **31**, 349–357.

Harari, D., Sarkarati, M., Gurwitz, J., McGlinchey-Berroth, G., Minaker, K. (1997). Constipation-related symptoms and bowel program concerning individuals with spinal cord injury. *Spinal Cord*, **35**, 394–401.

Hardy, A.G. (1976). Survival periods in traumatic tetraplegia. *Paraplegia*, **14**, 41–46.

Harrison, J., Glass, C.A., Owens, R.G., Soni, B.M. (1995). Factors associated with sexual functioning in women following spinal cord injury. *Paraplegia*, **33**, 687–692.

Hartkopp, A., Bronnum-Hansen, H., Seidenschnur, A.M., Biering-Sorensen, F. (1998). Suicide in a spinal cord injured population: its relation to functional status. *Arch Phys Med Rehab* **79**, 1356–1361.

Harvey, C., Rothschild, B.B., Asmann, A.J., Stripling, T.E. (1990). New estimates of traumatic SCI prevalence: a survey-based approach. *Paraplegia*, **28**, 537–544.

Harvey, C., Wilson, S.E., Greene, C.G., Berkowitz, M., Stripling, T.E. (1992). New estimates of direct costs of traumatic spinal cord injuries: results from a nationwide survey. *Paraplegia*, **30**, 834–850.

Heinemann, A.W., Doll, M.D., Armstrong, K.J., Schnoll, S., Yarkony, G.M. (1991). Substance use and receipt of treatment by persons with long-term spinal cord injuries. *Arch Phys Med Rehab* **72**, 482–487.

Heinemann, A., Donahoe, R., Keen, M., Scholl, S. (1988). Alcohol use by persons with recent spinal cord injuries. *Arch Phys Med Rehab* **69**, 619–624.

Heinemann, A.W., Hawkins, D. (1995). Substance abuse and medical complications following spinal cord injury. *Rehab Psychol* **40**, 125–140.

Heinemann, A.W., Linacre, J.M., Wright, B.D., Hamilton, B.B., Granger, C. (1993). Relationships between impairment and physical disability as measured by the functional independence measure. *Arch Phys Med Rehab* **74**, 566–573.

Hickman, J.K. (1993). *Spinal Cord Injury in Virginia: A Statistical Fact Sheet*. Fisherville, VA: Virginia Department of Rehabilitative Services.

Hinderer, S.R., Gupta, S. (1996). Functional outcome measures to assess interventions for spasticity. *Arch Phys Med Rehab* **77**, 1083–1089.

Holmgren, E., Giuliano, F., Hulting, C. (1998). Sildenafil (Viagra®) in the treatment of erectile dysfunction caused by spinal cord injury: a double blind, placebo-controlled, flexible dose, two-way crossover study [abstract]. *Neurology*, **50**, A127.

Hosack, K. (1998). The value of case management in catastrophic injury rehabilitation and long-term management. *J Case Mgmt* **4**, 58–67.

House, J.G., Stiens, S.A. (1997). Pharmacologically initiated defecation for persons with spinal cord injury: effectiveness of three agents. *Arch Phys Med Rehab* **78**, 1062–1065.

Hu, S.S., Cressy, J.M. (1992). Paraplegia and quadriplegia. In M.G. Brodwin, F.A. Tellez, S.K. Brodwin (eds.), *Medical, Psychosocial, and Vocational Aspects of Disability* (pp. 369–391). Athens, GA: Elliott and Fitzpatrick, Inc.

Hughes, S.J., Short, D.J., Usherwood, M.M., Tebbutt, H. (1991). Management of the pregnant woman with spinal cord injuries. *British Journal of Obstetrics and Gynecology*, **98**, 513–518.

Hutchinson, J.T., McGuckin, M. (1990). Occlusive dressings: a microbiologic and clinical review. *American Journal of Infection Control*, **18**, 257–268.

Injury Prevention Service. (1993). *Summary of Reportable Injuries in Oklahoma, 1988–1992*. Oklahoma City, OK: Oklahoma State Department of Health.

Ivie, C.S., DeVivo, M.J. (1994). Predicting unplanned hospitalizations in persons with spinal cord injury. *Arch Phys Med Rehab* **75**, 1182–1188.

Jackson, A.B. (1995). Medical management of women with spinal cord injury: a review. *Topics in Spinal Cord Injury Rehabilitation*, **1**, 11–26.

Jackson, A.B. (1996). Pregnancy and delivery. In D.M. Krotoski, M.A. Nosek, M.A. Turk (eds.), *Women with Physical Disabilities: Achieving and Maintaining Health and Well-being* (pp. 91–99). Baltimore: Paul H. Brooks Publishing Co.

Jackson, A.B., DeVivo, M. (1992). Urological long-term follow-up in women with spinal cord injuries. *Arch Phys Med Rehab* **73**, 1029–1035.

Jackson, A.B., Groomes, T.E. (1994). Incidence of respiratory complications following spinal cord injury. *Arch Phys Med Rehab* **75**, 270–275.

Jackson, A.B., Wadley, V. (1999). A multicenter study of women's self-reported reproductive health after spinal cord injury. *Arch Phys Med Rehab* **80**, 1420–1428.

Jackson, R.H. (1994). Home modifications for people with disabilities. In G.M. Yarkony (ed.), *Spinal Cord Injury: Medical Management and Rehabilitation* (pp. 183–203). Gaithersburg, MD: Aspen Publishers, Inc.

James, M., DeVivo, M.J., Richards, J.S. (1993). Postinjury employment outcomes among African-American and white persons with spinal cord injury. *Rehab Psychol* **38**, 151–164.

Janssen, T.W.J., Van Oers, C.A., Van Kamp, G.J., Ten Voorde, B.J., Van derWoude, L.A., Hollander, A.P. (1997). Coronary heart disease risk indications, aerobic power, and physical activity in men with spinal cord injuries. *Arch Phys Med Rehab* **78**, 697–705.

Johnston, B. (1982). Pregnancy and childbirth in women with spinal cord injuries: a review of literature. *Maternal Child Nursing Journal*, **21**, 41–46.

Johnson, R.L., Brooks, C.A., Whiteneck, G.G. (1996). Cost of traumatic spinal cord injury in a population-based registry. *Spinal Cord*, **34**, 470–480.

Kantor, A.F., Hartge, P., Hoover, R.N., Narayana, A.S., Sullivan, J.W., Fraumeni, J.F. (1984). Urinary tract infections and risk of bladder cancer. *Am J Epidemiology* **11**, 510–515.

Kapoor, V.K., Chahal, A.S., Jyoti, S.P., Mundkur, Y.J., Kotwal, S.V., Mehta, V.K. (1993). Intracavernous papaverine for impotence in spinal cord injured patients. *Paraplegia*, **31**, 675–677.

Kato, H., Inoue, T., Torii, S. (1998). A new postoperative management scheme for preventing sacral pressure sores in patients with spinal cord injuries. *Ann Plastic Surg* **40**, 39–43.

Katz, R.T. (1994). Management of spastic hypertonia after spinal cord injury. In G.M. Yarkony (ed.), *Spinal Cord Injury: Medical Management and Rehabilitation* (pp. 97–107). Gaithersburg, MD: Aspen Publishers, Inc.

Katz, J., Adler, J., Mazzarella, N., Ince, L. (1985). Psychological consequences of an exercise training program for a paraplegic man: a case study. *Rehab Psychol* **30**, 53–58.

Kaufman, J.M., Fam, B., Jacobs, S.J., Gabilondo, F., Yalla, S., Kane, J.P., Rossier, A.B. (1977). Bladder cancer and squamous metaplasia in the spinal cord injury patients. *J Urol* **9**, 317–320.

Kemp, B.J., Bauman, W.A., Adkins, R.H., Spungen, A.M., Krause, J.S. (1999). The relationship between serum lipid values, adiposity, and depressive symptomatology in persons aging with spinal cord injury. Manuscript submitted for publication.

Kemp, B., Krause, J.S., Adkins, R. (1999). Depression among African-Americans, Latinos, and Caucasians with spinal cord injury: an exploratory study. *Rehab Psychol* **44**, 235–247.

Kennedy, P., Frankel, H., Gardner, B., Nuseibeh, I. (1997). Factors associated with acute and chronic pain following traumatic spinal cord injuries. *Spinal Cord*, **35**, 814–817.

Kennedy, P., Lowe, R., Grey, N., Short, E. (1995). Traumatic spinal cord injury and psychological impact: a cross-sectional analysis of coping strategies. *Brit J Clin Psychol* **34**, 627–639.

Kerr, W., Thompson, M. (1972). Acceptance of disability of sudden onset in paraplegia. *Intl J Paraplegia* **10**, 94–102.

Kessler Institute for Rehabilitation. (1996). *Spinal Cord Injury Manual*. West Orange, NJ: Author.

Ketover, S., Ansel, H., Goldish, G., Roche, B., Gebhard, R. (1996). Gallstones in chronic spinal cord injury: is impaired gallbladder emptying a risk factor? *Arch Phys Med Rehab* **77**, 1136–1138.

Kettl, P., Zarefoss, S., Jacoby, K., Garman, C., Hulse, C., Rowley, F., Corey, R., Sredy, M., Bixler, E., Tyson, K. (1991). Female sexuality after spinal cord injury. *Sexuality and Disability*, **9**, 287–295.

Kewman, D.G., Tate, D.G. (1998). Suicide in SCI: a psychological autopsy. *Rehab Psychol* **43**, 143–151.

Kim, S.W., Charallel, J.T., Park. K.W., Bauerle, L.C., Shang, C.C., Gordon, S.K., Bauman, W.A. (1994). Prevalence of deep venous thrombosis in patients with chronic spinal cord injury. *Arch Phys Med Rehab* **75**, 965–968.

Kinney, W.B., Coyle, C.P. (1992). Predicting life satisfaction among adults with physical disabilities. *Arch Phys Med Rehab* **73**, 863–869.

Kitchener, K.S. (1984). Intuition, critical evaluation and ethical principles: the foundation for ethical decisions in counseling psychology. *Counseling Psychologist*, **12**, 43–55.

Kiwerski, J., Weiss, M., Chrostowska, T. (1981). Analysis of mortality of patients after cervical spine trauma. *Paraplegia*, **19**, 347–351.

Kocina, P. (1997). Body composition of spinal cord injured adults: review article. *Sports Medicine*, **23**, 48–60.

Komisarvk, B.R., Gerdes, C.A., Whipple, B. (1997). Complete spinal cord injury does not block perceptual responses to genital self-stimulation in women. *Arch Neurology* **54**, 1513–1520.

Kraus, J.F., Franti, C.E., Riggins, R.S., Richards, D., Borhani, N.O. (1975). Incidence of traumatic spinal cord lesions. *J Chron Dis* **28**, 471–492.

Krause, J.S. (1990). The relationship between productivity and adjustment following spinal cord injury. *Rehab Counsel Bull* **33**, 188–199.

Krause, J.S. (1991). Survival following spinal cord injury: a fifteen-year prospective study. *Rehab Psychol* **36**, 89–98.

Krause, J.S. (1992a). Adjustment to life after spinal cord injury: a comparison among three participant groups based on employment status. *Rehab Counsel Bull* **35**, 218–229.

Krause, J.S. (1992b). Employment after spinal cord injury. *Arch Phys Med Rehab* **73**, 163–169.

Krause, J.S. (1996). Employment after spinal cord injury: transition and life adjustment. *Rehab Counsel Bull* **39**, 244–255.

Krause, J.S. (1998a). Aging and life adjustment after spinal cord injury. *Spinal Cord*, **36**, 320–328.

Krause, J.S. (1998b). Skin sores after spinal cord injury: relationship to life adjustment. *Spinal Cord*, **36**, 51–56.

Krause, J.S. (1998c). Subjective well-being after spinal cord injury: relationship to gender, race/ethnicity, and chronological age. *Rehab Psychol* **43**, 282–296.

Krause, J.S. (1999). *Aging and Secondary Conditions after Spinal Cord Injury*. Manuscript submitted for publication.

Krause, J.S., Anson, C.A. (1996a). Employment after spinal cord injury: relationship to selected participant characteristics. *Arch Phys Med Rehab* **77**, 737–743.

Krause, J.S., Anson, C.A. (1996b). Self-perceived reasons for unemployment cited by persons with spinal cord injury: relationship to gender, race, age, and level of injury. *Rehab Counsel Bull* **39**, 217–227.

Krause, J.S., Crewe, N.M. (1987). Prediction of long-term survival of persons with spinal cord injury: an 11-year prospective study. *Rehab Psychol* **32**, 205–213.

Krause, J.S., Crewe, N.M. (1991). Chronologic age, time since injury, and time of measurement: effect on adjustment after spinal cord injury. *Arch Phys Med Rehab* **72**, 91–100.

Krause, J.S., Kemp, B.J., Coker, J.L. (1999). *Aging, Gender, Race/ethnicity, and Depression after Spinal Cord Injury: An analysis of the mediating roles of years of education and income*. Manuscript submitted for publication.

Krause, J.S., Kewman, D., DeVivo, M.J., Maynard, F., Coker, J., Roach, M.J., Ducharme, S. (1999). Employment after spinal cord injury: an analysis of cases from the model spinal cord injury systems. *Arch Phys Med Rehab* **80**, 1492–1500.

Krause, J.S., Dunn, K. *Subsequent Injuries Among Individuals with Pre-existing Spinal Cord Injury*. Manuscript in preparation.

Krause, J.S., Kjorsvig, J.M. (1992). Mortality after spinal cord injury: a 4-year prospective study. *Arch Phys Med Rehab* **73**, 558–564.

Krause, J.S., Saari, J.M., Dykstra, D. (1990). Quality of life and survival after spinal cord injury. *SCI Psychosocial Process*, **3**, 4–8.

Krause, J.S., Sternberg, M., Maides, J., Lottes, S. (1997a). Employment after spinal cord injury: differences related to geographic region, gender, and race. *Arch Phys Med Rehab* **79**, 615–624.

Krause, J.S., Sternberg, M., Maides, J., Lottes, S. (1997b). Mortality after spinal cord injury: an 11-year prospective study. *Arch Phys Med Rehab* **78**, 815–821.

Krause, J.S., Vines, C., Farley, T., Sniezak, J., Coker, J.L. (1999). *An Exploratory Study of Pressure Ulcers after Spinal Cord Injury: Relationship to protective and risk factors*. Manuscript submitted for publication.

Kreuter, M., Sullivan, M., Sivsteen, A. (1996). Sexual adjustment and quality of relationships in spinal paraplegia: a controlled study. *Arch Phys Med Rehab* **77**, 541–547.

Krotoski, D.M., Bennett, C.J. (1996). Managing bladder and bowel function. In D.M. Krotoski, M.A. Nosek, M.A. Turk (eds.), *Women with Physical Disabilities: Achieving and Maintaining Health and Well-being* (pp. 283–285). Baltimore: Paul H. Brookes Publishing Co.

Krotoski, D.M., Nosek, M.A., Turk, M.A. (1996). *Women with Physical Disabilities: Achieving and Maintaining Health and Well-being*. Baltimore: Paul H. Brookes Publishing Co.

Krum, H., Howes, L., Brown, D. (1992). Risk factors for cardiovascular disease in chronic spinal cord injury patients. *Paraplegia*, **30**, 381–388.

Kunkel, C.F., Scremin, A.M., Eisenberg, B., Garcia, J.F., Roberts, S., Martinez, S. (1993). Effect of "standing" on spasticity, contracture, and osteoporosis in paralyzed males. *Arch Phys Med Rehab* **74**, 73–78.

Kurtzke, J.F. (1975). Epidemiology of spinal cord injury. *Experimental Neurology*, **48**, 163–236.

Lal, S. (1998). Premature degenerative shoulder changes in spinal cord injury patients. *Spinal Cord*, **36**, 186–189.

Lammertse, D.P. (1993). The nervous system. In G.G. Whiteneck et al. (eds.), *Aging with Spinal Cord Injury* (pp. 129–137). New York: Demos Publications.

Lance, J.W. (1980). Symposium synopsis. In R.R. Young W.P. Koella (eds.), *Spasticity: Disordered Motor Control* (pp. 485–494). Chicago: Yearbook Medical Publishers.

Lanig, I.S. (1993). The genitourinary system. In G.G. Whiteneck et al. (eds.), *Aging with Spinal Cord Injury* (pp. 105–115). New York: Demos Publications.

Lanig, I.S., Chase, T.M., Butt, L.M., Hulse, K.L., Johnson, K.M.M. (1996). *A Practical Guide to Health Promotion after Spinal Cord Injury*. Gaithersburg, MD: Aspen Publishers, Inc.

Lanig, I.S., Lammertse, D.P. (1992). The respiratory system in spinal cord injury. *Phys Med Rehab Clin N Am* **3**, 725–740.

Lanig, I.S., Lammertse, D.P., Gerhart, K.A. (1993). *Durable Medical Equipment for the Patient with Spinal Cord Injury*. Chicago: American Spinal Injury Association.

Latham, L. (1994). When spinal cord injury complicates medical/surgical care. *Rehabilitation Nursing*, **57**, 26–29.

Lawrence, D.W., Bayakly, A.R., Mathison, J.B. (1992). *Traumatic Spinal Cord Injury in Louisiana: 1990 Annual Report*. New Orleans, LA: Louisiana Office of Public Health.

Lazar, R.B. (1994). Posttraumatic syringomyelia. In G.M. Yarkony (ed.), *Spinal Cord Injury: Medical Management and Rehabilitation* (pp. 109–112). Gaithersburg, MD: Aspen Publishers, Inc.

Lee, Y., Dattilo, J., Kleiber, D.A., Caldwell, L. (1996). Exploring the meaning of continuity of recreation activity in the early stages of adjustment for people with spinal cord injury. *Leisure Sciences*, **18**, 209–225.

Lemon, M.A. (1993). Sexual counseling and spinal cord injury. *Sexuality and Disability*, **11**, 73–97.

Leslie, D.P., Ahrendt, L. (1999). Managing severe spasticity with intrathecal Baclofen (ITB™) therapy. *Journal of Care Management* **5(5)**, 21–25.

Llang, H.W., Wang, Y.H., Wang, T.G., Lien, T.N. (1996). Clinical experience in rehabilitation of spinal cord injury associated with schizophrenia. *Arch Phys Med Rehab* **77**, 283–286.

Limke, J.C., Stiens, S.A. (1997). Carpal tunnel syndrome and/or median neuropathy of the wrist? In B.A. O'Young, M.A. Young, S.A. Stiens (eds.), *Physical Medicine and Rehabilitation Secrets: A Socratic Textbook* (pp. 184–189). Philadelphia: Hanley and Belfus.

Linsenmeyer, T.A. (1991). Evaluation and treatment of erectile dysfunction following spinal cord injury: A review. *J Am Paraplegia Soc* **14**, 43–51.

Linsenmeyer, T.A. (1997). Management of male infertility. In M.L. Sipski, C.J. Alexander (eds.), *Sexual Function in People with Disability and Chronic Illness: A Health Professionals Guide* (pp. 487–509). Gaithersburg, MD: Aspen Publishers, Inc.

Linsenmeyer, T.A., Perkash, I. (1991). Infertility in men with spinal cord injury. *Arch Phys Med Rehab* **72**, 747–754.

Linsenmeyer, T.A., Stone, J.M. (1993). Neurogenic bladder and bowel dysfunction. In J.A. DeLisa, et al. (eds.), *Rehabilitation Medicine: Principles and Practice* (2nd ed., pp. 733–758). Philadelphia: J.B. Lippincott Company.

Little, J.W. (1998). Neurologic system. In M.C. Hammond (ed.), *Medical Care of Persons with Spinal Cord Injury* (pp. 81–87). Washington, DC: Department of Veterans Affairs.

Little, J.W., Massagli, T.L. (1993). Spasticity and associated abnormalities of muscle tone. In J.A. DeLisa (ed.), *Rehabilitation Medicine: Principles and Practice* (2nd ed., pp. 666–677). Philadelphia: J.B. Lippincott Company.

Lloyd, L.K., Richards, J.S. (1989). Intracavernous pharmacotherapy for management of erectile dysfunction in spinal cord injury. *Paraplegia*, **27**, 457–464.

Locke, J.R., Hill, D.E., Walzer, Y. (1985). Incidence of squamous cell carcinoma in patients with long-term catheter drainage. *J Urol* **133**, 1034–1035.

Loubser, P.G., Donovan, W.H. (1996). Chronic pain associated with spinal cord injury. In R.K. Narayan, J.E. Wilberger, J.T. Povlishock (eds.), *Neurotrauma* (pp. 1311–1322). New York: McGraw Hill.

Louisiana Office of Public Health. (1999). *Traumatic Brain and Spinal Cord Injury in Louisiana: 1997 Annual Surveillance Report*. Author.

Macleod, A.D. (1988). Self-neglect of spinal injured patients. *Paraplegia*, **26**, 340–349.

Madorsky, J.G. (1995). Influence of disability on pregnancy and motherhood. *West J Med* **162**, 153–155.

Manns, P.J., Chad, K. (1999). Determining the relationship between quality of life, handicap, fitness, and physical activity for persons with spinal cord innury. *Arch Phys Med Rehab* **80**, 1566–1571.

Mariano, A.J. (1992). Chronic pain and spinal cord injury. *Clin J Pain* **8**, 87–92.

Martinez-Arizala, A., Brackett, N.L. (1994). Sexual dysfunction in spinal injury. In C. Singer, W.J. Weiner (eds.), *Sexual Dysfunction: A Neuro-medical Approach* (pp. 135–153). Armonk, NY: Futura Publishing Company, Inc.

Mawson, A.R., Biando, J.J, Neville, P., Linares, H.A., Winchester, Y., Lopez, A. (1988). Risk factors for early occurring ulcers following spinal cord injury. *Am J Phys Med Rehab* **67**, 123–127.

Maynard, F.M. (1993). Changing care needs. In G.G. Whiteneck et al. (eds.), *Aging with Spinal Cord Injury* (pp. 191–198). New York: Demos Publications.

Maynard, F.M., Karunas, R.S., Adkins, R.H., Richards, J.S., Waring, W.P. (1995). Management of the neuromusculoskeletal systems. In S.L. Stover et al. (eds.), *Spinal Cord Injury: Clinical Outcomes from the Model Systems* (pp. 145–169). Gaithersburg, MD: Aspen Publishers, Inc.

Maynard, F.M., Weingarden, S. (1990). Secondary complications of spinal cord injury. In D.F. Apple, L.M. Hudson (eds.), Spinal Cord Injury: The Model (pp. 57–65). Atlanta, GA: The Georgia Regional Spinal Cord Injury Care System Shepard Center for Treatment of Spinal Injuries, Inc.

McAlonan, S. (1996). Improving sexual rehabilitation services: The patient's perspective. *Am J Occupat Therapy* **50**, 826–834.

McAweeney, M.J., Forchheimer, M., Tate, D.G. (1996). Identifying the unmet independent needs of persons with spinal cord injury. *J Rehab* **62**, 29–34.

McColl, M.A., Rosenthal, C. (1994). A model of resource needs of aging spinal cord injured men. *Paraplegia*, **32**, 261–270.

McCollom, P. (1999). Life care planning 101: an introduction to the process. *J Case Mgmt* **5(6)**, 24–27.

McKinley, W.O., Jackson, A.B., Cardenas, D.D., DeVivo, M.J. (1999). Long-term medical complications after traumatic spinal cord injury: a regional model systems analysis. *Arch Phys Med Rehab* **80**, 1402–1410.

Means, B.L., Bolton, B. (1994). Recommendations for expanding employability services provided by independent living programs. *J Rehab* **60**, 20–25.

Meara, N.M., Schmidt, L.D., Day, J.D. (1996). Principles and virtues: a foundation for ethical decisions, policies, and character. *Counseling Psychologist*, **24**, 4–77.

Menter, R.R. (1990). Aging and spinal cord injury: implications for existing model systems and future federal, state, and local health care policy. *Spinal Cord Injury: The Model*. Proceedings of the national consensus conference on catastrophic illness and injury, December 1989. Atlanta, GA: Georgia Regional Spinal Cord Injury Care System, Shepard Center for Treatment of Spinal Injuries, Inc.

Menter, R.R. (1993). Issues of aging with spinal cord injury. In G.G. Whiteneck et al. (eds.), *Aging with Spinal Cord Injury* (pp. 1–8). New York: Demos Publications.

Menter, R.R., Hudson, L.M. (1995). Effects of age at injury and the aging process. In S.L. Stover et al. (eds.), *Spinal Cord Injury: Clinical Outcomes from the Model Systems* (pp. 272–288). Gaithersburg, MD: Aspen Publishers, Inc.

Menter, R., Weitzenkamp, D., Cooper, D., Bingley, J., Charlifue, S., and Whiteneck, G. (1997). Bowel management outcomes in individuals with long-term spinal cord injuries. *Spinal Cord*, **35**, 608–612.

Menter, R.R., Whiteneck, G.G., Charlifue, S.W., Gerhart, K., Solnick, S.J., Brooks, C.A., Hughes, L. (1991). Impairment, disability, handicap and medical expenses of persons aging with spinal cord injury. *Paraplegia*, **29**, 613–619.

Merli, G.J. (1992). Management of deep vein thrombosis in spinal cord injury. *Chest*, **102**, S652–657.

Merli, G.J., Herbison, G.J., Ditunno, J.F., Weitz, H.H., Henzes, J.H., Park, C.H., Jaweed, M.M., Heltzel, J. (1988). Deep vein thrombosis: prophylaxis in acute spinal cord injured patients. *Arch Phys Med Rehab* **69**, 661–664.

Mesard, L., Carmody, A., Mannarino, E., Ruge, D. (1978). Survival after spinal cord trauma. *Arch Neurology* **35**, 78–83.

Michals, E.A., Ramsey, R.G. (1996). Syringomyelia. *Orthopedic Nursing*, **15**, 33–41.

Monga, M., Bernie, J., Rajasekaran, M. (1999). Male infertility and erectile dysfunction in spinal cord injury: a review. *Arch Phys Med Rehab* **80**, 1331–1339.

Moonka, R., Stiens, S.A., Eubank, W.B., Stelzner, M. (1999). The presentation of gallstones and results of biliary surgery in a spinal cord injured population. *Am J Surg* **178**, 246–250.

Morris, J., Roth, E.J. (1994). Cognitive dysfunction in spinal cord injury. In G.M. Yarkony (ed.), *Spinal Cord Injury: Medical Management and Rehabilitation* (pp. 113–127). Gaithersburg, MD: Aspen Publishers, Inc.

Mourer, S.A. (1999). Abstracts in summary: the suicidal client in SCI. *SCI Psychosocial Process*, **12(1)**, 26–27.

Murphy, K.P., Kliener, E.M., Moore, M.J. (1994). The voiding alert system: a new application in the treatment of incontinence. *Arch Phys Med Rehab* **75**, 924–927.

Mutton, D.L., Scremin, A.M., Barstow, T.J., Scott, M.D., Kunkel, C.F., Cagle, T.G. (1997). Physiologic responses during functional electrical stimulation leg cycling and hybrid exercise in spinal cord injured subjects. *Arch Phys Med Rehab* **78**, 712–718.

Nance, P.W., Schryvers, O., Leslie, W., Ludwig, S., Krahn, J., Uebelhart, D. (1999). Intravenous pamidronate attenuates bone density loss after acute spinal cord injury. *Arch Phys Med Rehab* **80**, 243–251.

National Guideline Clearinghouse. (1998). *Detection and selection of evidence-based guidelines and related materials*. Available: www.guideline.gov.

National Spinal Cord Injury Association. (1996). *Common Questions about Spinal Cord Injury*. Woburn, MA: Author.

National Spinal Cord Injury Statistical Center. (1997). *Annual Report for the Model Spinal Cord Injury System*. Birmingham, AL: University of Alabama.

National Spinal Cord Injury Statistical Center. (2000). *Spinal Cord Injury: Facts and Figures at a Glance—January, 2000*. Birmingham, AL: University of Alabama.

Neff, W. (1971). Rehabilitation and work. In W. Neff (ed.), *Rehab Psychol* (pp. 109–142). Washington, DC: American Psychological Association.

Nehemkis, A., Groot, H. (1980). Indirect self-destructive behavior in spinal cord injury. In N. Farberow (ed.), *The Many Faces of Suicide* (pp. 99–115). New York: McGraw Hill.

Nehra, A., Werner, M.A., Bastuba, M., Title, C., Oates, R.D. (1996). Vibratory stimulation and rectal probe electroejaculation as therapy for patients with spinal cord injury: semen parameters and pregnancy rates. *J Urol* **155**, 554–559.

Neumayer, L.A., Bull, D.A., Mohr, J.D., Putnam, C.W. (1990). The acutely affected abdomen in paraplegic spinal cord injury patients. *Annals of Surgery*, **212**, 561–566.

Niazi, S.B.M., Salzberg, C.A., Byrne, D.W., Viehbeck, M. (1997). Recurrence of initial pressure ulcer in persons with spinal cord injuries. *Journal for Prevention and Healing*, **10**, 38–43.

Nobunaga, A.J., Go, B.K., Karunas, R.B. (1999). Recent demographic and injury trends in people served by the model spinal cord injury care systems. *Arch Phys Med Rehab* **80**, 1372–1382.

Northwest Regional Spinal Cord Injury System. (1994). *Syrinxes*. Seattle, WA: Author.

Northwest Regional Spinal Cord Injury System. (1996a). *Sexual Function and Fertility after SCI: Part 1: Men*. Seattle, WA: Author.

Northwest Regional Spinal Cord Injury System. (1996b). *Sexual Function and Fertility after SCI: Part 2: Women*. Seattle, WA: Author.

Northwest Regional Spinal Cord Injury System. (1997). *Aging and SCI*. Seattle, WA: Author.

Nosek, M.A. (1993). Personal assistance: its effect on the long-term health of a rehabilitation hospital population. *Arch Phys Med Rehab* **74**, 127–132.

Nosek, M.A., Howland, C.A. (1997). Breast and cervical cancer screening among women with physical disabilities. *Arch Phys Med Rehab* **78**, S39–44.

Nosek, M.A., Rintala, D.H., Young, M.E., Howland, C.A., Foley, C.C., Rossi, D., Chanpong, G. (1996). Sexual functioning among women with physical disabilities. *Arch Phys Med Rehab* **77**, 107–115.

Nosek, M.A., Stiens, S. (1996). Medical update part 2: latest information on reproductive health for women with spinal cord injuries: Neurogenic bowel dysfunction after spinal cord injury. *Paraplegia News*, **50**, 62–66.

Nyquist, R.H., Bors, E. (1967). Mortality and survival in traumatic myelopathy during nineteen years, from 1946 to 1965. *Paraplegia*, **5**, 22–48.

Ohry, A., Peleg, D., Goldman, J., David, A., Rozin, R. (1978). Sexual function, pregnancy and delivery in spinal cord injured women. *Gynecologic Obstetric Investigation*, **9**, 281–291.

Oklahoma State Department of Health. (1998). *Spinal Cord Injuries in Oklahoma, 1988–1997*. Oklahoma City, OK: Author.

Paralyzed Veterans of America. (1997). *A Guide to Wheelchair Sports and Recreation* (3rd ed.). Washington, DC: Author.

Pearson, E., Nance, P.W., Leslie, W.D., Ludwig, S. (1997). Cyclical etidronate: its effect on bone density in patients with acute spinal cord injury. *Arch Phys Med Rehab* **78**, 269–272.

Pentland, W.E., McColl, M.A., Rosenthal, C. (1995). The effects of aging and duration of disability on long term health outcomes following spinal cord injury. *Paraplegia*, **33**, 367–373.

Pope, K.S., Vasquez, M.J. (1991). *Ethics in Psychotherapy and Counseling: A Practical Guide for Psychologists*. San Francisco: Jossey-Bass.

Price, M. (1973). Causes of death in 11 of 227 patients with traumatic spinal cord injury over a period of nine years. *Paraplegia*, **11**, 217–220.

Priebe, M.M., Sherwood, A.M., Thornby, J.I., Kharas, N.F., Markowski, J. (1996). Clinical assessment of spasticity in spinal cord injury: a multidimensional problem. *Arch Phys Med Rehab* **77**, 713–716.

Pryor, J.L., LeRoy, S.C., Nagel, T.C., Hensleigh, H.C. (1995). Vibratory stimulation for treatment of an ejaculation in quadriplegic men. *Arch Phys Med Rehab* **76**, 59–64.

Quigley, M.C. (1995). Impact of spinal cord injury on the life roles of women. *Am J Occupat Therapy* **49**, 780–786.

Quill, T.E., & Brody, H. (1996). Physician recommendations and patient autonomy: Finding a balance between physician power and patient choice. *Annals of Internal Medicine*, **125**, 763–769.

Ragnarsson, K.T. (1993). The cardiovascular system. In G.G. Whiteneck et al. (eds.), *Aging with Spinal Cord Injury* (pp. 73–92). New York: Demos Publications.

Ragnarsson, K.T., Sell, G.H. (1981). Lower extremity fractures after spinal cord injury: a retrospective study. *Arch Phys Med Rehab* **62**, 418–423.

Ragnarsson, K.T., Hall, K.M., Wilmot, C.B., Carter, R.E. (1995). Management of pulmonary, cardiovascular, and metabolic conditions after spinal cord injury. In S.L. Stover et al. (eds.), *Spinal Cord Injury: Clinical Outcomes from the Model Systems* (pp. 79–99). Gaithersburg, MD: Aspen Publishers, Inc.

Ravesloot, C., Seekins, T., Walsh, J. (1997). A structural analysis of secondary conditions experienced by people with physical disabilities. *Rehab Psychol* **42**, 3–16.

Ravichandron, G., Silver, J.R. (1982). Survival following traumatic tetraplegia. *Paraplegia*, **20**, 264–269.

Ray, C., West, J. (1984). Social, sexual and personal implications of paraplegia. *Paraplegia*, **22**, 75–86.

Reame, N.E. (1992). A prospective study of the menstrual cycle and spinal cord injury. *Am J Phys Med Rehabilitation* **71**, 15–21.

Research and Training Center on Independent Living. (1993a). *Chronic Pain Management*. Lawrence, KS: University of Kansas.

Research and Training Center on Independent Living. (1993b). *Pressure Sores*. Lawrence, KS: University of Kansas.

Research and Training Center on Independent Living, (1994). *SCI & Aging*. Lawrence, KS: University of Kansas.

Research and Training Center on Independent Living, (1996). *Joint Problems*. Lawrence, KS: University of Kansas.

Reynolds, G.G. (1993). Becoming successful health care consumers. In G.G. Whiteneck et al. (eds.), *Aging with Spinal Cord Injury* (pp. 229–238). New York: Demos Publications.

Richards, J.S., Brown, L., Hagglund, K., Bua, G., Reeder, K. (1988). Spinal cord injury and concomitant traumatic brain injury: results of a longitudinal investigation. *Am J Phys Med Rehabilitation* **67**, 211–216.

Richards, J.S., Osuna, F.J., Jaworski, T., Novack, T.A., Leli, D., Boll, T.J. (1991). The effectiveness of different methods of defining traumatic brain injury in predicting post-discharge adjustment in a spinal cord injury population. *Arch Phys Med Rehab* **72**, 275–279.

Rintala, D.H. (1997, April). Identifying and utilizing community resources to maintain SCI survivors' long-term health, *Issues of post-acute spinal cord injury survivors*. Preconference workshop conducted at NARPPS annual conference, New Orleans, LA.

Rintala, D.H., Loubser, P.G., Castro, J., Hart, K.A., Fuhrer, M.J. (1998). Chronic pain in a community-based sample of men with spinal cord injury: prevalence, severity, and relationship with impairment, disability, handicap, and subjective well-being. *Arch Phys Med Rehab* **79**, 604–614.

Rohe, D.E., Athelston, G.T. (1982). Vocational interests of persons with spinal cord injury. Journal of Counseling Psychology, **29**, 283–291.

Rohe, D.E., Athelstan, G.T. (1985). Change in vocational interests after spinal cord injury. *Rehab Psychol* **30**, 131–143.

Rohe, D., Krause, J.S. (1998). Stability of interests after severe physical disability: an 11-year longitudinal study. *Journal of Vocational Behavior*, **52**, 45–58.

Rose, M., Robinson, J.E., Ells, P., Cole, J.D. (1988). Pain following spinal cord injury: results from a postal survey. *Pain*, **34**, 101–102.

Rossier, A.B., Fam, B.A. (1984). Indication and results of semirigid penile prostheses in spinal cord injury patients: long-term followup. *J Urol* **131**, 59–62.

Rossier, A.B., Foo, D., Shillito, J., Dyro, F.M. (1985). Post-traumatic syringomyelia: incidence, clinical presentation, electrophysiological studies, syrinx protein and results of conservative and operative treatment. *Brain*, **108**, 439–461.

Roth, E.J. (1994). Pain in spinal cord injury. In G.M. Yarkony (ed.), *Spinal Cord Injury: Medical Management and Rehabilitation* (pp. 141–158). Gaithersburg, MD: Aspen Publishers, Inc.

Roth, E.J., Lovell, L., Heinemann, A.W., Lee, M.Y., Yarkony, G.M. (1992). The older adult with a spinal cord injury. *Paraplegia*, **30**, 520–526.

Rubin, S.E., Wilson, C.A., Fischer, J., Vaughn, B. (1992). *Ethical Practices in Rehabilitation*. Carbondale, IL: Southern Illinois University-Carbondale.

Rutkowski, S.B., Middleton, J.W., Truman, G., Hagen, D.L., Ryan, J.P. (1995). The influence of bladder management on fertility in spinal cord injured males. *Paraplegia*, **33**, 824–826.

Salzberg, C.A., Byrne, D.W., Cayten, C.G., Niewerburgh, P.V., Murphy, J.G., Viehbeck, M.A. (1996). New pressure ulcer risk assessment scale for individuals with spinal cord injury. *Am J Phys Med Rehabilitation* **75**, 96–104.

Samsa, G., Patrick, C.H., Fuessner, J.R. (1993). Long-term survival of veterans with traumatic spinal cord injury. *Arch Neurology* **50**, 909–914.

Sauer, P.M., Harvey, C.J. (1993). Spinal cord injury and pregnancy. *Journal of Perinatal and Neonatal Nursing*, **7**, 22–34.

Schmitt, J., Midha, M., Mckenzie, N. (1995). *Diagnosis and Management of Disorders of the Spinal Cord*. Philadelphia: W.B. Saunders Company.

Seftel, A., Bodner, D., Krueger, B. (1998). Muse for erectile dysfunction in spinal cord injured patients. *J Spinal Cord Med* **21**, 381.

Selzman, A.A., Hampel, N. (1993). Urologic complications of spinal cord injury. *Urol Clin N Am* **20**, 453–464.

Shamberg, S., Stiens, S.A., Shamberg, A. (1997). Personal enablement through environmental modifications. In B.A. O'Young, M.A. Young, S.A. Stiens (eds.), *Physical Medicine and Rehabilitation Secrets* (pp. 86–93). Philadelphia: Hanley and Belfus.

Sherman, A.L., Cardena, D.D., Shredberg, S. (1997). Management of traumatic optic neuropathy with coexistent spinal cord injury: a case report. *Arch Phys Med Rehab* **78**, 1012–1014.

Sie, I.H., Waters, R.L., Adkins, R.H., Gellman, H. (1992). Upper extremity pain in the postrehabilitation spinal cord injured patient. *Arch Phys Med Rehab* **73**, 44–48.

Sims, B., Manley, S., Richardson, G. (1993). A model of lifetime services. In G.G. Whiteneck et al. (eds.), *Aging with Spinal Cord Injury* (pp. 353–360). New York: Demos Publications.

Sipski, M.L. (1991). The impact of spinal cord injury on female sexuality, menstruation, and pregnancy: a review of the literature. *J Am Paraplegia Soc* **14**, 122–126.

Sipski, M.L. (1997). Spinal cord injury and sexual function: an educational model. In M.L. Sipski, C.J. Alexander (eds.), *Sexual Function in People with Disability and Chronic illness: A Health Professionals Guide* (pp. 149–176). Gaithersburg, MD: Aspen Publishers, Inc.

Sipski, M.L., Alexander, C.J. (1992). Sexual function and dysfunction after spinal cord injury. *Phys Med Rehab Clin N Am* **3**, 811–828.

Sipski, M.L., Alexander, C.J., Rosen, R.C. (1995). Orgasm in women with spinal cord injuries: a laboratory-based assessment. *Arch Phys Med Rehab* **76**, 1097–1102.

Soderstrom, G., Ducker, T. (1985). Increased susceptibility of patients with cervical cord lesions to peptic gastrointestinal complications. *J Trauma Injury Infect Crit Care* **25**, 1030–1038.

Sonksen, J., Sommer, P., Biering-Sorensen, F., Ziebe, S., Lindhard, A., Loft, A., Andersen, A.N., Kristensen, J.K. (1997). Pregnancy after assisted ejaculation procedures in men with spinal cord injury. *Arch Phys Med Rehab* **78**, 1059–1061.

Spica, M.M. (1989). Sexual counseling standards for the spinal cord injured. *Journal of Neuroscience Nursing*, **21**, 56–60.

Spira, A. (1986). Epidemiology of human reproduction: mini review. *Human Reproduction*, **1**, 111–115.

Staas, W.E., Formal, C.S., Gershkoff, A.M., Hirschwald, J.F., Schmidt, M., Schultz, A.R., Smith, J. (1993). Rehabilitation of the spinal cord injured patient. In J.A. DeLisa et al. (eds.), *Rehabilitation Medicine: Principles and Practice* (2nd ed., pp. 886–915). Philadelphia: J.B. Lippincott Company.

Stampfer, M.J., Sacks, F.M., Salvini, S., Willett, W.C., Hennekens, C.H. (1991). A prospective study of cholesterol, apolipoproteins, and the risk of myocardial infarction. *N Eng J Med* **325**, 373–381.

Stewart, M., Brown, J.B., Weston, W.W., McWhinney, I.R., McWilliam, C.L., & Freeman, T.R. (1995). *Patient-centered medicine: Transforming the clinical method*. Thousand Oaks, CA: SAGE Publications.

Stiens, S.A. (1995). Reductions in bowel program intervals with polyethylene glycol based suppositories. *Arch Phys Med Rehab* **76**, 674–677.

Stiens, S.A. (1998a). Cardiovascular system. In M.C. Hammond (ed.), *Medical Care of Persons with Spinal Cord Injury* (pp. 43–50). Washington, DC: Department of Veterans Affairs.

Stiens, S.A. (1998b). Gastrointestinal system. In M.C. Hammond (ed.), *Medical Care of Persons with Spinal Cord Injury* (pp. 51–60). Washington, DC: Department of Veterans Affairs.

Stiens, S.A. (1998c). Personhood, disablement, and mobility technology. In D.B. Gray, L.A. Quatrano, M.L. Lieberman (eds.), *Designing and Using Assistive Technology: The Human Perspective* (pp. 29–49). Baltimore: Paul H. Brookes Publishing Co.

Stiens, S.A., Bierner-Bergman, S., Formal, C.S. (1997). Spinal cord injury rehabilitation: 4. Individual experience, personal adaptation, and social perspectives. *Arch Phys Med Rehab* **78**, 579–583.

Stiens, S.A., & Berkin, D. (1997). A clinical rehabilitation course for college undergraduates provides an introduction to biopsychosocial interventions that minimize disablement. *American Journal of Physical Medicine and Rehabilitation*, **76**, 462–470.

Stiens, S., Bierner-Bergman, S., Goetz, L. (1997). Neurogenic bowel dysfunction after spinal cord injury: clinical evaluation and rehabilitative management. *Arch Phys Med Rehab* **78**, S86–102.

Stiens, S.A., Haselkorn, J.K., Peters, J., Goldstein, B. (1996). Rehabilitation intervention for patients with upper extremity dysfunction: challenges of outcome evaluation. *American Journal of Industrial Medicine*, **29**, 590–601.

Stiens, S.A., Johnson, M.C. III, Lyman, P.J. (1995). Cardiac rehabilitation in patients with spinal cord injuries. *Phys Med Rehab Clin N Am* **6**, 263–296.

Stiens, S.A., Westheimer, R.K., Young, M.A. (1997). Satisfying sexuality despite disability. In B.A. O'Young, M.A. Young, S.A. Stiens (eds.), *Physical Medicine and Rehabilitation Secrets* (pp. 62–67). Philadelphia: Hanley and Belfus.

Stinneford, J.G., Keshavarzian, A., Nemchasky, A., Doria, M., Durkin, M. (1993). Esophagitis and esophageal motor abnormalities in patients with chronic spinal cord injury. *Paraplegia*, **31**, 384–392.

Stone, J. Nino-Murcia, M., Wolfe, V., Perkash, I. (1990). Chronic gastrointestinal problems in spinal cord injury patients: a prospective analysis. *Am J Gastroenterology* **9**, 1114–1119.

Stotts, K.M. (1986). Health maintenance: paraplegic athletes and nonathletes. *Arch Phys Med Rehab* **67**, 109–114.

Stover, S.L., DeLisa, J.A., Whiteneck, G.G. (1995). *Spinal Cord Injury: Clinical Outcomes from the Model Systems*. Gaithersburg, MD: Aspen Publishers, Inc.

Stover, S.L., DeVivo, M.J., Go, B.K. (1999). History, implementation, and current status of the national spinal cord injury database. *Arch Phys Med Rehab* **80**, 1365–1371.

Stover, S.L., Fine, P.R. (eds.). (1986). *Spinal Cord Injury: The Facts and Figures*. Birmingham, AL: University of Alabama at Birmingham.

Stover, S.L., Hale, A.M., Buell, A.B. (1994). Skin complications other than pressure ulcers following spinal cord injury. *Arch Phys Med Rehab* **75**, 987–993.

Stover, S.L., Hall, K.M., DeLisa, J.A., Donovan, W.H. (1995). Systems benefits. In S.L. Stover et al. (eds.), *Spinal Cord Injury: Clinical Outcomes from the Model Systems* (pp. 317–326). Gaithersburg, MD: Aspen Publishers, Inc.

Stover, S.L., Niemann, K.M., Tulloss, J.R. (1991). Experience with surgical resection of heterotopic bone in spinal cord injury patients. *Clin Ortho Rel Res* **263**, 71–77.

Szasz, G. (1992). Sexual health care. In C.P. Zejdlik (ed.), *Management of Spinal Cord Injury* (2nd ed., pp. 175–201). Boston: Jones and Bartlett Publishers.

Szollar, S. (1997). Osteoporosis in men with spinal cord injuries. *West J Med* **166**, 270–271.

Szollar, S.M., Martin, E.M.E., Parthemore, J.G., Sartoris, D.J., Deftos, L.J. (1997). Demineralization in tetraplegic and paraplegic men over time. *Spinal Cord*, **35**, 223–228.

Szollar, S.M., Martin, E.M.E., Sartoris, D.J., Parthemore, J.G., Deftos, L.J. (1998). Bone mineral density and indexes of bone metabolism in spinal cord injury. *Am J Phys Med Rehabilitation* **77**, 28–35.

Tarvydas, V.M. (1987). Decision-making models in ethics: models for increased clarity and wisdom. *Journal of Applied Rehabilitation Counseling*, **18**, 50–52.

Tate, D.G., Riley, B.B., Perna, R., Roller, S. (1997). Quality life issues among women with physical disabilities or breast cancer. *Arch Phys Med Rehab* **78**, S18–25.

Taylor, G. (1967) *Predicted versus Actual Response to Spinal Cord Injury: A Psychological Study*. Doctoral dissertation, University of Minneapolis: Minneapolis, MN.

Taylor, L.P., McGruder, J.E. (1996). The meaning of sea kayaking for persons with spinal cord injuries. *Am J Occupat Therapy* **50**, 39–46.

Tepper, M.S. (1992). Sexual education in spinal cord injury rehabilitation: Current trends and recommendations. *Sexuality and Disability*, **10**, 15–31.

Thomas, J.P. (1995). The model spinal cord injury concept: development and implementation. In S.L. Stover et al. (eds.), *Spinal Cord Injury: Clinical Outcomes from the Model Systems* (pp. 1–9). Gaithersburg, MD: Aspen Publishers, Inc.

Thompson, L. (1998, September). *Functional Changes with Spinal Cord Injury*. Paper presented at the Forty-Fourth Annual Conference of the American Paraplegia Society, Las Vegas, NV.

Thurman, D.J., Sniezek, J.E., Johnson, D., Greenspan, A., Smith, S.M. (1995). *Guidelines for Surveillance of Central Nervous System Injury*. Atlanta, GA: Centers for Disease Control and Prevention.

Trieschmann, R.B. (1988). *Spinal Cord Injuries: Psychological, Social and Vocational Rehabilitation* (2nd ed.). New York: Demos Publications.

Triolo, R.J., Bieri, C., Uhlir, J., Kobetic, R., Scheiner, A., Marsolais, E.B. (1996). Implanted functional neuromuscular stimulation systems for individuals with cervical cord injuries: clinical case reports. *Arch Phys Med Rehab* **77**, 1119–1128.

Umbach, I., Heilporn, A. (1991). Review article: post-spinal cord injury syringomyelia. *Paraplegia*, **29**, 219–221.

Uniform Data System for Medical Rehabilitation (1998). *WeeFIM System*^SM *Clinical Guide: Version 5*. Buffalo, NY: State University of New York at Buffalo.

Uniform Data System for Medical Rehabilitation (1997). *Guide for the Uniform Data Set for Medical Rehabilitation (including the FIM*™ *instrument), Version 5.1*. Buffalo, NY: State University of New York at Buffalo.

U.S. Bureau of the Census. (1992). *Statistical Abstract of the United States (112th ed.)*. Washington, DC: U.S. Department of Commerce.

U.S. Department of Justice. (1996). *A Guide to Disability Rights Laws*. Author.

U.S. Preventive Health Services Task Force. (1989). *Guide to Clinical Preventive Services: An assessment of the effectiveness of 169 interventions*. Baltimore: Author.

Utah Department of Health. (1993). *Utah Spinal Cord Injury Surveillance Summary, 1989–1991*, Salt Lake City, UT: Author.

VanderSluis, C.K., TenDuis, H.J., Geertzen, J.H.B. (1995). Multiple injuries: an overview of the outcome. *J Trauma Injury Infect Crit Care* **38**, 681–686.

Verduyn, W.H. (1986). Spinal cord injured women, pregnancy and delivery. *Paraplegia*, **24**, 231–240.

Vernon, J.D., Silver, J.R., Ohry, A. (1982). Post-traumatic syringomyelia. *Paraplegia*, **20**, 339–364.

Waites, K.B., Canupp, K.C., DeVivo, M.J. (1993). Epidemiology and risk factors for urinary tract infection following spinal cord injury. *Arch Phys Med Rehab* **74**, 691–695.

Walker, B.C., Holstein, S.S. (1994). Vocational rehabilitation and spinal cord injury. In G.M. Yarkony (ed.), *Spinal Cord Injury: Medical Management and Rehabilitation* (pp. 217–222). Gaithersburg, MD: Aspen Publishers, Inc.

Wanner, M.B., Rageth, C.J., Zach, G.A. (1987). Pregnancy and autonomic hyperreflexia in patients with spinal cord lesions. *Paraplegia*, **25**, 482–490.

Warnemuende, R. (1986). Misconceptions and attitudes about disability and the need for awareness. *Journal of Applied Rehabilitation Counseling*, **17**, 50–51.

Waters, R.L., Adkins, R.H. (1997). Firearm versus motor vehicle related spinal cord injury: preinjury factors, injury characteristics, and initial outcome comparisons among ethically diverse groups. *Arch Phys Med Rehab* **78**, 150–155.

Waters, R.L., Adkins, R.H., Yakura, J.S. (1991). Definition of complete spinal cord injury. *Paraplegia*, **29**, 573–581.

Waters, R., Adkins, R., Yakura, J., Sie, I. (1993). Motor and sensory recovery following complete tetraplegia. *Arch Phys Med Rehab* **74**, 242–247.

Waters, R., Adkins, R., Yakura, J., Sie, I. (1994a). Motor and sensory recovery following incomplete paraplegia. *Arch Phys Med Rehab* **75**, 67–72.

Waters, R., Adkins, R., Yakura, J., Sie, I. (1994b). Motor and sensory recovery following incomplete tetraplegia. *Arch Phys Med Rehab* **75**, 306–311.

Waters, R.L., Sie, I.H., Adkins, R.H. (1993). The musculoskeletal system. In G.G. Whiteneck et al. (eds.), *Aging with Spinal Cord Injury* (pp. 53–71). New York: Demos Publications.

Waters, R., Yakura, J., Adkins, R., Sie, I. (1992). Recovery following complete paraplegia. *Arch Phys Med Rehab* **73**, 784–789.

Watson, N. (1981). Late ileus in paraplegia. *Paraplegia*, **19**, 13–16.

Weed, R.O. (1999). Life care planning: past, present, and future. In R.O. Weed (ed.), *Life Care Planning and Case Management Handbook* (pp. 1–11). Boca Raton, FL: CRC Press.

Weingarden, S. (1992). The gastrointestinal system and spinal cord injury. *Phys Med Rehab Clin N Am* **3**, 765–781.

Weitzenkamp, D.A., Gerhart, K.A., Charlifue, S.W. (1997). Fatigue: precursors and impact among long-term spinal cord injury survivors [Abstract]. *Arch Phys Med Rehab* **78**, 896.

Weitzenkamp, D.A., Gerhart, K.A., Charlifue, S.W., Whiteneck, G.G., Savic, G. (1997). Spouses of spinal cord injury survivors: the added impact of caregiving. *Arch Phys Med Rehab* **78**, 822–827.

Welner, S. (1993). Treatment of sexually transmitted diseases in the physically disabled woman. In F.B. Haseltine, S.S. Cole, D.B. Gray (eds.), *Reproductive Issues for Persons with Physical Disabilities* (pp. 275–290). Baltimore: Paul H. Brookes Publishing Co.

Welner, S. (1996). Contraception, sexually transmitted diseases, and menopause. In D.M. Krotoski, M.A. Nosek, M.A. Turk (eds.), *Women with Physical Disabilities: Achieving and Maintaining Health and Well-being* (pp. 81–90). Baltimore: Paul H. Brookes Publishing Co.

Westgren, N., Hultling, C., Levi, R., Seiger, A., Westgren, N. (1997). Sexuality in women with traumatic spinal cord injury. *Acta Obstetr Gynecol Scand*, **76**, 977–983.

Whipple, B., Richards, E., Tepper, M., Komisarak, B. (1996). Sexual response in women with complete spinal cord injury. In D.M. Krotoski, M.A. Nosek, M.A. Turk (eds.), *Women with Physical Disabilities: Achieving and Maintaining Health and Well-being* (pp. 69–80). Baltimore: Paul H. Brooks Publishing Co.

White, M.J., Rintala, D.H., Hart, K.A., Fuhrer, M.J. (1993). Sexual activities, concerns, and interests of women with spinal cord injury living in the community. *Am J Phys Med Rehabilitation* **72**, 372–378.

Whiteneck, G.G. (1993). Learning from recent empirical investigations. In G.G. Whiteneck et al. (eds.), *Aging with Spinal Cord Injury* (pp. 23–37). New York Demos Publications.

Whiteneck, G.G., Charlifue, S.W., Frankel, H.L., Fraser, M.H., Gardner, B.P., Gerhart, K.A., Krishnan, K.R., Menter, R.R., Nusebieh, I., Short, D.J., Silver, J.R. (1992). Mortality, morbidity, and psychosocial outcomes of persons spinal cord injured more than 20 years ago. *Paraplegia*, **30**, 617–630.

Whiteneck, G.G., Charlifue, S.W., Gerhart, K.A., Lammertse, D.P., Manley, S., Menter, R.R., Seedroft, K.R. (1993). *Aging with Spinal Cord Injury*. New York: Demos Publications.

Whiteneck, G.G., Menter, R.R. (1993). Where do we go from here? In G.G. Whiteneck et al. (eds.), *Aging with Spinal Cord Injury* (pp. 361–369). New York: Demos Publications.

Whiteneck, G., Tate, D., Charlifue, S. (1999). Predicting community reintegration after spinal cord injury from demographic and injury characteristics. *Arch Phys Med Rehab* **80**, 1485–1491.

Widerstrom-Noga, F.G., Felipe-Cuervo, E., Broton, J.G., Duncan, R.C., Yezierski, R.P. (1999). Perceived difficulty in dealing with consequences of spinal cord injury. *Arch Phys Med Rehab* **80**, 580–586.

Wilkerson, D.L., Johnston, M.V. (1997). Clinical program monitoring systems: current and future directions. In M.J. Fuhrer (ed.), *Assessing Medical Rehabilitation Practices: The Promise of Outcomes Research* (pp. 275–305). Baltimore: Paul H. Brookes Publishing Co.

Wilmot, C.B., Cope, D.N., Hall, K.M., Acker, M. (1985). Occult head injury: its incidence in spinal cord injury. *Arch Phys Med Rehab* **66**, 227–231.

Wilmot, C.B., Hall, K.M. (1993). The respiratory system. In G.G. Whiteneck, et al. (eds.), *Aging with Spinal Cord Injury* (pp. 93–104). New York: Demos Publications.

Winkler, T. (1990, May). *Squamous Cell Carcinoma in a Decubitus Ulcer—A Fatal Sequela.* Poster session presented at the annual meeting of the American Spinal Injury Association, Orlando, FL.

Winkler, T. (1999). Spinal cord injury and life care planning. In P.M. Deutsch, H.W. Sawyer (eds.), *A Guide to Rehabilitation* (pp. 16-1-16-127). Purchase, NY: AHAB Press, Inc.

Winkler, T., Weed, R.O. (1999). Life care planning for spinal cord injury. In R.O. Weed (ed.), *Life Care Planning and Case Management Handbook* (pp. 297–324). Boca Raton, FL: CRC Press.

Witkowski, J.A., Parish, L.C. (1992). Debridement of cutaneous ulcers: medical and surgical aspects. *Clinics in Dermatology*, **9**, 585–591.

Wong, H.D., Millard, R.P. (1992). Ethical dilemmas encountered by independent living service providers. *J Rehab* **58**, 10–15.

Woolsey, R.M. (1986). Chronic pain following spinal cord injury. *J Am Paraplegia Soc* **9**, 39–41.

World Health Organization. (1999). *International classification of functioning and disability. Beta-2 draft, full version.* Geneva, Switzerland: Author.

Wylie, E.F., Chakera, T.M.H. (1988). Degenerative joint abnormalities in patients with paraplegia of duration greater than 20 years. *Paraplegia*, **26**, 101–106.

Yarkony, G.M. (1993). Aging skin, pressure ulcerations, and spinal cord injury. In G.G. Whiteneck et al. (eds.), *Aging with Spinal Cord Injury* (pp. 39–52). New York: Demos Publications.

Yarkony, G.M. (ed.). (1994a). *Spinal Cord Injury: Medical Management and Rehabilitation.* Gaithersburg, MD: Aspen Publishers, Inc.

Yarkony, G.M. (1994b). Medical and physical complications of spinal cord injury. In G.M. Yarkony (ed.), *Spinal Cord Injury: Medical Management and Rehabilitation* (pp. 17–25). Gaithersburg, MD: Aspen Publishers, Inc.

Yarkony, G.M. (1994c). Pressure ulcers: medical management. In G.M. Yarkony (ed.), *Spinal Cord Injury: Medical Management and Rehabilitation* (pp. 77–83). Gaithersburg, MD: Aspen Publishers, Inc.

Yarkony, G.M., Formal, C.S., Crawley, M.F. (1997). Body composition of spinal cord injured adults. *Sports Medicine*, **23**, 48–60.

Yarkony, G.M., Heinemann, A.W. (1995). Pressure ulcers. In S.L. Stover et al. (eds.), *Spinal Cord Injury: Clinical Outcomes from the Model Systems* (pp. 100–119). Gaithersburg, MD: Aspen Publishers, Inc.

Yarkony, G.M., Roth, E.L., Heinemann, A.W., Lovell, L.L. (1988). Spinal cord injury rehabilitation outcome: the impact of age. *Journal of Clinical Epidemiology*, **41**, 173–177.

Yarkony, G.M., Roth, E.J., Heinemann, A.W., Wu, Y.C., Katz, R.T., Lovell, L. (1987). Benefits of rehabilitation for traumatic spinal cord injury: multivariate analysis of 711 patients. *Arch Neurology* **44**, 93–96.

Yasukawa, L., Stevens, S., Ueberfluss, J. (1994). Wheelchairs. In G.M. Yarkony (ed.), *Spinal Cord Injury: Medical Management and Rehabilitation* (pp. 169–174). Gaithersburg, MD: Aspen Publishers, Inc.

Yekutiel, M., Brooks, M.E., Ohry, A., Yarom, J., Carel, R.S. (1989). The prevalence of hypertension, ischemic heart disease and diabetes in traumatic spinal cord injured patients and amputees. *Paraplegia*, **27**, 58–62.

Young, J.S., Burns, P.E., Bowen, A.M., McCutchen, R. (1982). *Spinal Cord Injury Statistics: Experience of the Regional Spinal Cord Injury Systems*. Phoenix, AZ: Good Samaritan Medical Center.

Young, M.E., Rintala, D.H., Rossi, C.D., Hart, K.A., Fuhrer, M.J. (1995). Alcohol and marijuana use in a community-based sample of persons with spinal cord injury. *Arch Phys Med Rehab* **76**, 525–532.

Young, R.R. (Fall, 1996). What to do about spasticity. *Spinal Cord Injury Life*, 10–11, 21–22.

Zasler, N.D. (1991). Sexuality in neurologic disability: an overview. *Sexuality and Disability*, **9**, 11–27.

Zejdlik, C.P. (1992). Reestablishing bowel control. In C.P. Zejdlik (ed.), *Management of Spinal Cord Injury* (2nd ed., pp. 397–416). Boston: Jones and Bartlett.

Glossary

A

abduction	Movement of an arm or leg away from the body.
acute SCI	The early stages of a SCI; first three months to a year.
acute care	The phase of managing health problems that is conducted in a hospital for individuals needing medical attention. In SCI medicine, this is the period of medical stabilization and initial rehabilitation.
activities of daily living (ADLs)	Routine activities carried out for personal hygiene and health (including bathing, dressing, feeding) and for operating a household.
adaptive behavior	The ability to function as independently as possible and the ability to meet culturally imposed demands of personal and social responsibility.
adaptive equipment	Any equipment that enables a person with a disability to function more independently.
adduction	Movement of an arm or leg toward the body.
afferent	Nerves that carry sensory impulses to the central nervous system.
akinesia	General weakness and poverty of movement.
ambulation	"Walking" with braces and/or crutches. Also movement from place to place with any device, manual or power wheelchair.
amenorrhea	Absence of menstruation.
anal sphincter	Either of two muscles controlling the closing of the anus.
ankle-foot-orthosis (AFO)	A brace applied to the ankle and calf area to compensate for joint instability.
ankylosis	Bone-to-bone fixation of a joint leading to immobility because of ossification, or bony deposits of calcium, at joints.
ANS	Autonomic nervous system
anterograde amnesia	Difficulty retaining new information after traumatic brain injury (TBI); difficulty with new learning.
aptitudes	Specific abilities required of an individual to perform a given work or avocational activity.
areflexic	Without reflexes.
arrhythmia	Any deviation from the normal pattern of the heartbeat.
ascending pathways	Nerve pathways that go upward from the spinal cord toward the brain and carry sensory information from the body.
ASIA	American Spinal Injury Association
ASIA impairment scale	The current scale recommended by ASIA to classify people with SCI into functional categories based on the amount of sensory and motor sparing.
ASIA A	Complete: No motor or sensory function is preserved in the sacral segments S4–S5.
ASIA B	Incomplete: Sensory but not motor function is preserved below the neurologic level, including the sacral segments S4–S5.
ASIA C	Incomplete: Motor function is preserved below the neurologic level, and more than half of key muscles below the neurologic level have a muscle grade less than 3.

ASIA D	Incomplete: Motor function is preserved below the neurologic level, and at least half of key muscles below the neurologic level have a muscle grade of 3 or more.
ASIA E	Normal: History of SCI with full clinical recovery, motor and sensory examination is within normal limits.
aspiration	Entry of fluid or food into the lungs through the windpipe. Can cause a lung infection or pneumonia.
assisted	Physical aid required for completion of an activity.
assistive devices	Equipment, ranging from the very simple devices to complex electronics, that aids in the control of fine and gross motor functioning, ambulation, and balance. Includes items such as wheelchairs, braces, splints, and aids that monitor and control bodily functions.
assistive technology	A broad term that refers to the application of technology to assist individuals with SCI and other disabilities achieve independence by providing access to computers, communication devices, and environmental controls.
atelectasis	Loss of breathing function characterized by collapsed lung tissue.
atony	Lacking normal muscle tone.
atrophy	A wasting away or decrease in size of a cell, tissue, organ, or part of the body caused by lack of nourishment, inactivity, or loss of nerve supply. Atrophy is most common after lower motor neuron injuries.
augmentive and alternative communication	Forms of communication that supplement or enhance speech or writing, including electronic devices, picture boards, and sign language.
Autonomic nervous system (ANS)	The part of the nervous system that controls involuntary activities, including heart muscle, glands, smooth muscle tissue.
auxiliary aids	Devices or services that compensate for a disabling condition.
axon	Part of neuron that conducts impulses away from the cell body.

B

Babinski sign	Reflex indicative of neurological pathology. Elicited by firmly pressing a blunt instrument, such as a key, on the lateral side of the sole of the foot and running it up towards the toes. In a normal person the toes curl downward. In an upper motor neuron lesion the toes move upward and spread apart.
bactiuria	Presence of bacteria in the urine.
balanced-forearm-orthosis	A wheelchair device that, by supporting the forearm, eliminates the force of gravity, thus enabling the person with limited arm function to perform such tasks as feeding and keyboarding.
barrier-free environment	Containing no obstacles to accessibility and usability by people with disabilities.
bedsore	See *decubitus ulcer*.
BFO	Balanced forearm orthosis
bilateral sensory stimulation	Stimulation of both sides of the body simultaneously, using touch, hearing, or vision, to determine whether an individual perceives the stimulus on one side or the other.
bladder management	A comprehensive plan for maintaining continence, preventing infection, and retaining renal function.

bladder training	Methods for training a neurogenic bladder to empty (micturition) without the use of an indwelling catheter. For example, drinking measured amounts of fluid and timing the intervals for accomplishing urination.
bowel program	A comprehensive treatment plan designed to minimize or eliminate the occurrence of unplanned or difficult evacuations, to evacuate stool at a regular, predictable time within 60 minutes of bowel care, and to minimize gastrointestinal complications experienced by persons with a neurogenic bowel.
brace	An appliance utilized to support a part of the body to facilitate or improve function.
bradycardia	Slow heart rate, usually fewer than 60 beats per minute.
brain injury	A more specific term than head injury. Damage to the brain that results in impairments in one or more functions, including: arousal, attention, language, memory, reasoning, abstract thinking, judgment, problem-solving, sensory abilities, perceptual abilities, motor abilities, psychosocial behavior, information processing, and speech.

C

calculi, renal	Stones that may form in either kidney or bladder.
cardiovascular system	The heart and the various conducting vessels (arteries, veins, and capillaries) which supply the body.
case management	A collaborative process that assesses, plans, implements, coordinates, monitors, and evaluates options and services to meet an individual's health needs through coordination of available resources to promote quality, cost-effective outcomes.
catheter	A flexible tube for withdrawing fluids from, or introducing fluids into, a cavity of the body, most often the bladder.
cauda equina	The collection of spinal roots descending from the lower part of the spinal cord at vertebral level S1 and occupying the sacral vertebral canal below the spinal cord.
CCM	Certified Case Manager
CDMS	Certified Disability Management Specialist
central nervous system (CNS)	The brain, spinal cord, and their nerve endings.
cervical	Pertaining to the neck, especially the vertebrae in the neck or that segment of the spinal cord.
chemoprophylaxis	The prevention of disease by the use of chemicals or drugs.
cholelithiasis	The presence of gallstones in the gallbladder.
CLCP	Certified Life Care Planner
clearinghouse	An operation that disseminates a wide range of information sources.
clinical trials	Systematic studies in human subjects aimed at determining the safety and effectiveness of new or unproven therapies.
cognitive impairment	Difficulty with one or more of the basic functions of the brain: perception, memory, attentional abilities, and reasoning skills.
cohort	A group of persons who have characteristics in common and who are studied over a long period of time. A cohort study is a longitudinal study.
cohort, historical	A group of study participants characterized by archival data (medical records, family histories, and so on), as opposed to data collected prospectively.

colitis	Inflammation of the colon.
coma	A state of unconsciousness from which the person cannot be aroused, even by powerful stimulation.
community living skills	Includes money handling, wheelchair mobility, shopping, recreational, vocational and educational activities, and transportation.
complete recovery	A complete return of all motor and sensory function, but may still have abnormal reflexes.
complication	An added difficulty or problem not directly or inevitably related to a disease or injury, which exacerbates the outcome of the original primary diagnosis.
condom catheter	A synthetic sheath with an attached tube, which is worn over the penis for the purpose of urinary collection.
consumer	One who uses a commodity or service; persons who are clients of rehabilitation service agencies, or a relative or spouse who represents the interests of that individual.
contralateral	Opposite side.
conus medularis	Lower end of spinal cord.
CPT	Current procedural terminology
CRC	Certified Rehabilitation Counselor
Crede maneuver	Mechanical suprapubic abdominal pressure used to expel urine from the bladder.
cross-sectional study	A survey or screening test administered at a strategic or single point in time.
CT scan	Computerized Tomography
cumulative survival rate	Proportion of persons surviving longer than a survival rate given time period.
current procedural terminology	A system developed by the American Medical Association for standardizing the terminology and coding used to describe medical services and procedures.
curvilinear trend	A trend in which a graphic representation of the data yields a curved line.
CVE	Certified Vocational Evaluation Specialist
cystitis	Inflammation of a bladder, especially the urinary bladder.
cystogram	A radiographic test of the bladder after the administration of dye.
cystoscopy	Test performed by the urologist to examine the inside of the bladder and ureter, which is done with a lighted instrument called a *cystoscope*.
cystourethrogram	A radiographic test of the bladder and urethra, using an injection of dye.
cytology	The study of cells.

D

day care	A service provided during ordinary working hours for the person who requires supervision, including assistance with medication, meal preparation, dressing, or moving about.
debride	To remove foreign material and dead or damaged tissue from a wound or ulcer.
decubitus ulcer	Skin lesion usually resulting from prolonged pressure over a bony prominence.

deep tendon reflex	Tendon reflexes or muscle stretch reflexes are contrasted with reflexes of a superficial type. In muscle stretch reflexes, the tendon or insertion of a muscle is briskly tapped with a reflex hammer and the resulting contraction of the muscle is graded from 0 (no response) to 4+ (maximal response with spreading to other muscles or clonus).
demographic study	The study of a sample of a population group that may represent a typical cross-section of that population.
dendrite	Part of the neuron that conducts impulses to the cell body.
dependent	An individual who requires another person for either supervision or physical assistance to perform an activity.
depot wheelchair	A basic manual wheelchair typically used in airports, hospitals, or nursing homes. Depot wheelchairs are not designed for active people who use wheelchairs for personal mobility.
depression, reactive	A mood disturbance characterized by feelings of sadness, despair, and discouragement resulting from and normally proportionate to some personal loss or tragedy.
dermatome	Anatomical representation of levels of the spinal cord corresponding to the spinal innervation of different parts of the skin. Dermatome represents sensation.
descending pathways	Nerve pathways that go down the spinal cord and allow the brain to control movement of the body below the head.
diagnostic related groups (DRGs)	A classification of illness conditions expected to have similar hospital resource use. Medicare uses this classification to pay for inpatient hospital care. The groupings are based on diagnoses, procedures, age, sex, and the presence of complications or comorbidities.
diaphragm pacing	Surgical implantation of a pacemaker to stimulate a damaged phrenic nerve to function without use of a mechanical respirator or ventilator.
digital stimulation	Manual rectal stimulation for individuals with tetraplegia or high paraplegia with limited trunk mobility and balance.
direct costs	Charges that are the direct result of the injury, incurred either by the person with SCI or his or her responsible third party, regardless of the amount that is actually paid.
disability	Any restriction or lack of ability (resulting from an impairment) to perform any activity in the manner or within the range considered normal for a human being.
discharge planning	An interdisciplinary process to assist the individual and family in the development of post-hospital plans that ensure continuity of care and services consistent with the maximum level of independent functioning in the least restrictive environment.
discount rate	Assumed rate of return on investments over and above the rate of inflation, which is used to convert future charges or losses into current dollars.
distention	The act of or state of being abnormally stretched beyond capacity.
diverticulosis	The presence of a number of pouches or sac openings from a tubular or saccular organ, such as the colon or bladder.

Doppler	An ultrasonic flow detector used to diagnose phlebitis by determining whether a change in venous blood flow occurs during ventilation.
DSM-IV	The Diagnostic and Statistical Manual of the American Psychiatric Association, Fourth Edition; the standard guide to the classification of mental disorders.
durable medical equipment	Specialized equipment that is necessary for individuals with physical disabilities to maximize their independence (includes wheelchairs, wheelchair cushions and accessories, positioning equipment, bath equipment, standing frames, walkers, hand splints, and leg braces).
dysesthesia	A common effect of SCI characterized by sensations of numbness, tingling, burning, or pain felt below the level of lesion.
dyspepsia	A vague feeling of epigastric discomfort, felt after eating.

E

ECG	Electrocardiogram (EKG)
ECU	Environmental Control Unit
edema	Swelling; common in legs and feet.
efferent	Nerves that carry motor impulses from the central nervous system to muscles or glands.
egress	A means or place of going out; exit.
electrocardiogram	The recording made by electrode pads located on the individual's chest to monitor heart rate and rhythm.
electroejaculation	A method of collecting semen from men with ejaculatory dysfunction. Uses an electrical probe in the rectum. The sperm can be used to fertilize eggs in the uterus or in the test tube.
electromyography	An insertion of needle electrodes into muscles to study the electrical activity of muscle and nerve fibers. Helps diagnose damage to nerves or muscles.
EMG	Electromyography
environmental control unit (ECU)	Electronic unit that assists people who cannot control unit use their hands. Switches initiated by voice, breath, shoulder, or eye control monitors for devices that aid in the usage of lights, telephone, appliances, computer, etc.
epidemiology	The study of the occurrence, distribution, and causes of diseases in humans.
epididymitis	Inflammation of the sperm storage tube that runs along the posterior surface of the testis.
erythema	A reddened area on the skin surface.
estradiol	The most potent naturally occurring human estrogen.
etiology	The study of all factors that may be involved in the development of a disease.
evidence-based guidelines	Clinical practice guidelines that have been developed using research findings that have been graded for scientific strength.
evidence tables	Charts, developed by methodologists to support guideline development, that describe scientific literature citations and the type and quality of the reported research for use in developing clinical practice guidelines.
extension	The act of straightening out a joint after flexing it.

F

FIM^{TM} *instrument*	A standardized instrument for measuring burden of care.
flaccid	Absence of muscle contraction.
flexion	The act of bending a joint.
follow-up	The process of comprehensive reevaluations of the medical, rehabilitative, and psychosocial status of the individual with SCI. Reevaluations are scheduled on a routine basis, as well as when emergent needs arise.
Frankel Grade	The previous classification scheme used for categorizing individuals with SCI based on the amount of preserved neurologic function below the "zone" of injury. This Frankel Grading System was replaced by the ASIA Impairment Scale in 1993.
Frankel Grade A	Complete: No sensory or motor function is preserved below the level of lesion.
Frankel Grade B	Incomplete: Preserved sensation only. Preservation of any demonstrable sensation, excluding phantom sensations. Voluntary motor function is absent.
Frankel Grade C	Incomplete: Preserved motor capacity (nonfunctional). Preservation of voluntary motor function that performs no useful purpose except psychologically. Sensory function may or may not be preserved.
Frankel Grade D	Incomplete: Preserved motor capacity (functional). Preservation of voluntary motor function that is functionally useful.
Frankel Grade E	Complete recovery: Complete return of all motor and sensory function, but reflexes may still be abnormal.
FSH	Follicle-stimulating hormone
functional electrical stimulation (FES)	The application of low-level computer-controlled electric current to the neuromuscular system, including paralyzed muscles, to enhance or produce function (walking, bike exercise, etc.) FES has been used in experiments to facilitate grip for individuals with tetraplegia, using a switch activated by shoulder shrug. Other uses include correction of scoliosis, bladder and bowel control, electroejaculation, and phrenic nerve stimulation.
functional level	Level of motor capacity in persons with SCI or other impairments that allows the individual to perform various activities.
functional limitations	A limitation in function that results from physical, mental, and emotional disabilities, which adversely affect the individual's capacity to function.
fusion	Surgical procedure that stabilizes two or more vertebrae by constructing bone and/or hardware connections between them.

G

gait training	Instruction in walking, with or without equipment; also called *ambulation training*.
gastritis	Inflammation of the stomach.
gastrointestinal system	Pertains to the organs of the gastrointestinal tract, from mouth to anus.
genitourinary system	Includes all of the organs involved in the secretion and elimination of urine. These include the kidneys, ureters, bladder, and urethra.

Glasgow coma scale   A standardized system used to assess the degree of brain impairment and to identify the seriousness of injury in relation to outcome. The system involves three determinants: eye opening, verbal responses, and motor response, all of which are evaluated independently according to a numerical value that indicates the level of consciousness and degree of dysfunction. Scores run from a high of 15 to a low of 3. Persons are considered to have sustained a "mild" brain injury when their score is 13 to 15.

H

hand controls   Adaptive equipment that allows persons with limited use of their extremities to drive motor vehicles.

handicap   A disadvantage for a given individual, resulting from an impairment or disability, that limits or prevents the fulfillment of a normal role normal (depending on age, sex, and social and cultural factors) for that individual.

hemiparesis   Partial paralysis or weakness of one side of the body.

HO   Heterotopic Ossification

hospital charges   The amount of money billed for hospital expenses. The amount billed does not necessarily reflect the actual costs of providing any of the services and/or items provided nor does it necessarily equal the amount ultimately collected or paid. In cases of SCI, hospital charges represent approximately 80 percent of the total initial expenses.

hydronephrosis   A kidney distended with urine to the point that its function is impaired.

hypalgesia   Diminished sensitivity to pain.

hypesthesia   Diminished sensation to touch.

hypotension   Abnormally low blood pressure.

hypotonic bladder   Muscles in the bladder stay relaxed due to spinal cord damage and contractions are not strong enough to empty the bladder.

I

ICP   Intermittent catheterization program

ICD-9-CM   International Classification of Diseases — 9th Revision Clinical Modification

ideographic methodology   Study of the individual case, emphasizing the uniqueness of each personality.

ileus   An obstruction of the intestines.

impairment   Any loss or abnormality of psychological, physiological, or anatomical structure or function.

incidence   Number of new cases of SCI occurring in the United States each year.

incontinent   Unable to control bowel and bladder functions.

independent   Activity can be completed without aid of equipment or physical assistance.

independent living program   A federal–state initiative to improve access to community-based and integrated residential services for individuals with disabilities. Provides community-based advocacy and peer counseling, case management, personal assistance and counseling services, information and referral, independent living skill development, and emergency services.

independent with equipment   No physical assistance necessary for setup or completion of activity including equipment application.

independent with equipment and setup	No physical assistance necessary to complete the activity. Physical setup of person and equipment is necessary before the activity is carried out.
independent with orthosis	Person utilizes orthosis for activity, without other equipment.
indirect costs	Forgone wages and associated fringe benefits that directly result from the SCI.
indwelling catheter	A flexible tube retained in the bladder by some retention catheter device for purpose of continuous urinary drainage.
ingress	A means or place of entering.
innervate	To supply a body part or organ with nerves or nervous stimuli.
interdisciplinary team approach	A method of diagnosis, evaluation, and individual program planning in which two or more specialists, such as medical doctors, psychologists, rehabilitation counselors, occupational or physical therapists, nurses, recreational therapists, social workers, etc., participate as a team, contributing their skills, competencies, insights, and perspectives to focus on identifying the comprehensive rehabilitation needs of the person with a SCI and on devising ways to meet those needs.
intermittent catheterization program	Bladder training program in which a catheter is inserted to empty the bladder at regular time intervals (usually every 3 to 6 hours).
International Classification of Diseases 9th Revision, Clinical Modification	A classification system adapted by the U.S. from the World Health Organization in coding diagnosis and procedures for clinical and research purposes, medical records and billing, inpatient, outpatient, and community programs. The ICD-9-CM consists of over 12,000 diagnosis codes and 3,500 procedure codes.
interquartile range	The range of values containing the central half of observations; that is, the range between the 25th and 75th percentile.
intravenous pyelogram	A radiographic profile of the kidneys. Routinely included in SCI evaluations to check for damage to the kidneys.
ipsilateral	Same side of the body.
ischemia	A severe reduction in the supply of blood to particular body tissues, such as brain, heart, lungs, and kidneys.
IVP	Intravenous pyelogram

J

job analysis	The systematic study of an occupation in terms of what the worker does in relation to data, people, and things; the methods and techniques employed; the machines, tools, equipment, and work aids used; the materials, products, subject matter, or services which result; and the traits required of the worker.
job seeking skills	Those skills that enable a person to seek out job vacancies and apply for them. Includes knowledge of self, capabilities, and job requirements, where to find information about job openings, how to fill out an application, how to take employment tests, and how to handle a job interview.

K

kinesthetic awareness	Awareness of body position and movement in space.

knee-ankle-foot orthosis (KAFO)	A brace that stabilizes or facilitates movement at the knee, ankle, and foot joints.

L

laminectomy	A surgical procedure done to remove the vertebral arch to gain access to and dorsally decompress the spinal cord.
LCP	Life Care Plan
LE	Lower extremity
leg bag	A small, thick plastic bag that can be secured to the leg to collect urine. It is connected by tubing to a catheter inserted into the urinary bladder or over the penis.
leisure skills	The ability to participate in recreational activities and to plan for and make effective use of one's leisure time and opportunities.
lesion	A broad term for traumatic or pathological discontinuity of tissue. Specifically, any pathologic or traumatic injury to the spinal cord.
life care plan	A comprehensive, interdisciplinary document that systematically addresses the medical and nonmedical needs of a person with a catastrophic injury or illness and projects the costs of needed goods and services over the person's estimated lifespan. Along with the costs associated with the disabling condition, replacement schedules and frequency of treatments are also delineated. The Life Care Plan is specific to the person and not generalized to a type of injury or disability.
life expectancy table	The length of time that a person of a given age and sex is expected to live according to statistical (i.e., actuarial) tables.
lightweight wheelchair	A manual wheelchair with minimal adjustments designed for individual or institutional use.
longitudinal study	A study that follows subjects over a period of time.
lower extremity	Referring to the legs.
lower motor neuron	Nerve fibers that originate in the spinal cord and travel out of the central nervous system to muscles in the body. An injury to these nerve cells can destroy reflexes and may also affect bowel, bladder, and sexual functions.
LPC	Licensed Professional Counselor
LRC	Licensed Professional Vocational Rehabilitation Counselor
lumbar	Pertaining to that area immediately below the thoracic spine; the strongest part of the spine, the lower back.

M

magnetic resonance imaging (MRI)	A type of diagnostic imaging that relies upon the interactions of magnetic fields and radio frequency radiation with body tissues. The MRI is better than CT scans for viewing soft tissue.
mammogram	An x-ray film of the soft tissues of the breast.
median survival time	Point at which 50 percent of a given population has died.
mental status examination	A generic term (i.e., numerous articles, texts, and guidebooks present different outlines for conducting the examination) that describes a structured observation and interview technique in which the examiner evaluates a comprehensive set of characteristics (e.g., appearance, orientation, attention, concentration, memory, and insight) related to the individual's current mental status.

meta-analysis	A statistical technique for combining the results of many studies, giving greater weight to the final conclusion.
methylprednisolone	A steroid, administered within 8 hours of acute spinal cord trauma; it is the first drug shown to improve recovery from SCI.
micturition	Voiding, urinating.
mild increase in tone	Some resistance to passive stretch is noted, but increases in tone do not interfere with ROM or function.
mobility limitations	Restricted ability to get from one place to another; may be caused either by physical disability or environmental barriers.
moderate increase in tone	More resistance to passive stretch is noted, and increase in tone may make ranging more difficult; however, ROM remains within normal limits. Individual is still able to perform the ADL, but the quality of the performance may be impaired.
morbidity	The rate at which an illness occurs in a population.
mortality	The condition of being subject to death.
motoneuron	(Motor neuron) A nerve cell whose cell body is located in the brain or spinal cord and whose axons leave the central nervous system by way of cranial nerves or spinal roots. Motoneurons supply innervation to muscles. A *motor unit* is the combination of the motoneuron and the set of muscle fibers it innervates.
motor functional	A neurologically incomplete SCI with preservation of useful voluntary motor function below the level of lesion.
motor level	The most caudal segment of the spinal cord with normal motor function on both sides of the body.
motor nonfunctional	A neurologically incomplete lesion with some preservation of voluntary motor function, which performs no useful purpose except psychologically.
motor skills	That which is necessary to impart motion (i.e., ROM, strength, sensation, coordination) capabilities for particular tasks.
mouth sticks	Sticks of variable lengths that, when held in the mouth and manipulated by a person with tetraplegia, serve to facilitate functional activities, such as keyboarding, page turning, dialing a phone.
MRI	Magnetic resonance imaging
muscle tone	Used in clinical practice to describe the resistance of a muscle to being stretched.
musculoskeletal system	All of the muscles, bones, joints, and related structures, such as the tendons and connective tissue, that function in the movement of the parts and organs of the body.
myotome	Those muscles controlled by a single spinal segment.

N

nebulizer	A device used to reduce liquid medication to an extremely finely divided cloud; useful in delivering medication to the deep part of the respiratory tract.
necrosis	Death and subsequent deterioration of tissue.
nephron	Structural and functional unit of the kidney.
nerve	A large cordlike structure made up of connective tissue and several nerve fibers that convey neural impulses between some part of the body and the central nervous system.

nervous system	The extensive, intricate network of structures that activates, coordinates, and controls all the functions of the body.
neurogenic	Having origin in the nervous tissue.
neurogenic bladder	The interference in bladder function (i.e., storage and voiding) resulting from damage to the central or peripheral nervous system.
neurogenic bowel	Colonic dysfunction (constipation, incontinence, and difficulty with evacuation) caused by lack of nervous control of the colon, pelvic floor, and anal sphincters.
neurologic level	The most caudal segment of the spinal cord with normal sensory and motor function on both sides of the body.
neuron	A nerve cell that can receive and send information by way of synaptic connections.
nonambulatory	Not able to walk.
nursing home	A residential facility for individuals who require supervision in all activities, including assistance with medication, meal preparation, bathing, dressing, and moving about; the patient may also require special nursing care and/or ongoing therapy. There are nursing homes that provide minimal to maximum care; also called *extended care facilities*.

O

orthosis	A splint or brace designed to improve function or to provide stability or support to a body part.
osteomyelitis	Infection of bone.
ostomy	An opening to the skin from an organ. For example, a suprapubic catheter drainage (cystostomy), for elimination of intestinal contents (colostomy or ileostomy) or for passage of air (tracheostomy).
OT	Occupational therapist

P

paraparesis	Partial paralysis affecting the lower extremities.
paraplegia	Loss of neurologic function at any level below the cervical spinal cord segments.
passive standing	Use of a padded frame to support a person with SCI in standing.
PCA	Personal care attendant
pelvic inflammatory disease (PID)	An infection anywhere in a woman's genital tract above disease the cervix.
peripheral nervous system	Nerves outside the spinal cord and brain of the central nervous system. If damaged, peripheral nerves have the ability to regenerate.
peristalsis	The movement of the intestine, characterized by waves of alternate circular contraction and relaxation by which contents are propelled forward.
personal assistance services	Assistance provided by an individual to assist a person assistance with SCI to perform activities of daily living, fulfill services responsibilities, and reach personal goals. This may include personal, household, communication, and mobility services.
phrenic nerve stimulation	Electrical stimulation of the nerves that go from C3–C5 level spinal cord to the diaphragm, facilitating breathing in people with C1 and C2 level tetraplegia. Uses an implanted electrode and receiver, controlled by a wheelchair-mounted transmitter.

physical demands (exertional)	One of the primary strength activities (walk, stand, sit, lift, carry, push, pull), which define a level of work.
physical demands (nonexertional)	Those activities (climb, balance, stoop, kneel, crouch, crawl, reach, handle, finger, feel, talk, hear, taste/smell, vision) other than primary strength activities, which define a level of work.
placebo	An inert substance or inactive treatment given to the control group in an experiment instead of a therapy that is being evaluated.
pneumonia	Inflammation of the lung.
population-based study	The study of a group of individuals that is collectively distinguished by a particular trait or situation, e.g., SCI.
prehension	Use of the hands and fingers to grasp or pick up objects.
preserved sensation only	A neurologically incomplete lesion with preservation of any demonstrable sensation, excluding subjective phantom sensations. Voluntary motor function is absent.
pressure sore	See *decubitus ulcer*.
pressure sore grades	A four-point scale used to assess the severity of grades pressure sores: Grade One sores are limited to the superficial layers of the skin. Grade Two sores extend into the fatty tissues under the skin. Grade Three sores extend through the skin and underlying fat and involve the muscle tissue. Grade Four sores contain extensive soft tissue damage as well as extending into the bone.
prevalence	Number of existing cases of SCI in the United States at any given time.
priapism	A dangerous condition wherein the penis remains erect for a prolonged period because of retention of blood in the corpora. This can cause ischemic damage to the penis.
prokinetic medications	Medications prescribed to stimulate gastrointestinal motility.
proprioception	Awareness of the static position and movement of body parts.
prospective study	A study that is planned in advance of data collection.
prosthesis	Replacement device for a body part, for example, an artificial limb.
PVA	Paralyzed Veterans of America
psychogenic erection	Penile erection evoked by visual, olfactory, and other psychic stimuli such as fantasies.
psychosocial	Pertaining to the psychological and social aspects of human function.
psychotherapy	A treatment for personality, emotional, behavioral, and psychiatric diagnoses that utilizes primarily verbal and non-verbal communication, rather than medical or surgical treatment, to effect a cure or remission.
PT	Physical therapist
pulmonary embolism	Obstruction or occlusion of the pulmonary artery or branch vessel by a transported clot or vegetation, a mass of bacteria, or other foreign material of the pulmonary arteries, most frequently by detached fragments of thrombus from a leg or pelvic vein, especially when thrombosis has followed an operation or confinement to bed.
pulmonary function tests	Series of tests used to evaluate ventilatory diffusion and perfusion abilities.
pyelogram	An x-ray picture of the kidneys and ureters.

Q

quadriparesis	Weakness of all four extremities.
quadriplegia	Loss of neurologic function of any injured or diseased cervical spinal cord segment, affecting all four body limbs. Being replaced with the term *tetraplegia* (which is technically more accurate, combing tetra + plegia, both from the Greek, rather than quadri + plegia, a Latin/Greek amalgam).
quality of life	A subjective concept by which one defines the degree of life satisfaction. It is based on the many dimensions of life experience and personal values. Critical factors include independence, social support, activity, control, and health. Common dimensions identified by Americans include physical and material well-being; relationships with other people; participation in social, community, and civic activities; personal development and fulfillment; and recreation.

R

radiogram	An x-ray image.
range of motion (ROM)	The normal range of movement of any body joint; also refers to exercises designed to maintain this range and prevent contractures.
range of motion active	The muscles around the joint do the work to move it.
range of motion passive	Movement of a joint by means other than contraction of the muscles around that joint; e.g., someone else moves the joint.
rectal stimulation	Manual stimulation of the rectum to facilitate evacuation of the lower bowel.
rectosigmoidoscopy	The examination of the rectum and pelvic colon with a sigmoidoscope.
reflex	An involuntary response to a stimulus involving nerves not under control of the brain. In some types of paralysis, reflexes cannot be inhibited by the brain; they become exaggerated and thereby cause spasms.
reflexogenic erection	Penile erection evoked by tactile stimulation.
rehabilitation	The process of providing a program of coordinated services, with the full participation of the individual with SCI, to achieve physical, psychological, social, economic, and vocational potential. Rehabilitation is a dynamic process of learning to live with a disability in an individual's own environment, beginning at the moment of injury and continuing for the duration of the person's life.
rehabilitation technology	Compensatory strategies and adaptive equipment to increase or improve functional capabilities of persons with disabilities; used to enhance vocational, educational, and/or independent living opportunities for persons with disabilities; technological methods of achieving practical outcomes in the rehabilitation process.
residual functional capacity	Remaining physical and mental work potential and capacity for person with a disability.
residual urine	Urine that remains in bladder after voiding. Too much left can lead to a bladder infection.
respiratory system	The complex of organs and structures that performs the pulmonary ventilation of the body and the exchange of oxygen and carbon dioxide between the ambient air and the blood circulating through the lungs.

respite care	A substitute who for takes over the care of an individual temporarily (a few hours up to a few days) to provide a period of relief for the primary care giver.
retrograde pyelogram	Insertion of contrast material directly into kidney through an instrument. Used to study kidney function.
retrospective study	A study that starts with the present condition of a population of individuals and collects data about their past history to explain their present condition.
robotics	Various types of technology used apart from the individual to perform tasks that otherwise could not be completed by the person with a disability (e.g., using a robotic arm for feeding self).
ROM	Range of motion

S

sacral	Refers to the fused segments of the lower vertebrae or lowest spinal cord segments below the lumbar level.
sacral sparing	Incomplete lesion in which sensation is intact in the sacral area. Paralysis and loss of sensation are complete in all other areas below lesion level.
SCI	Spinal cord injury
SCI care system	An organized, multidisciplinary system of care that provides initial acute treatment and rehabilitation as well as lifetime follow-up services for individuals with SCI.
secondary disability	Additional disability that is directly or indirectly the result of the primary disability or develops separately from the primary disability.
secondary impairment	Any loss or abnormality (anatomical, physiological, or psychological) that occurs in an individual with preexisting impairments.
selective placement	Work situation where provisions are made by the employer to meet the special needs of an individual with a handicapping condition.
self-catheterization	Intermittent catheterization, the goal of which is to empty the bladder as needed, on one's own, to minimize risk of infection.
sensation	Feeling stimuli that activate sensory organs of the body, such as touch, temperature, pressure, and pain.
sensory level	The most caudal segment of the spinal cord with normal sensory function on both sides of the body.
severe increase in tone	Tone is increased to the point where ROM can no longer be maintained within normal limits. ADLs will be decreased secondary to tone.
sexuality counseling	Using supportive techniques and special methods to help persons with SCI and their families deal with special and intimate relationship issues.
sheltered workshop	A work setting certified as such by the wage and hour division. It provides transitional and/or long-term employment in a controlled and protected working environment for those who are unable either to compete or to function in the open job market due to their disabilities. May provide vocational evaluation and work adjustment services.
shunt	A tube to drain a cavity; in the spinal cord, used to treat a syrinx by equalizing pressures between the syrinx and the spinal fluids.

sigmoidoscopy	An examination of the part of the colon called the *sigmoid flexure*. The test is done with a tube called a *sigmoidoscope*.
skeletal level	The level at which, by radiographic examination, the greatest vertebral damage is found.
SMR	Standardized Mortality Ratio
social assessment	General background data collected by a case worker; includes a brief description of family or other support group resources and the individual's position and role in the family (child, parent, spouse); emotional, financial and environmental resources and their availability to the individual with a disability; educational and employment history.
social skills	A component of rehabilitation in which the individual with SCI learns effective communication techniques and adaptive behaviors for a variety of social situations.
sonogram	The process of imaging deep structures of the body by measuring and recording the reflection of pulsed or continuous high-frequency sound waves.
spasm	Involuntary muscle contraction that may interfere with function.
sphincter	A small muscle that can open or occlude a passageway, for instance in the urethra or anus.
sphincterotomy	Cutting of bladder sphincter muscle, to reduce urinary outflow obstruction and improve voiding efficiency.
spinal cord	The solid cord extending from the bottom of the brain stem to the conus medullaris at the L1 level in the lumbar spine.
spinal nerve	Any of 30 pairs of nerves arising from the spinal cord and innervating other parts of the body.
SSDI	Social Security Disability Insurance
SSI	Supplemental Security Income
standardized mortality ratio	Ratio of the actual number of deaths occurring in a group of individuals in a given time period to the expected number of deaths in that same group over the same time period. The ratio is based on the age, sex, and race of the group members coupled with general population mortality rates.
suctioning	Removal of mucus and secretions from lungs; important for individuals with high level tetraplegia who lack ability to cough.
supported employment	Paid work in a variety of settings, particularly regular work sites, specially designed for individuals with disabilities 1) for whom competitive employment has not traditionally occurred, and 2) who, because of their disabilities, need intensive or ongoing support to perform in a work setting.
support hose	Anti-embolic stockings. Tight knee- or thigh-high stockings that support the leg muscles and thus help prevent pooling of blood in veins of the legs.
suprapubic catheterization	A catheter that is inserted above the pelvic bone. This catheter is placed through the abdomen above the pubic area into the bladder. A hole is surgically made in the abdomen and the bladder to create openings for the catheter.

suprapubic cystostomy	A small opening made in the bladder and through the abdomen, sometimes to remove large stones, more commonly to establish a catheter urinary drain.

T

tachycardia	Rapid beating of the heart, conventionally applied to rates over 100 per minute.
task analysis	Breakdown of a particular job into its component tasks.
temperament	Adaptability requirements made on the worker by specific types of jobs.
tenodesis	(Hand splint) Metal or plastic support for hand, wrist, and/or fingers. Used to facilitate greater function to a disabled hand by transferring wrist extension into grip and finger control.
third-party funding	Reimbursement for services rendered to a person in which an entity other than the recipient of the services is responsible for the payments, e.g., an insurance company.
thoracic	Pertaining to the chest, vertebrae, or spinal cord segments between the cervical and lumbar areas.
timed voiding	Bladder training program in which the person goes to the toilet at regular intervals whether feeling the urge to urinate or not. The goal is bladder continence through prevention of overfilling.
tone, muscle	The tension in resting muscles and the amount of resistance that is felt when a muscle is stretched.
tonometry	The measurement of intraocular pressure by determining the resistance of the eyeball to indentation by an applied force.
topical agents	A broad category of creams, lotions, and skin preparations applied externally.
tracheostomy	A temporary surgical opening at the front of the throat to provide access to the trachea or windpipe to assist in breathing.
transfer	Method of moving the body from one surface to another (e.g., bed to wheelchair, wheelchair to shower, etc.).

U

UE	Upper extremity
ultralight wheelchair	An adjustable manual wheelchair designed for an individual's use as a long-term mobility aid.
UMN	Upper motor neuron
upper extremity	The area above the waist and below the neck, including the arms.
upper motor neuron	Long nerve cells that originate in the brain and travel in tracts through the spinal cord. Any injury to these nerves cuts off contact and brain control. Reflex activity is still intact, however, resulting in spasticity. For men with upper motor neuron injuries, reflex erections are still possible.
urinary tract	All organs and ducts involved in the secretion and elimination of urine from the body.
ureter	Tube connecting each kidney to the bladder.
urethra	Tube which carries urine from the bladder outside the body.

V

validity	The extent to which a test measurement or other device measures what it is intended to measure.

Valsalva maneuver	Any forced expiratory effort (strain) against a closed glottis.
ventilator	Mechanical device to facilitate breathing in persons with impaired diaphragm function.
vertebrae	Any one of the 33 bones of the spinal column. There are 7 cervical, 12 thoracic, 5 lumbar, 5 sacral, and 4 coccygeal vertebrae.
vital capacity	Maximum volume of air in an exhaled breath; an important measure of ventilatory function for individuals with high tetraplegia.
vocational evaluation	A comprehensive process that systematically utilizes work, real or simulated, as the focal point for assessment and vocational exploration, the purpose of which is to assist individuals in vocational development. Vocational evaluation incorporates medical, psychological, social, vocational, educational, cultural, and economic data in the attainment of the goals of the evaluation process.
vocational rehabilitation process	The sequence of comprehensive services deemed appropriate to the needs of a person with a disability and designed to achieve objectives directed toward the realization of the individual's maximum physical, social, mental, and vocational potential.

W

weaning	Gradual removal of mechanical ventilation, as individual's respiratory muscle strength improves and the vital capacity increases.
work adjustment	An individualized, structured, and planned, closely adjustment supervised, remedial work experience designed to promote the acquisition of good work habits, to increase physical and emotional tolerance for work activity and interpersonal relationships, and to modify aptitudes and behaviors that inhibit the satisfactory performance of work.

Z

zone of partial preservation	Those dermatomes and myotomes, caudal to the neurologic level, which remain partially innervated in SCI. When some impaired sensory and/or motor function is found below the lowest normal segment, the exact number of segments so affected should be recorded for both sides as the ZPP. The term is used only with complete injuries.

Index

Note: boldface numbers indicate illustrations; italic *t* indicates a table.